Fitness Management

A Comprehensive Resource
for
Developing, Leading, Managing, and Operating
a
Successful Health/Fitness Club

Stephen Tharrett, M.S.
Dallas, Texas

James A. Peterson, Ph.D., FACSM
Monterey, California

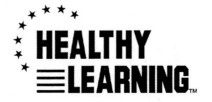

HEALTHY LEARNING

ISBN: 1-58518-940-5
Library of Congress Control Number: 2005936093
Cover design: Jeanne Hamilton
Book layout: Jeanne Hamilton

Front cover photo credits: Ed LaCasse: pool, spa, Pilates; Dennis Dal Covey/Covey Media: racquetball, strength training, treadmill, group exercises, locker room.

Healthy Learning
P.O. Box 1828
Monterey, CA 93942
www.healthylearning.com

This book is dedicated to my family. To my wife, Denise, who has stood by me for over 28 years, providing support, inspiration, patience, and love. To my children, Alyssa and Travis, for their love and support and for teaching me so much about what is required to be a leader. Finally to my father, John Tharrett, who passed away over a decade ago and who was my hero growing up. While this project was a labor of love, I could not have done so without the unconditional love provided by my family.

S.T.

This book is dedicated to every individual who has helped make the joy of exercise a reality for another person.

J.P.

Dedication

Acknowledgments

I want to acknowledge all of the incredible people in this industry who have shared their passion and wisdom with me about the business of operating a successful health/fitness club.

First, I would like to thank the leaders and peers who served with me for 21 years at ClubCorp, including Robert Dedman Sr., Richard Poole, Bob Johnson, Doug Howe, Frank Gore, Murray Siegel, and Steve Plakotoris, each of whom it was my honor to work with, and who gave me the opportunity to learn and grow by freely sharing their knowledge and love of the business. Next, I would like to acknowledge the incredible members of the ClubCorp athletic and tennis committees, over 40 strong dedicated and passionate leaders. Each of these special people (particularly the committee leaders, such as Gordon Collins, Billy Freer, Tommy English, Nony Michulka, Rich Andrae, Jill Bauman, Vicki McGrath, Frank Martin, Mike Saldivar, Pam Koch, Jim Swieter, and Bill Johnston) never hesitated to share their wisdom or heart. Finally, I would like to express my appreciation to the over 5,000 employees who worked in the athletic and tennis arena at ClubCorp, including my wonderful assistant, Michele Arnette, who, without knowing it, taught me the real "in and outs" of the business.

I would also like to acknowledge the industry leaders who have been so open and willing to share their knowledge and insights about the industry. Frankly, there are so many to thank in this regard that I cannot begin to mention everyone who has impacted my professional life in a positive manner. On the other hand, I would like to personally thank those individuals who have served as role models for me during my tenure in the industry. With over 2,000 years of experience, these exceptional industry individuals are what the industry is about. The list of those individuals to whom I am eternally grateful in this regard include people such as Rick Caro of Management Vision, Norm Cates of the *Club Insider*, Frank Napolitano of TSI, Spencer Garrett of Pierpont Racquet Club, Rob Goldman of the Columbia Association, Gary Klencheski of Fitcorp, Mitch Wald of Sport and Health, Carl Porter of the Michigan Athletic Club, Gale Landers of Fitness Formula, Steve Schwartz of Tennis Corporation of America, Tim Rhode of the Maryland Athletic Club, Jill Kinney of Club One, Red Lerille of Red's, Rudy Riska, who spent more than four decades as the executive director of the Downtown Athletic Club in New York, Jim Gerber of Western Athletic Clubs, Annbeth Eschbach of Exhale, Robert Chaiken and the esteemed members of the Faust Group, and the many others with whom it was my honor and pleasure to serve during my involvement with the industry. In addition to the aforementioned industry leaders, I would also like to give very special thanks to John McCarthy, executive director of IHRSA, who has been a mentor over the years and provided valuable insight into the writing of this book. Finally, thanks to the entire team at IHRSA, particularly Herman Rutgers, for their incredible efforts in advancing our industry over the past two decades.

I also would like to acknowledge the wonderful and talented people involved in other aspects of the industry who have shared a wealth of information with me over the years. In particular, I would like to thank Andy Richters of Star Trac, Gary Klein of Keiser, Bob Taggert of T2 Fitness, Mike Zinda of Life Fitness, Stan Peterman formerly of Quinton, Ken Germano and Dr. Cedric Bryant of ACE, Hervey Lavoie of Ohlson Lavoie, and Brian Davidson, formerly of Life Fitness. Frankly, space does not permit me to list everyone who has been a trusted friend and business associate over the past 20 years. It goes without saying that your assistance has been invaluable.

A special thanks to Dr. Dee Edington, former dean of the School of Kinesiology at the University of Michigan and director of the Wellness Research Center at the University, and Dr. Tom Sattler, former professor at the University of Illinois at Chicago, for their mentorship over the years. A very special thanks to my co-author, Jim Peterson, former director of sports medicine at StairMaster Sports/Medical Products, Inc. and retired professor of physical education at the United States Military Academy at West Point. Over the years, Jim has helped set a professional course for me to follow, and has always been there to provide a helping hand. Finally, a special and heartfelt thanks to my daughter, Alyssa, who helped immensely in pulling together the materials for this book. One final note, an extended and very special thank you to Jill Bauman, former manager of the Athletic and Swim Club in New York, who reviewed each draft of the manuscript and provided recommendations that played a significant role in shaping the final version of this book.

Unfortunately, I am sure I have missed more names than I have mentioned. On the other hand, hopefully, all of the wonderful and talented people with whom I have been blessed to share this journey are aware of how grateful I am for the positive impact that they have had on my life. One key point is inescapable…we are all in an incredible business!

S.T.

Special thanks to Kris Heath and Kristi Huelsing for their invaluable assistance in this project.

J.P.

Contents

This book is designed to serve three distinct target populations. One group is the upper-level undergraduate and graduate students who are seeking to embark on a career in the fitness, health, racquet, and sport club industry. Another are young professionals who are already working in the industry and who are seeking information and insights that can help them expand their professional horizons and possibly move into management. Finally, the book is intended for seasoned industry professionals who want to know more about areas in which they may not have as much experience or knowledge as they would like to have.

As you read this book, keep in mind that the fitness, health, racquet, and sport club industry is currently in its adolescence and slowly approaching maturity. As the industry has matured and expanded over the years, the demand for professionals with both strong business acumen and a passion and understanding of the dynamics of the industry has become paramount to health/fitness club owners and investors. Thirty years ago, this industry was in its infancy, developed, operated, and pushed forward by entrepreneurs who had a passion for fitness and what they were doing. Circumstances forced these industry pioneers to focus on surviving first and creating an industry second.

Over the past three decades, as the industry has begun to mature, many of the dynamics of the club business have changed. For example, in recent years, financial markets have and will continue to invest in the industry. Concurrently, major industry figures are creating national and international health/fitness club companies and franchises. This maturation process has resulted in a shortage of leaders and managers who can take the industry to the next level, and help it to continue to grow profitability on an ever-changing playing field. Much of this situation can be attributed to the fact that the industry has not established (at this point at least) a formal educational process for bringing professionals into the industry.

Over the years, one of the most pressing issues that other health/fitness club owners have brought to my attention is the critical need for a reliable mechanism for sharing the information that is needed to help better develop the future business leaders for the industry. This book is my attempt to help address that void. I have chosen to write it as a means of sharing with the readers the wealth of knowledge and passion that I have garnered from 25 years of working with the most incredible people in the industry. In reality, this book presents the insights and wisdom of industry leaders who collectively have over 5,000 years of experience in the industry.

Preface

This book is separated into seven distinct sections, based on the skill sets needed to succeed as a leader and manager in this industry. Section I introduces the reader to the fitness, health, racquet, and sport club industry by touching on the history of the industry, the current practices and trends in the industry, and the attitudes and attributes of the consumer who chooses to be a member of a club. Section II focuses on health/fitness club membership, starting with a discussion of the differences between a member and a consumer, and progressing into the marketing and sales practices necessary to succeed in the business.

Part III provides an overview of member retention and the process of utilizing great service and great programming to create memorable member experiences. Section IV reviews the administrative business functions of the industry, beginning with the formation of a legal business entity, progressing to the financial standards and processes, and concluding with an examination of the key issues involved in buying, leasing, and selling a club. Section V looks at the employee side of the health/fitness club business, starting with a detailed overview of the people-related requirements, and concluding with a discussion of the essential aspects of leadership within the industry.

Part VI addresses the facility and equipment side of the business, covering topics ranging from facility design to equipment selection. Part VII details the key operational issues within a health/fitness facility, beginning with an overview of the risk management practices in the industry and progressing through the most essential operating practices for both front-of-the-house and behind-the-house club operations.

Part VIII provides an overview of the international health/fitness club market. Part IX offers a picture of what the future may hold for our industry. Part X presents case studies of unusual management experiences, ranging from customer and member-related scenarios to employee and big business scenarios. Each case study provides an overview of an unusual or unexpected business event and the actions taken by the respective clubs and their leaders.

This book also features several appendices that contain examples of various operating policies and practices that can be implemented within a health/fitness facility from day one.

In conclusion, our primary goal in writing this book is to expand the horizons of its readers and provide them with a valuable resource that can help them in their professional development. If the publication of this book has a positive impact on the key issues attendant to the fitness, health, racquet, and sport club industry, then the effort involved in writing it will have been more than worthwhile.

—S.T.

INTRODUCTION TO THE HEALTH/FITNESS INDUSTRY

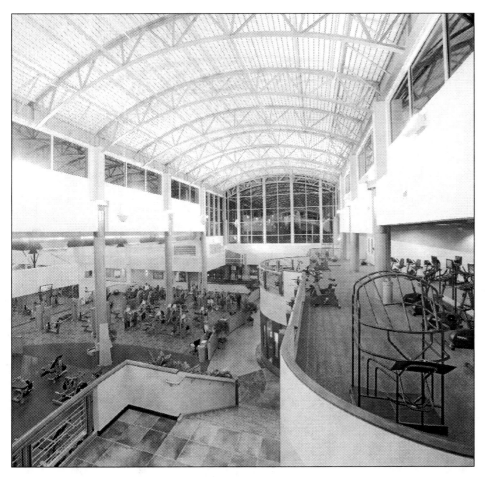

- Chapter 1: The Health/Fitness Club Industry: Challenge and Change
- Chapter 2: The Physical Activity Beliefs and Behaviors of Americans and Their Implications for Health/Fitness Clubs
- Chapter 3: Consumer Attitudes Toward Health/Fitness Clubs That Affect Their Reasons for Joining and Staying

Part One

1

The Health/Fitness Club Industry: Challenge and Change

Chapter Objectives

The primary objective of this chapter is to present an overview of the culture of the health/fitness industry. The chapter begins by reviewing (pre-1980) the industry's history in order to provide insight into the cultural roots of the industry. This discussion is followed by a section that features a more in-depth look at the modern history of the industry (from 1980 forward), with particular emphasis on the state of the industry as of 2005. The chapter concludes by offering a review of likely industry trends that will occur over the next ten-to-15 years.

The Early Years (Pre-1980)

The health/fitness club industry as is generally known today has its roots in an industry culture that emanated from male-oriented social and sport clubs and institutes of physical culture. During the 1800s, a small network of men's athletic clubs, such as New York Athletic Club, existed which were founded on bringing together men who were interested in both the pursuit of sport and the social status perceived to be a by-product of membership in such clubs.

These early athletic clubs were created to foster social relationships and business relationships. They had facilities that provided an environment for actively pursuing social networking and engaging in sport activities. As a rule, these early clubs had swimming pools, gymnasiums, billiard rooms, racquet courts, locker rooms, and social quarters that included dining spaces and lodging. In most cases, these clubs served as an avenue for networking with peers and a venue for friendly athletic competition.

During this same time period (the 1800s), a small number of "gyms" opened in Europe and later in the United States. These gyms included Gymnase Triat, which opened in Paris in 1847, and Turnvereins, which opened

> The health/fitness club industry as is generally known today has its roots in an industry culture that emanated from male-oriented social and sport clubs and institutes of physical culture.

In 1875, the Boston YMCA became one of the first official health clubs

in New York, Boston, and Philadelphia in the 1850s. In 1875, the Boston YMCA became one of the first official health clubs in the United States. Nineteen years later, Louis Durlacher opened one of the first commercial health/fitness clubs in New York City.

By the early part of the twentieth century, this type of athletic club became even more prevalent, with expansion of the number of these clubs in several major U.S. markets, including New York, Chicago, Los Angeles, and New Orleans. Concurrently, an evolution of health/fitness clubs similar to the facility operated by Louis Durlacher occurred. For example, during the early 1900s, the primary concern of many men who might otherwise be interested in joining a health/fitness club was the pursuit of feats of strength and physique. In response, gyms began to arise that provided an environment for these men to pursue activities (e.g., weightlifting, gymnastics, and acrobatic arts) that focused on physical development. These gyms appealed to a relatively small audience of men whose fitness and sports goals differed considerably from the men who joined the socially oriented athletic clubs. Among the earliest efforts in this regard was a facility developed by John Fritze who opened a gym in the 1930s in Philadelphia, PA, called Germantown, which was later followed on the West Coast by one built by Vic Tanny, which opened in 1939.

By the 1940s, the development of these "bodybuilding and weightlifting" gyms had come into vogue. One of the most renowned was Leo Stern's in 1946, followed shortly thereafter by Eastman's in 1947, and Harold Zinkin's in 1948. Relatively small, these original gyms offered memberships for around $60 annually. By the early 1950s, additional gyms had sprouted up across the west, including Bill Pearl's in 1953 and York's in the East. During this same time period, Joe Gold, who later earned recognition for both Gold's Gym and World Gym, entered the club business. About this same time, the first health/fitness club chain, "American Health/Silhouette," was created by Ray Wilson. Over the next several years, the concept of one organization offering multiple clubs would spread. One event of special consequence (for the health/fitness industry) that occurred during this period was the invention of the first prototype of the Universal Gym (i.e., a multi-station weight training machine) by Harold Zinkin in the late 1950s in a back room of his Palm Avenue gym in Fresno, California.

Bodybuilding gyms continued to flourish in the 1960s. These gyms were owned and operated by physical-culture enthusiasts whose primary interest was to offer their peers a customized environment for pursuing their physical culture and strength training interests. These early West Coast gyms were developed by individuals such as Vince Girondi, Bill Pearl, and Jack LaLanne, as well as the original pioneers of the gym genre. Similar gyms subsequently opened on the East Coast, thereby creating a bi-coastal opportunity for those individuals interested in the pursuit of physical culture.

One person who facilitated the aforementioned trend was Bob Hoffman, who founded York Barbell in 1938. In the process, he established an industry powerhouse. York became the first fitness manufacturer to take root in the industry. Hoffman's efforts helped further expand interest in weight training and physical culture. It is important to keep in mind that during this time period, the pursuit of structured physical activity was primarily a male-oriented pursuit.

In the 1960s, however, that situation was changed by Jack LaLanne, who gave the fitness, health, and sport club industry a huge promotional lift. Using the new (at the time) medium of television to reach out to millions of Americans everywhere with his gospel message of "get up, work out, and feel better," LaLanne brought the benefits of physical conditioning into the American consciousness. The Jack LaLanne Show, which started in the early 1950s, brought physical activity to televisions nationwide. In the process, LaLanne created a demand for knowledge about the pursuit of physical activity.

Subsequently, Jack LaLanne founded his own chain of health/fitness centers, which over the next decade became one of the largest chains of health clubs in the nation. During this period, the equipment in fitness centers consisted mostly of free weights (York), free weight benches (York or homemade), stationary bicycles, self-propelled walking machines (treadmills), vibrating belts, and pulley machines. During the 1960s, the health/fitness industry received a huge boost from the roll-out of the Universal Gym. The original Universal Gym was a multi-station machine, whose system of weight stacks and pulleys brought resistance training to the masses by offering a relatively safe, easy, and fast approach to training.

During the 1960s, the health/fitness industry received a huge boost from the roll-out of the Universal Gym.

The next decade saw the dawn of the modern health/fitness industry, sparked by both scientific investigations and marketing research that opened up a new segment of consumers for the health/fitness industry. During the 1960s, a new type of health/fitness facility originated—the racquet club. Some of the earliest examples of this genre included the Saw Mill Racquet Club in upstate New York, the Midtown Tennis Club in Chicago, and the University Club in Houston.

While the athletic clubs and the gyms that were popular in the previous periods continued to grow, it was the introduction of the racquet club that brought an entirely new audience to the industry. These racquet clubs consisted mainly of individually owned businesses that were operated by people who had a passion for the pursuit of racquet sports and physical activity. These facilities primarily consisted of indoor tennis courts, racquetball and handball courts, swimming pools, and small fitness centers. During this period, two industry-related associations formed—one representing indoor tennis clubs and one representing racquetball clubs. Concurrent with the growth of racquet clubs was the continued expansion and evolution of gyms and club chains, such as Jack LaLanne's, Holiday Health Spas, Scandinavian Health Spas, and Family Fitness Centers.

During the 1970s, four landmark events occurred that would forever change the landscape of the health/fitness industry and push it into its modern period beginning in the 1980s. The first notable occurrence was the development of Nautilus machines in the early 1970s by Arthur Jones, an unconventional eccentric who was at the forefront of an effort that questioned many of the standard prescription guidelines for training. Based on the principle of variable resistance, these resistance machines took the young industry by storm. For the first time ever, average Americans had equipment that they could use to muscularly condition themselves in a relatively short period of time. In the process, Nautilus became the standard piece of equipment for health/fitness facilities and began appearing in almost every gym, YMCA, athletic club, and racquet club in the United States. The popularity of this equipment led many racquet clubs and athletic clubs to convert one or more of their racquet courts into a "Nautilus Center," for which they charged additional fees to access the equipment.

The second landmark event was the introduction of the Lifecycle. Conceptually developed by Ray Wilson and sold by a future industry legend, Augie Nieto, the Lifecycle become the first commercial, electronically operated stationary bicycle. The Lifecycle helped enhance the young industry by motivating people to engage in stationary cycling by providing a user-friendly, fun way to perform cardiovascular exercise.

The third significant event was the groundbreaking work of Kenneth Cooper, MD, who conducted ground-breaking research on the benefits of aerobic exercise. In his best-selling book, *Aerobics*, Dr. Cooper introduced the world to an easy-to-complete way to quantify the aerobic impact of physical activity and to the medical and health benefits of aerobic activity. Dr. Cooper's research and his resulting book produced a surge of interest in both exercise and health/fitness clubs that would springboard the industry into the mainstream of public life.

ACSM, a renowned professional association of sports medicine, medical, and exercise science specialists, led the way in developing and disseminating the first set of nationally recognized guidelines for exercise testing and prescription.

The fourth and final landmark development involved the efforts of the American College of Sports Medicine (ACSM). ACSM, a renowned professional association of sports medicine, medical, and exercise science specialists, led the way in developing and disseminating the first set of nationally recognized guidelines for exercise testing and prescription. First printed in 1975, these guidelines would subsequently serve as a benchmark for all health/fitness professionals for prescribing exercise and assessing fitness.

In addition to the aforementioned landmark events, two other individuals also had a substantial impact on the industry in the 1970s—Arnold Schwarzenegger and Jane Fonda. A former Mr. Universe, Schwarzenegger became the face of Gold's Gym (and later World Gym) and, through movies, such as Pumping Iron, introduced an entirely new generation to the benefits of weight training. Concurrently, Fonda was featured on a series of exercise videos that helped to popularize "aerobic" exercise classes.

As a result of the aforementioned landmark events, the advent of the modern health/fitness and sport club industry occurred. During this notable period, the racquet-club industry grew quickly, while at the same time, new types of health/fitness clubs were introduced to the marketplace. Another significant occurrence during this time period was the creation of the largest chain of health/fitness clubs in the nation—Bally's. Bally's was one of the first organizations to consolidate several existing health/fitness club chains into one large national brand (Holiday, Scandinavian, etc.). A national chain of franchised Nautilus health clubs and a series of Cardio Fitness Centers in New York City also opened during this period.

The Modern Period (1980-2000)

The 1980s

In 1981, the International Sports and Racquet Association (IRSA) was formed by the merging of the National Racquet Club Association and the National Tennis Club Association. The formation of IRSA represented the first landmark event of the modern era. The early founders of IRSA, Rick Caro, Norm Cates, Curt Buesman, and others, had no idea at the time that the association they created in 1981 would go on, under the leadership of its founding director, John McCarthy, to become the leading voice for the health/fitness industry and would serve as a compelling factor in the emerging recognition of this industry as an essential part of the American culture.

In 1981, the International Sports and Racquet Association (IRSA) was formed by the merging of the National Racquet Club Association and the National Tennis Club Association.

According to early research conducted by IRSA, there were a total of approximately 6,200 clubs in 1982. By the end of the decade, eight years later, that number would rise to 13,854 clubs, servicing approximately 21 million Americans or 7.4% of the total population. This figure represented an increase of over 100% in the number of health, fitness, and sport clubs (Figures 1.1) over the eight-year period from 1982 to 1990. The 100% plus growth in the number of health/fitness clubs during the 1980s and the corresponding growth in the number of health/fitness club users (up to approximately 21 million) were fueled by several landmark activities, as well as the continued popularity of health/fitness facilities that was sparked by the landmark events of the 1970s.

The 6,200 clubs that started the decade of the 1980s and the 13,854 clubs that brought the decade to a close represented a real mix. First, the racquet and tennis clubs began to diversify, creating fitness centers out of existing racquet courts, as more consumers expressed an interest in engaging in cardiovascular and resistance training. Individually owned and operated health/fitness clubs, commonly called "Mom & Pop" clubs, sprouted rapidly. Many of these clubs incorporated the term "Nautilus" in their commercial name as a means of attracting a wider audience. During this time period, Bally's became the industry leader, through its consolidation of many of the smaller chains.

In the process, Bally's became the face of the industry, much to the dismay of IRSA, which focused on representing health/fitness clubs that were committed to operating in a prudent, ethical manner. The emergence of Bally's was seen as both a positive and negative for the industry. On one hand, Bally's brought consumers to the industry; on the other hand, Bally's occasionally generated a degree of negative publicity through its aggressive business practices.

In addition to commercial health/fitness clubs, the 1980s saw the emergence of the corporate fitness center industry. Because research showed that employee-based fitness programs brought a return for the company, many corporations began to actively integrate on-site heath/fitness facilities into their employee offerings. One of the first was the Pepsi Center in Purchase, New York, under the leadership of Dr. Dennis Colacino. Eventually, corporations such as Exxon, Monsanto, and Johnson and Johnson became the benchmarks for this new segment of the industry during this period.

Cardio Fitness of New York, which initially arose in the late 1970s, was the first club chain in the 1980s to focus its efforts on offering its clients the opportunity to achieve scientific and medically based cardiovascular fitness, targeting corporate executives. Another institutional entry during the 1980s was the Fitness Company of New York, which was developed on both a scientific and corporate health model of fitness. The Sports Training Institute (STI) of New York, founded by Dr. Michael O'Shea, was the first club group to bring a personal training model to the market. While STI eventually closed, its organizational structure and approach would become a model for the entire industry and one of the landmark events of the 1980s. Subsequently, club chains, such as Family Fitness in Southern California and 24 Hour Fitness in Northern California, became major players in the low-dues dollar business segment of the industry. In later years, they joined together to become the largest organizational player in the industry—24 Hour Fitness.

Tennis Corporation of America (TCA), originally founded by Allan Schwartz as a tennis club, became a leading operator of both tennis clubs and sports clubs. The Midtown Tennis Club, TCA's first club, which was opened in the 1960s, was the largest indoor tennis club at the time. Several other highly regarded industry-based companies, including Fitcorp of Boston, a corporate fitness based company, and Club Sports International of Denver, an operator of high-end sports clubs, were also established during this period. About this time, women's-only clubs began to flourish, with chains such as Lucille Robert's and Living Well Lady. As the 1980s came to a close and the number of clubs had reached in excess of 13,000 facilities, the diversity of club offerings had expanded to include such facilities as pure racquet/tennis clubs, multipurpose sports clubs, fitness clubs, YMCAs, and corporate fitness centers.

As the number of clubs grew in the 1980s, so did the number of members who used the clubs and the manner in which they used them.

As the number of clubs grew in the 1980s, so did the number of members who used the clubs and the manner in which they used them. While no accurate estimate of club patronage was available in 1980, by 1987 the industry was able to estimate that it served 17 million members, who on average used the club 72 times a year (about 1.4x a week) (Figures 1.2 and 1.3). The research also indicated that out of the 17 million members, approximately 30.6 percent (5.3 million) could be considered core members (i.e., individuals who use a particular club at least 100x a year) (Figure 1.4). This figure indicated that about one-third of all members actually were participating at their club at least twice a week.

The rapid growth in the number of clubs and members during the 1980s was fueled by both documented data that supported both the need for and the value of engaging in physical activity on a regular basis and the impact that targeted programming had on popular culture. An out-pouring of new research continued to show the "exercise is medicine" connection. Study after study linked regular exercise with a reduction in cardiovascular disease, as well as almost every other health-related disorder, including diabetes, high blood pressure, cancer, and obesity. While such data definitely played a role in helping bring more people to the clubs, a more likely factor in that regard was the introduction of programming that emphasized the trends of the popular culture.

Study after study linked regular exercise with a reduction in cardiovascular disease, as well as almost every other health-related disorder, including diabetes, high blood pressure, cancer, and obesity.

Programming innovations were a main factor in club growth in the 1980s. The biggest program trend to influence the industry and a landmark event by itself was the introduction of aerobic, group-exercise classes (commonly referred to as "aerobics"). The advent of aerobics introduced an entirely new market to health/fitness clubs—women. The primary appeal of aerobics to women was its dance orientation and, arguably more importantly, its socialization of exercise. Jacki Sorensen and her aerobic dancing program, along with Judy Misset and her jazzercise, took the country by storm. These popular exercise modalities were soon followed by high-impact aerobics and then low-impact aerobics, which were popularized in the mid-1980s by the movie "Perfect," with Jaime Lee Curtis. By the end of the 1980s, aerobic classes were bringing more people to clubs than any other activity.

In the mid-1980s, personal training became a program trend in the industry, particularly on the east and west coast. Concurrently, racquet sports also played a significant role in the growing movement by facilities to become more program driven.

The 1980s also saw the industry make a strong push toward raising the professional credibility of its instructors. In that regard, the American College of Sports Medicine undertook the preeminent role in the effort to certify health/fitness professionals. Joining ACSM in the effort were organizations such as the American Fitness and Aerobics Association (AFAA), The American Council on Exercise (ACE), The International Dance Exercise Association (IDEA), and the National Strength and Conditioning Association (NSCA). In response, each of these organizations offered educational and/or certification programs to support the growing demand by the industry for qualified health/fitness professionals.

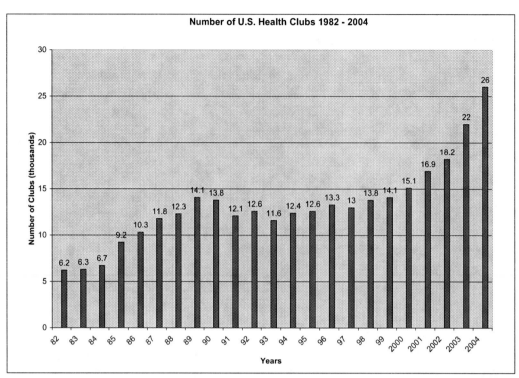

Figure 1.1. The number of health/fitness clubs in the United States 1982-2004

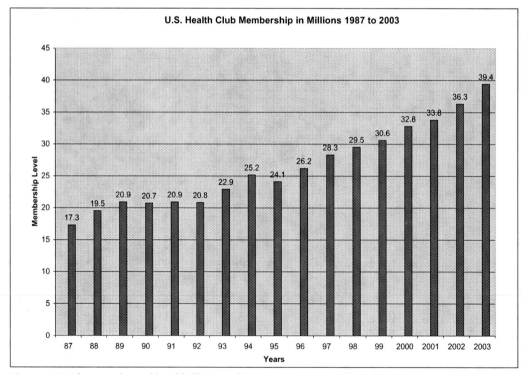

Figure 1.2. The number of health/fitness club members (in millions)

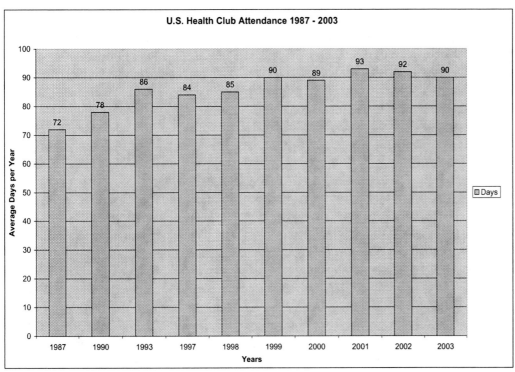

Figure 1.3. Average number of days a health/fitness club member uses the club annually

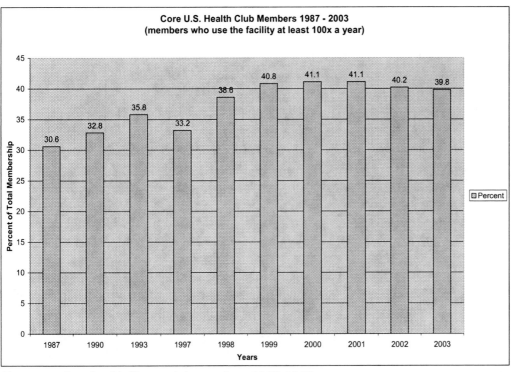

Figure 1.4. Core health/fitness club members 1987-2003

Another significant occurrence in the 1980s was the rapid growth of a new factor in the health/fitness industry—fitness equipment manufacturers. While Nautilus continued to flourish as a manufacturer and distributor of resistance training equipment, new competitors arose to serve the emerging market. For example, during this period, Eagle, later to become Cybex, became a significant player in the resistance equipment business. Joining Cybex were companies such as BodyMasters, Paramount, and Universal. On the cardiovascular side of the equipment equation, Life Fitness, founded by Augie Nieto of Lifecycle fame, led the way. Through the introduction of the Lifecycle, the Liferower, and later the Lifestep, and the Lifetreadmill, Life Fitness took the lead in the manufacture and sales of cardiovascular equipment. StairMaster was another successful equipment manufacturing company that originated in the 1980s under the visionary leadership of Randy Peterson and Nicholas Orlando. StairMaster evolved from the landmark creation, manufacturing, and marketing of the StairMaster—the first mechanical stairclimbing machine. It could safely be argued that the StairMaster was the industry's signature product during the 1980s and might have been the most popular form of cardiovascular training equipment in the United States during this period. The success of Life Fitness and StairMaster led other companies, such as Trotter, Unisen, and Precor, to enter the fitness equipment industry. During this decade, the motorized treadmill was even further popularized by companies such as Quinton and Trotter and later blossomed under the efforts of companies such as Precor, Unisen, and Life Fitness.

The 1990s

At the beginning of the decade, a total of 13,854 clubs were operating in the United States. By the end of the decade, that total had grown to approximately 16,000 clubs, an overall increase of 15% (Figures 1.1). Concurrently, the number of club members increased by 36% from 21 million members at the beginning of the decade to 33 million by the end of the decade (Figure 1.2). During this period, the number of core members in health/fitness clubs increased by 100%, from just less than seven million to nearly 14 million. Interestingly, the average club member at the end of the decade used the club on average 89 times a year, up from an average of 72 times a year ten years earlier (Figure 1.3). In a similar vein, the percentage of Americans who were members of clubs grew from just over seven percent of the total population of the United States at the beginning of the decade to 13% of the population at the end of the decade. All of the aforementioned data indicates that the industry grew more in terms of both the number of members using clubs and how frequently these members used the clubs, rather than being simply a by-product of the proliferation in the number of clubs. In other words, demand was growing faster than supply, a positive indicator for the continued growth of the industry.

> It could safely be argued that the StairMaster was the industry's signature product during the 1980s and might have been the most popular form of cardiovascular training equipment in the United States during this period.

A significant change in the market demographics of the average club member also occurred in the 1990s. During the growth period of the 70s and 80s, the typical member of a health/fitness club was a male between the ages of 18 and 34, with an annual income under $50,000. As the industry progressed during the decade, however, the demographics of club members changed. The primary market for membership became individuals who were older (35 to 54), as well as more affluent ($50,000 to $75,000). By the end of the decade, the average age and household income of prospects continued to climb. At that point, a member was most likely to be between 35-54, equally likely to be male or female, and likely to be someone making in excess of $75,000 annually.

The aforementioned demographic swing, along with the new focus on family, would cause significant changes in the industry during the decade. It should be noted that during the 1990s, the total amount of retail spending in the industry had grown from around $6.5 billion in the early 1990s to $11.6 billion by the end of the decade, an increase of over 50% in consumer spending on health/fitness memberships (Figure 1.5).

As a result of both the under supply of health/fitness clubs and the growing financial performance of these commercial entities, the investment world began to look at the health/fitness club industry as a viable investment option. The movement of substantial equity into the industry from non-industry sources, such as equity groups, merchant banks, etc., represents one of the landmark occurrences in the 1990s for the industry. In fact, this influx of investment was a precursor of many of the changes that would take place in the 21st century.

It should be noted that during the 1990s, the total amount of retail spending in the industry had grown from around $6.5 billion in the early 1990s to $11.6 billion by the end of the decade, an increase of over 50% in consumer spending on health/fitness memberships.

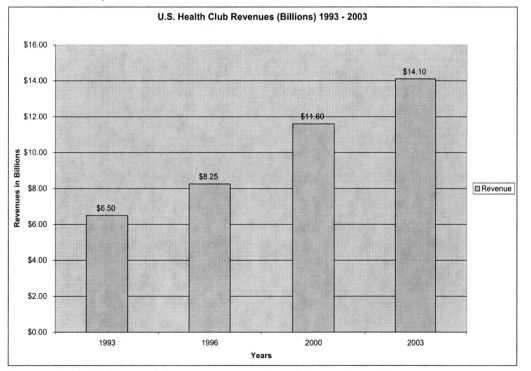

Figure 1.5. Health/fitness club revenues in the United States 1993-2003

The 1990s also served as host to some of the most significant program and service trends to hit the industry since its earliest years.

From a club and facility perspective, the 1990s brought several significant changes, including:

- Consolidation and the formation of larger multi-club operators on a local, regional, and national scale (e.g., Bally's, 24 Hour Fitness, Town Sports International, Wellbridge, Sport & Health, Lifetime Fitness, Five Seasons, Club One, etc.)

- The establishment of fitness centers (i.e., fitness- and exercise-only centers with no sports component)

- The development of large suburban multipurpose clubs that focused primarily on the family (e.g., Lifetime Fitness, WAC, etc.)

- The creation of multiple-modailty studios (aerobics, spinning, and Yoga)

- The dawn of the club-based spa

- The creation of distinct club brands (e.g., Bally's, Crunch, Equinox, 24 Hour Fitness, etc.)

- The entry of hospital-based facilities into the industry, in large part driven by the aging population and the realization of the medical community that "prevention" should be an integral part of the medical business model

- The entry of expensive large-scale, community-owned and operated recreation centers, which would compete in the industry on a not-for-profit basis

- The expansion of the number of YMCAs and JCCs into a more competitive position in an attempt to serve the fitness market

- The development of apartment- and hotel-based fitness centers

The aforementioned changes in the types of health/fitness facilities and operations were driven by the evolving demographics, alterations in popular culture, additional research on the benefits of exercise, and the maturing of the industry from a purely business perspective.

The 1990s also served as host to some of the most significant program and service trends to hit the industry since its earliest years. Among the more influential trends and program practices to arise during this period were the following:

- Spinning. Introduced by Johnny G and Schwinn, spinning became the rage during the early to mid-90s and has continued to be one of the industry's most sought-after programs. Spinning involves group-based cycling that is done to music.

- Yoga and Pilates. As the average age of the club members continued to increase in the 1990s, classes in yoga and Pilates became mainstays of the industry. The trend was toward softer activity that emphasized stretching and movement, rather than aerobics. Yoga is an Eastern form of moving meditation that combines stretching with breathing. Pilates is a form of exercise that is based on principles that were developed by Joseph Pilates in the 1920s.

- Weight training. Research showing the beneficial effects of resistance training on bone health, weight control, and overall health led to an enormous increase in the popularity of weight training.

- Personal training. The public's perception of personal training changed dramatically in the 1990s. Once considered a fringe program that appealed to a very small audience of affluent members, personal training became the primary program thrust of the industry during this period, as even more individuals recognized the value of receiving personalized attention and instruction.

- Packaged group exercise. In the 1990s, the focus on "aerobics" had generally been replaced in the industry with "group exercise," and with it, an emphasis on having more diversity in group-exercise programming. In the process, programs such as STEP, Body Pump, Spinning, Precision Cycling, Body Rage, and Kickbox Fitness, among others, became household programs in the industry.

- Kids' programming. By the end of the decade, most suburban clubs had come to realize that their ability to successfully attract a sufficient number of members would, in large part, be driven by their ability to offer a variety of youth-oriented programs.

- Seniors' programming. In the 1990s, the ever-increasing age level of the average club member, in part driven by the aging of the baby boomers, created a need for an entirely new focus of programming that was geared towards providing exercise alternatives for those individuals over the age of 50. For example, the development of Wellbridge was in response to this particular program trend.

- Day spas. By the end of the decade, the day-spa concept had taken hold in the industry, as many members perceived spa treatments to be an integral part of their overall approach to improving their level of well-being.

In 1996, possibly the most important landmark for the health and fitness industry ever to occur happened when the U.S. government released the U.S. Surgeon General's Report on Physical Activity and Health.

In 1996, possibly the most important landmark for the health and fitness industry ever to occur happened when the U.S. government released the U.S. Surgeon General's Report on Physical Activity and Health. In this report, the U.S. Surgeon General provided the American public with a clear, yet critical, message: Americans would benefit immensely from a regular program of physical activity. In essence, the message detailed the fact that engaging in physical activity on a regular basis contributes significantly to reductions in many health-related disorders. Furthermore, if specific activity guidelines were followed, individuals could improve their health and prolong the quality of their life. The full impact of this report has yet to be completely realized, since most Americans have not fully embraced the significance of the report. Nonetheless, the impact of this particular report on the industry was very significant.

The 1990s also served as a springboard for some of the most significant equipment innovations in the industry since the development of StairMaster, Lifecycle, and Nautilus machines. Among the equipment innovations that occurred during this period were the following:

- The elliptical trainer. Precor introduced the concept of elliptical training in the early 90s. Named the EFX, the Precor elliptical trainer changed the face of equipment-based training forever. The elliptical trainer provided a low-impact, comfortable approach to training that would slowly lead to a significant decrease in the popularity of such activities as indoor cycling and mechanical stairclimbing.

- Spinning bike. The introduction of the spinning bike was a new twist on the bicycle ergometers of the 70s and 80s, such as those that were made by Body Guard and Monarch. The spinning bike allowed members to train in social groups, while simultaneously controlling the intensity level of their training.

- Plate-loaded resistance equipment. First introduced by Hammer in the late 1980s, but subsequently even more popularized in the 1990s, plate-loaded equipment combined the safety features of selectorized machines with the impact of free-weight training.

- Treadmills. While treadmills have been around for over 40 years, companies such as Star Trac, Life Fitness, Quinton, and Precor brought new dynamics to this particular type of equipment in the 1990s. In the process, treadmills became one of the most popular pieces of equipment in the industry, as manufacturers included programming options and audio and visual entertainment as a basic feature on their products—all at a reasonable cost.

- Pilates-based equipment. While Pilates equipment has been around since the 1920s, it was essentially introduced to the club industry during the 1990s. By the end of the decade, Pilates equipment would continue to grow in popularity.

- Personal entertainment systems. The development of Cardio Theater (and later Broadcast Vision) by Tony Deleede was a landmark occurrence in the industry. For many consumers, the introduction of Cardio Theater changed the way that they evaluated their club experience.

The 1990s also witnessed an oversupply in the number of organizations that attempted to provide education and certification support to the industry. By the end of the decade, over 200 organizations laid claim to being the health/fitness professional certification of choice, leaving both the industry and consumers to wonder, "Which certification really insures that the recipient is a qualified fitness professional?"

The final landmark change that occurred in the 1990s was the change in direction taken by the International Health, Racquet, and Sportclub Association

> The 1990s also served as a springboard for some of the most significant equipment innovations in the industry since the development of StairMaster, Lifecycle, and Nautilus machines.

(IHRSA). From its inception and through the first half of the 1990s, IHRSA (formerly IRSA) had focused on being an association of quality clubs. This focus allowed it to develop resources to upgrade the professionalism of its membership. During the later half of the 1990s, however, IHRSA made a conscious shift in strategy. In the process, IHRSA became an industry trade association, one that focused on public advocacy for the industry and expanded its role in the growing international market. This change in direction allowed IHRSA to partner with other organizations in an attempt to establish a more significant voice for the industry in public policy and industry promotion.

Not only has the industry mix become more diverse, so has the size of club facility that the industry markets to the consumer.

The Early 21st Century (2000-2005)

At the beginning of the new century, there were 15,900 health/fitness clubs in the United States, serving approximately 33 million members. In only four years, the number of clubs had grown to just over 26,000, serving just over 41 million members (Figures 1.1-1.2). During this period, the percentage of Americans who were members of clubs increased from approximately 13% of the population to 14% of the population. In only four short years, the number of clubs had increased by nearly 35%, while the number of club members had grown by slightly over 18%.

The aforementioned trend is the polar opposite of what occurred during the 1990s, when the growth in membership outpaced the growth in clubs, and demand exceeded supply. A review of available data as far back as 1987 shows that the average number of members per facility had dropped from over 2,000 per club to approximately 1,500 per club. What occurred during the early part of the new century is an over-development in the number of clubs, as compared to the growth in membership. In other words, the industry began to carve the pie into smaller pieces, rather than grow the size of the pie. Club growth had created saturation in several significant markets, such as New York, Los Angeles, Chicago, and other major metropolitan markets. In these areas, the number of clubs far surpassed the growth in market demand. Most of this shift in supply and demand was fueled by the influx of investment capital and the growth strategies of various regional and national club chains, including Bally's, 24 Hour Fitness, LA Fitness, Equinox, Sports Club/LA, Town Sports International, and Life Time Fitness, among others. The supply-and-demand equation has been further tilted by the fact that most of the club growth has occurred in what is commonly termed "fitness boxes," club models that look and feel the same and which lack any real brand differentiation. In reality, all of the blame for this oversupply cannot be attributed purely to the growth in the number of commercial clubs. By 2004, the industry mix was very diverse as reflected in Figure 1.6, which is based on the *2003 Health Club Trend Report* by American Sports Data.

Not only has the industry mix become more diverse, so has the size of club facility that the industry markets to the consumer. According to the *2005*

The industry
currently faces the
twin challenges of
having an oversupply
of clubs and a lack
of product
differentiation.

Club/Facility Type	Percentage of the Market
Commercial Clubs	47%
YMCA/JCC	17%
University-Based Facilities	65
Hospital-Based Facilities	5%
Residential Facilities	5%
Corporate Facilities	4%
Municipal Facilities	4%
Military Facilities	2%
Hotel/Resort Facilities	2%
Country Club Facilities	2%
Private Studios	1%

Figure 1.6. Industry mix of various types of clubs and facilities

Club Size	Percentage of the Market
Under 20,000 S.F.	20%
20,000 to 35,000 S.F.	26%
35,000 to 60,000 S.F.	20%
Greater than 60,000 S.F.	34%

Figure 1.7. Club size as a percentage of the club market

Health Club Trend Report, underwritten by IHRSA, clubs can be categorized into one of four categories, with each representing a given percentage of the market. Figure 1.7 provides an overview of that mix. Most recently, the newest segment of the market that has shown incredible growth is the number of small clubs under 3,000 square feet, illustrated by entities such as Curves for women and Cuts for men.

Looking closer at industry research as reflected in *IHRSA's 2004 Global Report* and the *2004 Health Club Trend Report* produced by American Sports Data, it is evident that during the first four years of the new century, the industry has had more success generating usage from its existing members, rather than attracting new members to the market. In 1990, the average club member used their club 79 times a year, while by 2005, that usage figure had increased to just over 90 times a year. Furthermore, the number of core members (i.e., those individuals who used the club more than 100 times a year) had increased to 16 million, or approximately 40% of the total membership base. In fact, the most active club members were those individuals who were over the age of 55. The available statistics indicate that by 2005, the industry had managed to elicit greater usage from its membership, more than it had been able to drive additional non-members into the clubs. As a result, the industry currently faces the twin challenges of having an oversupply of clubs and a lack of product differentiation.

In 2004, the profile of a club member was shifting radically. By 2004, the industry consumer profile was as follows:

- Fifty-two percent of members were women.

- The 55-and-over population had become its fastest growing segment. As of 2004, this group represented 19% of the overall membership (up from under 10% only 15 years earlier).

- The 35-to-54 age group was the largest segment of membership at 37%, having gown by over 140% in the last 15 years.

- While those individuals who are 18 to 34 years of age still represent 34% of the membership, this group had the least growth in the past 15 years.

- The number of members under the age of 18 was growing rapidly, second only to those over age 55.

- Membership penetration is highest for women 35 to 44 and men 25 to 34.

- Ten percent of all adults over the age of 55 are members of clubs, while 16% of those ages who are 35 to 54 are members.

- The average household income for club members had reached $76,000 annually.

- Over half of all club members had a four-year college degree.

Future Industry Trends

By 2005, a number of industry trends had shifted, as the facilities, equipment, and programs employed in the industry reflected the new demographics and psychographics of the American population. These trends represent the true state of the health/fitness club industry as of 2005 and are the precursors for what the industry can likely expect over the next ten years. Among the most significant of these trends are the following:

Facilities:
- Aquatic entertainment facilities with zero-depth pools, water slides, and water features

- Day spas and salons

- Mind/body studios focused on Pilates, yoga, and other Eastern arts

- Personal training studios

- Mega-clubs offering every facility option possible

- Youth centers with dedicated fitness and activity areas

Equipment:
- Treadmills with features such as televisions and fans

- Elliptical trainers

Ten percent of all adults over the age of 55 are members of clubs, while 16% of those ages who are 35 to 54 are members.

- Recumbent bicycles
- Personal entertainment centers on equipment
- Functional fitness equipment

Programs and Services:

- Yoga, especially non-traditional styles such as "Bikram yoga, power yoga, and western yoga
- Group classes in a box (Body Pump, Body Rage, Body Flow, etc.)
- Fusion fitness (blend of styles such as spin/yoga, Pilates/pump, kickbox fitness, yoga/Pilates, etc.)
- Extreme fitness (boot camp, SWAT fitness, combat conditioning, etc.)
- Core and functional fitness (focus on the core muscle groups and personal performance activities)
- Youth sports performance conditioning
- Pre-packaged weight-loss programs
- Spa services
- Pilates and gyrotonics

As a consequence of IHRSA's and the industry's efforts to have the industry accepted as a mainstream entity and the maturation of the industry into a $14 billion undertaking, the public and government began to place new demands on the level of accountability of both the industry and the professionals involved in the delivery of fitness services.

In 2005, the industry also was faced with the challenges brought on by an increasing demand from the public for professional accountability. As a consequence of IHRSA's and the industry's efforts to have the industry accepted as a mainstream entity and the maturation of the industry into a $14 billion undertaking, the public and government began to place new demands on the level of accountability of both the industry and the professionals involved in the delivery of fitness services. Examples of some of the public and government expectations that have either occurred or are about to happen include:

- State-level legislation that mandates the placement of automated external defibrillators in every health club (as of 2005, five states have passed legislation)
- State-level legislation that mandates the registration or licensing of personal trainers
- State-level legislation governing the operation of spa services
- Higher expectations by the public for business practices grounded in integrity from all health/fitness club operators
- Expectations from the financial world for greater accountability and standardization of accounting practices in health/fitness clubs
- Expectations from investors for quarterly earnings performances similar to Wall Street expectations

- Expectations by the public that the franchising of health/fitness clubs will continue. In that regard, beginning in 2003 and continuing through 2005, the industry has witnessed a substantial growth in the level of franchising groups such as Gold's, Powerhouse, and newcomers, such as Curves, Workout Express, Butterfly Lite, and Cuts, either expanded their efforts or entered the market during this period.

2

The Physical Activity Beliefs and Behaviors of Americans and Their Implications for Health/Fitness Clubs

In fact, the success of the health and fitness club business is extremely dependent upon the physical activity beliefs and behaviors of Americans.

Chapter Objectives

In order to gain a greater understanding of the physical activity practices of Americans and ultimately their potential suitability as health/fitness club members, it is important to understand the values and attitudes that Americans have toward physical activity. In that regard, research has shown that the values and attitudes held by individuals are the major determinants of their behavior. In other words, the core determinant of a person's actions is that individual's core values, which are at the heart of the attitudes they have. In fact, the success of the health and fitness club business is extremely dependent upon the physical activity beliefs and behaviors of Americans. This chapter provides an overview of the available research pertaining to both the attitudes of Americans toward physical activity and their actual physical activity behavior. The information in the chapter is designated to help club owners and operators better position their clubs for success by enabling them to more fully understand the beliefs and behaviors of their potential clients.

Core American Values Toward Physical Activity and Health

When Americans are asked to rank their core values and how those values align with their overall satisfaction with life, health and fitness are an integral part of their response. According to research conducted by Roper Starch for IHRSA in 2001 and additional research conducted in 2003 by American Sports Data, Americans rank health as the third most important value behind family and spouse. Concurrently, they rank fitness seventh among their top eight values (family, spouse, health, friends, career, diet, fitness, and money). It is interesting to note that both health and fitness are rated as more important than money (refer to Figure 2-1).

On the other hand, when indicating the importance of each value to their overall level of satisfaction with life, health and fitness seem far less relevant to Americans than values such as family, spouse, and money. Taken at face value, it is evident that when Americans prioritize their values, that health and fitness are important, but when measured as a contributor to their overall level of satisfaction with life, health and fitness fall lower on the scale.

When Americans are questioned in greater depth about their attitude toward the importance of health and fitness, they share the following:

- 97% of Americans say it is essential and/or important to maintain good health.

- 91% of Americans say it is essential and/or important to keep up their physical appearance.

When indicating the importance of each value to their overall level of satisfaction with life, health and fitness seem far less relevant to Americans than values such as family, spouse, and money.

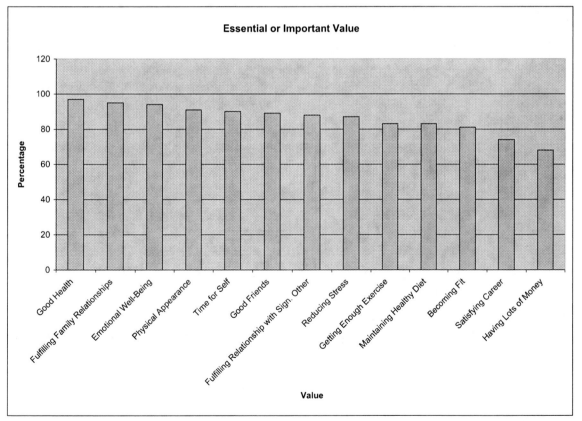

Figure 2.1. Priority ranking of American values

- 83% of American's say it is essential and/or important to get enough exercise.

- 81% of American's say it is essential to become physically fit.

- Women are far more likely than men to say fitness is important to health (nearly 60% of women versus 30% for men). Women are also more likely (40% to 30%) than men to say fitness is important to appearance.

- 74% of Americans are satisfied with their physical health, while 61% are satisfied with their physical appearance. Only 49% are satisfied with the amount of physical activity they get.

- Younger men seem more satisfied than younger women with their health and appearance, but as both groups age, men become less satisfied and women more satisfied.

When this data and the supporting research are examined, the following conclusions can be drawn:

- Americans understand the importance of being healthy and fit, yet they don't see as much value in actually exercising to obtain the health and fitness that they say they value so much.

- Women, more than men, understand the importance of fitness to health and wellbeing.

- Americans as a rule, and men more than women, are generally satisfied with their health, appearance, and fitness. As a result, they already see themselves as having met the value equation when it comes to health and fitness and are less likely to see themselves as having a need to actually engage in activity such as exercise.

Americans understand the importance of being healthy and fit, yet they don't see as much value in actually exercising to obtain the health and fitness that they say they value so much.

What Active Americans Say Are the Reasons They Participate in Exercise and Sports

When men and women are asked for the reasons why they engage in physical activity (exercise and sports), their responses indicate that there are multiple variables that influence their actual behavior. Figure 2.2, based on research conducted by Roper Starch on behalf of the International Health, Racquet, and Sportclub Association (IHRSA) in 2001, provides a concise overview of the multiplicity of reasons Americans give for exercising.

It is clear from looking at Figure 2.2 that men and women have different reasons for exercising. This information is important because understanding these gender-related differences can assist club owners/managers in developing club-based programs that can help attract and retain club members. For example, men are far more inclined than women to claim fun, enjoyment, personal challenge, and competition as driving forces for their exercise habits. Women, in turn, are far more inclined to see losing weight,

Reason for Exercising	Men's Response Percentage	Women's Response Percentage
To remain fit	63%	70%
For fun and enjoyment	56%	44%
To lose weight	26%	54%
To assist with a medical condition	21%	33%
For the personal challenge	29%	16%
Prevention of health problems	30%	42%
For competition	27%	9%

Figure 2.2. The reasons Americans give for exercising

Americans can be classified in one of four categories of fitness consciousness: non-believers, indifferent, uninitiated believers, and hard-core participants.

Non-Believers 2% of the population	Indifferent 16% of the population	Uninitiated Believers 63% of the population	Hard-Core Participants 17% of the population
Do not embrace the fitness lifestyle	No real interest in fitness	Believe fitness has value	Embrace fitness
Don't believe exercise is importantand	Negative attitude toward fitness	25% are sedentary and 26% are very active	Doers and believers; apostles of exercise
Sedentary lifestyle	Likely to claim they are not healthy	70% claim to be overweight	Regard their health as excellent
Male dominated	Equally likely to be male or female	More likely to be a woman and younger	57% male
Least educated	Low income and education	37% are college educated	49% are college educated and 38% are making in excess of $75K

Figure 2.3. Traits attributed to each of the basic categories of fitness consciousness

staying fit, and helping prevent or assist with health-related conditions as a reason for their exercising.

The Level of Fitness Consciousness Among Americans as a Predictor of Joining and Staying with Exercise

According to the research conducted by American Sports Data in 2003 and supported by the work of Dr. Rod Dishman, Americans can be classified in one of four categories of fitness consciousness: non-believers, indifferent, uninitiated believers, and hard-core participants. Understanding these categories and the accompanying traits and characteristics can assist clubs both in attracting new members and retaining existing ones. Figure 2.3 offers an overview of the traits associated with each basic category.

It is evident that those who are non-believers or indifferent are not good candidates for membership in a health/fitness club because the values and beliefs that they hold toward exercise would be very difficult to overcome when attempting to entice them to join a club. Even if they were sold a membership through "closing techniques," they would be unlikely to ever use their membership. The individuals who have hard-core, favorable attitudes toward fitness represent 16% of the population, a total which closely parallels the percentage of Americans who are currently health club members (14%). This would indicate that as an industry, we are close to extracting all of the low hanging fruit and need to develop strategies that will attract the uninitiated segment (63%) of the population if we are to continue to grow the membership market.

What a Portrait of Those Who Exercise Can Mean to Clubs

In the work that Roper Starch conducted for IHRSA in 2001, exercisers and non-exercisers were identified by a set of personality or physcographic characteristics. Grasping the nuances of these classifications can help club operators better understand the dynamics of how to develop and deliver a personalized club experience that can help attract and retain members. According to Roper's research, there are a total of six classifications: balanced holistics, conscientious preventors, social competitors, abracadabras, woulda-shouldas, and sit-com skeptics. An overview of the key attributes that characterize each of these six different and important groups involves the following:

> The individuals who have hard-core, favorable attitudes toward fitness represent 16% of the population, a total which closely parallels the percentage of Americans who are currently health club members (14%).

❑ *Balanced Holistics (13%)*. These are individuals who see exercise as important to both their emotional and physical health. They exercise regularly and focus on reaching a state of internal harmony. They are twice as likely to be club members in comparison to the average American. They define themselves as socially confident, goal-oriented, energetic, and intelligent. They are more likely to be female (58%), college educated (32%), have a higher household income (average of $42K), be married (69%), and younger (40) than the average American.

❑ *Conscientious Preventors (8%)*. This group takes a balanced approach to physical activity and sees exercise as an avenue for the prevention of health-related problems. They are twice as likely to be club members and describe themselves as health-conscious, family-oriented, religious, and perfectionists. They are more likely to be older women (60% female, average age of 55); college educated (32%), and have a higher income (average of $46K) than the average American.

❑ *Social Competitors (20%)*. These individuals prefer to spend their time in an environment that is social, engaging, and competitive. They are no more likely than other Americans to be club members. They describe themselves as professional, ambitious, risk-taking, and outgoing. They are also more likely to be male (60%) and single than the average American. They tend to fall within the average range when it comes to their level of college education and income, but are younger than the average American.

❑ *Woulda-Shouldas (12%)*. These are people who exercise, though not on a regular basis, and who tend to feel self conscious about themselves. They describe themselves as out of shape, emotional, shy, and professionally ambitious. They are most likely to be younger single males (62% male and 37% single) who have average earnings and slightly more college education than the general public.

❑ *Sit-Com Skeptics (33%)*. Members of this category see exercise as nothing more than a craze that is followed by self-absorbed individuals. They feel that a reasonable diet and clean living are the answer to good health. Generally speaking, they tend to be older married males (70% married and 56% male), with less education and less household income.

> **Sit-com skeptics see exercise as nothing more than a craze that is followed by self-absorbed individuals.**

At first glance, a question might arise concerning what value exists in being aware of the aforementioned information. In essence, the answer is fairly straightforward. If club owners/managers were to create a profile questionnaire for their member prospects and existing members and then categorize these individuals into one of the four groups categorized by Roper, then they would have the capability of creating programs and services that would allow them to better tailor the club experience to each group's needs and interests.

What Americans Are Actually Doing When it Comes to Physical Activity

Up to this point, much of this chapter has addressed the beliefs and values that Americans have about exercise and sports. As was previously stated, understanding those values and beliefs will help club operators and/or fitness professionals better understand how they can exert greater influence on changing the exercise and sports behavior of the public and, as a consequence, grow their membership base. This section of the chapter presents an overview of the actual reported physical-activity behavior of Americans. The information is designed to provide further insight into the relationship between values, beliefs, and behavior when it comes to exercise.

	1987	1990	1993	1997	2000	2003
Millions	42.3	51.5	50	52.6	51.7	50.9
% of total U.S. Population	19.7	23.2	21.8	21.8	20.8	19.8

Figure 2.4. Annual American involvement in physical fitness pursuits on an active basis

The number of core or active participants in physical-fitness activity has continued to grow over the past 15 years, but as a percentage of the population, it has remained flat.

In the 2002 American Sports Data (ASD) report on *Trends in U.S. Physical Fitness Behavior*, physical fitness activity was divided into three distinct categories: fitness, recreation, and outdoor activity. The fitness category included such activities as aerobics, aquatics, free weights, Pilates, yoga, etc. Recreation involved participating in such undertakings as basketball, football, ice-skating, tennis, racquet sports, volleyball, etc. Outdoor activity consisted of engaging in activities such as hiking, rock climbing, mountain biking, skiing, etc. According to Figure 2.4 (based on data compiled in the aforementioned 2002 American Sports Data Report), American involvement in physical-fitness activities on an active basis has increased from 42 million in 1987 to nearly 51 million in 2002 (it should be noted that "active" is defined as 100x in at least one activity annually).

A review of Figure 2.4 indicates that the percentage of Americans who report being actively involved in physical fitness activity (fitness, sports, outdoor) has continued to drop since 1990, falling to a level of below 20% of the population in 2003. It is interesting to note that participation in fitness -only activities has increased from just over 27 billion participation days in 1987 to 30 billion participation days in 2002, although the number of individuals participating in sports activity and outdoor activity has remained relatively flat at 8.3 billion participation days and just under 1.4 billion participation days, respectively (refer to Figure 2.5). This data, along with other statistics provided by the ASD's research, indicate the following macro trends in physical-fitness behavior:

- The number of core or active participants in physical-fitness activity has continued to grow over the past 15 years, but as a percentage of the population, it has remained flat.

- Women are more likely than men to be core or active participants.

- Those 55+ are the largest segment of active individuals.

- 34% of those individuals with college degrees are active, while just 13% of those individuals who do not have a college education are active.

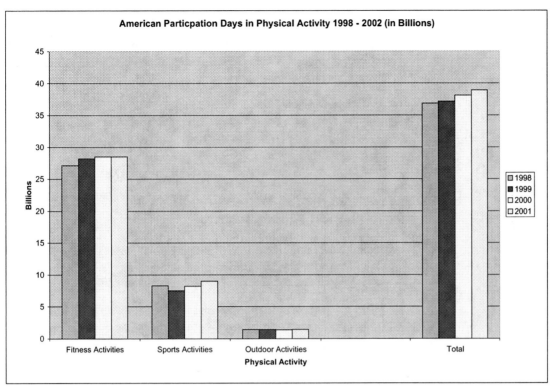

Figure 2.5. Total number of days in which Americans engage in physical activity

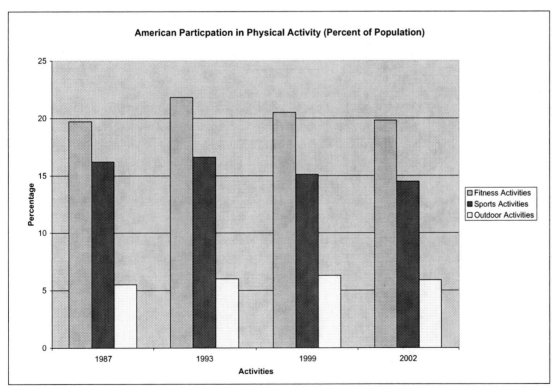

Figure 2.6. Percent of the American population that engages in selected physical activities

- Men are far more likely than women to be involved in outdoor activity.

- Over the past 10 years, participation in club-based activities, such as high-impact aerobics (40%), step aerobics (30%), mechanical stairclimbing (10%), and stationary cycling (30%), have all declined.

- During the past 10 years, the following activities have shown continuous growth in participation: spinning (10%), elliptical training (100%), free weight training (50%), yoga (100%), and Pilates (150%).

One key to attracting people to exercise and fitness is to better understand their personality dynamics and having the club tailoring its promotional and programming package to fit those dynamics.

Key Takeaways from the Research on American Beliefs and Behavior with Regard to Physical Fitness Behavior

- Americans, in general, understand and acknowledge that exercise and fitness are important to their health. Furthermore, they tend to see them as important values.

- While 80% of Americans claim that exercise is important, only 19% have adopted the appropriate behavior in some fashion.

- While the fitness consciousness of Americans is higher than ever before (according to the media and research), actual fitness behavior is at one of its lowest points in the past 20 years. A real disconnect seems to exist between what the brain knows and the body does.

- Physical fitness behavior is slowly becoming the domain of the older, more-educated, and more-affluent population.

- Health and leading a balanced life seem to be overtaking appearance as a prime factor in whether an individual engages in physical activity.

- One key to attracting people to exercise and fitness is to better understand their personality dynamics and having the club tailoring its promotional and programming package to fit those dynamics. For example, if someone is an uninitiated social competitor, then the club's package must be different for them than it might be for an uninitiated balanced holistic. Likewise, if club operators are core users who could be characterized as conscious preventors, they should not expect their target market to be attracted to those factors that attracts them.

It is important to be aware of the differences in what motivates women and men and how an individual's age, education, and background can affect that person's behavior. This understanding can help club operators to adapt their efforts accordingly.

3

Consumer Attitudes Toward Health/Fitness Clubs That Affect Their Reasons for Joining and Staying

Chapter Objectives

The heart and soul of any successful health/fitness club is its membership. Without a thriving membership base, a health/fitness club will never reach its operating and financial potential. Membership, therefore, must be the top priority when it comes to building a successful club. The first step in building club membership is to understand what consumers perceive about the club experience and what triggers influence their decision to join a particular facility. This chapter initially focuses on providing an overview of consumer perceptions of health/fitness clubs and then details the reasons why consumers actually join a health/fitness club.

The first step in building club membership is to understand what consumers perceive about the club experience and what triggers influence their decision to join a particular facility.

Consumer Attitudes about Health/Fitness Clubs

As discussed in the previous chapter, the attitudes and beliefs that consumers have about exercise are the primary drivers of their actual exercise behavior. This relationship also applies to consumer behavior with regard to actually joining a health/fitness club. What the consumers perceive about the health/fitness club experience has been shown to play a major role in their decision about whether to become a member. While more personally relevant needs and wants can alter the impact of consumer attitudes as they impact their decision whether to join a club, attitudes toward health/fitness clubs still play a very significant role in their decision whether to become a member of a and more importantly, which health/fitness club to join.

In 2001, Roper Starch, on behalf of IHRSA, studied the attitudes of both non-members, former club members, and existing club members to gain a more thorough grasp of the underlying attitudes about health/fitness clubs and why people join. This research was the first meaningful work in this arena since the 1985 study sponsored by IHRSA titled, "Why People Join." Among the key facts that Starch identified in his research are the following:

48% of consumers believe that health/fitness clubs are only for those who are physically fit and not for those individuals who are just beginning a fitness program.

- 66% of consumers feel that the purchase of a health-club membership is worth the expense.

- 60% of consumers agree that health/fitness clubs offer more knowledge and expertise on fitness than consumers can obtain on their own.

- 56% of consumers believe that health/fitness clubs are fun.

- 48% of consumers believe that health/fitness clubs are only for those who are physically fit and not for those individuals who are just beginning a fitness program.

- 45% of consumers see health/fitness clubs as being for young people.

- 31% of consumers believe that health/fitness clubs are places to go to "pick up" others.

- 62% of consumers believe that health/fitness clubs are overcrowded.

One point that can be deduced from Starch's data is that consumers, in general, place a value on the health/fitness club experience, primarily in the ability of the club to provide an environment of expertise and enjoyment. Concurrently, a perception also exists among the public that health/fitness clubs are overcrowded, are primarily entities for young people, and are particularly appropriate places to pick up dates. Obviously, these types of attitudes and beliefs present a challenge to any club that is attempting to attract prospects to its doors.

	Non-Members	Former Club Members	Current Club Members
Worth the Money	61%	85%	93%
Fun Place	52%	76%	78%
For Fit People	53%	40%	16%
Pick-up Places	33%	27%	14%
For Younger People	48%	37%	22%
Overcrowded	62%	75%	73%

Figure 3.1. Consumer attitudes toward health/fitness club membership

It should be kept in mind that the aforementioned highlighted findings are generalized across the three segments of the population that Starch studied— non-members, former club members, and current club members. When a closer look is taken at the attitudes by segment (refer to Figure 3.1), even greater understanding of the dynamics of consumer attitudes and their impact on health/fitness club membership can be gained.

Given the information presented in Figure 3.1, the health/fitness club operator could logically extrapolate the following concerning consumer attitudes about health/fitness clubs:

- The non-member is far less likely to see the value in a health/fitness club than either a member or a former member. From a club perspective, this determination means that clubs need to educate prospects better about the real value of the club experience.

- The non-member is far more likely to say a health/fitness club is not a fun place than either a former member or a member. From a club perspective, this conclusion suggests that clubs must do a better job of portraying the entertainment aspect of the health/fitness club experience.

- The non-member overwhelmingly believes, in comparison to former members and current members, that health/fitness clubs are for the fit and young, as well as a place to 'pick-up" someone. In light of the research presented in the first chapter that concluded that the average age of club members is getting older, this perception is not in touch with the actual reality. The pertinent questions have to be, "What are club operators doing to perpetuate these beliefs among the public or what can they do to change them?"

- Non-members, former members, and members all hold a similar view that health/fitness clubs are overcrowded. From the club operator's perspective, this viewpoint is one of the most challenging and possibly damaging perspectives the industry could present. Research has shown that if consumers feel the clubs are too crowded, they will be far less likely to join a health/fitness club.

Research has shown that if consumers feel the clubs are too crowded, they will be far less likely to join a health/fitness club.

The Reasons Members Give for Joining a Health/Fitness Club

While the previous section examined the attitudes that consumers hold about health/fitness clubs, this section reviews the reasons club members give for actually joining a particular club. Since approximately 14% of the population of the U.S. are health/fitness club members at the present time, the reasons given for joining only reflect a small percentage of the total consumer population. It should be kept in mind that when reviewing this information, that while these reasons can play a critical role in how a club markets itself to the public, these reasons—by themselves—will not help a club overcome the public perceptions of the health/fitness industry. Understanding and then acting on both the attitudes that individuals have toward clubs and the reasons members give for joining a club will be most useful and helpful when developing and implementing a successful health/fitness club operation. Figure 3.2 details the global reasons underlying why consumers become health/fitness club members.

If global reasons given by both men and women for joining a health/fitness club are considered in light of the information provided in the previous chapter on the attitudes that individuals hold toward physical fitness, some very important generalizations can be identified that might enhance the efforts of clubs to attract members, including:

Men are far less likely to see a club as being of value for them based on the need to be motivated to exercise or to establish relationships. Rather, men tend to be motivated by their need for a competitive and challenging environment.

- Men are driven by a need to have a place to exercise. Furthermore, they desire a competitive, engaging experience that challenges them.

- Men are far less likely to see a club as being of value for them based on the need to be motivated to exercise or to establish relationships. Rather, men tend to be motivated by their need for a competitive and challenging environment.

- Women also desire a place to exercise, but are equally as likely to exercise at home or in another environment.

- Women place far greater value on the club experience if their friends are also members and if they can interact with a friendly staff.

- Women place far greater value on the social aspect a club offers (e.g., group exercise classes), as well as on the opportunities within the club setting to establish relationships.

Beyond the aforementioned global motivators for joining a health/fitness club, other factors that are more holistic and personal exist concerning why individuals join a particular club. Understanding these more personal factors can assist club operators in personalizing (and thereby enhancing) the overall sales process:

- Current and former members all indicate that they feel better after a workout than before and see the experience as beneficial to their overall health.

Reason	Men	Women
Place to exercise	60%	50%
Need motivation to exercise	28%	38%
Friendly staff	17%	26%
Friends joined	17%	25%
Participate in classes	4%	20%

Figure 3.2. Why consumers become health/fitness club members

- Current and former members see the club experience as important to their emotional wellbeing and an opportunity to get centered.

Beyond the actual reasons given by the public for joining a health/fitness club, several factors influence the consumers' reasons for making the buying decision concerning club membership. When designing programs to attract members, clubs can enhance their efforts by considering these benchmark indicators. Figure 3-3 identifies the leading factors that indicate why men and women make the final decision to purchase a club membership.

The benchmarks in Figure 3.3 clearly indicate that women tend to be greatly influenced by factors that would not be relevant to most men and vice versa. Men seem to be influenced most by the type, quality, and availability of equipment, along with the existence of a competitive and challenging environment. Women, in turn, are more influenced in their buying decision by the cleanness of the facility, whether their friends are members, and the basic atmosphere that exists in the club. As such, the atmosphere for women needs to be non-intimidating, relaxed, friendly, and socially engaging.

Men	Women
Location of the club to home or work (within 12 to 15 minutes)	Location of the club to home or work (within 12 to 15 minutes)
Convenience (easy to get in and out)	Convenience (easy to get in and out)
Quality of the facility and equipment	Cleanliness of the facility
The price—value equation. Is it a good deal?	Friends are members
Availability of equipment	Non-intimidating environment
Staff quality and service	Group-exercise programs and kids' services
Competitive environment	Staff quality and service delivery

Figure 3.3. Benchmark indicators concerning purchasing a club membership

Reasons Why Members Either Stay in or Quit Clubs

Once a consumer decides to join a health/fitness club, the process of keeping that member involved begins. This process is referred to as membership retention. Similar to the factors attendant to the joining process, members have specific reasons that they give for quitting a club and/or remaining a member. This section reviews the reasons that members offer for leaving or staying with a health/fitness club that they have joined.

When former club members are questioned about their reasons for dropping their membership, the top seven responses given are as follows:

Similar to the factors attendant to the joining process, members have specific reasons that they give for quitting a club and/or remaining a member.

- They could not afford the membership   30%
- The facility was overcrowded   27%
- They didn't have time to use the club   26%
- The club's location was not convenient   18%
- They lost the motivation to use the club   17%
- They moved out of the area   16%
- They switched to outdoor exercise   15%

Of the reasons that members give for relinquishing their club membership, the most challenging for club operators is the statement by the former members that they could not afford it. In most cases, this reasoning really means they did not use the club enough to warrant the cost of the membership.

When these reasons are examined more closely, three of them are consistent with the factors that impact consumer attitudes about the club and their reasons for joining. The level of crowding, convenience, and motivation are all variables that not only influence whether consumers join a club, but also why they don't remain as members. It seems reasonable to assume that if members are indicating these are their primary drivers for foregoing their club membership, they did not perceive these factors as critical problems at the time they joined the club. Club operators need to understand the genesis of this disconnect. Of the reasons that members give for relinquishing their club membership, the most challenging for club operators is the statement by the former members that they could not afford it. In most cases, this reasoning really means they did not use the club enough to warrant the cost of the membership.

Research conducted on membership retention helps clarify the factors contributing to why individuals quit even further. When former members are asked in more depth about the "real reasons" for quitting, their responses can often be grouped into two major categories—facility-driven and personally-diven. Figure 3.4 details some of the reasons provided by former club members with regard to their facility-related and personal reasons for quitting.

Facility-Driven Reasons for Quitting	Personal Reasons for Quitting
Overcrowding	Did not use the facility enough
Dissatisfaction with the staff	Lost interest and motivation
Lack of attention from the staff	Did not have a partner
Dissatisfied with programs	Switched to exercising at home
Unresponsive management	Did not achieve desired results
Culture of the club	
Facility was not clean	
Dishonest business practices	

Figure 3.4. Why individuals forego their club membership

Variables Associated with Remaining a Member

When individuals are asked what factors impact their decision whether to remain a club member, their answers are very similar to those that individuals give for quitting a club, only the opposite. Among the primary reasons given by individuals for remaining a member of a health/fitness club are the following:

- Their relationship with the staff. The better the relationship, the more likely they are to remain with the club.

- Positive first impressions with the staff and the facility

- Their initial connection with the club, both with meeting other members and meeting staff

- Achieving their expressed fitness and health goals

What Should Clubs Learn from the Research on Consumer Attitudes Toward Clubs

As has been discussed in the first two sections of this chapter, multiple, mitigating reasons exist concerning why people join a club, many of which are different in nature from their actual perceptions of what a club is. In order to bring consumers into the club, operators must focus on overcoming any negative attitudes that prospects may initially hold toward the club. Even when these negative attitudes are reversed, the club must be able to offer an experience that is consistent with the reasons that consumers give for joining a particular facility. Finally, having brought new members into the club, club operators should try to better understand the basis for the reasons that members give for leaving and staying and how they can impact those reasons in a meaningful fashion. In this regard, it is interesting to note the disconnect between consumer attitudes about the health/fitness club business, their reasons for joining a club, and finally their reasons for leaving (refer to Figure 3.5).

The club must be able to offer an experience that is consistent with the reasons that consumers give for joining a particular facility.

Consumer Perceptions of Health/Fitness Clubs	Reasons Given for Joining Health/Fitness Clubs	Reasons Given for Relinquishing Membership in a Health/Fitness Club
Clubs are worth the money.	Good price	Didn't use the club enough to warrant the cost
Clubs are fun.	Group exercise programs	Poor programming
Club staff is knowledgeable.	Staff quality	Lack of attention from the staff
Clubs are for the young.	Friends are members.	No partner
Clubs are overcrowded.	Non-intimidating environment	Overcrowded
Clubs are for those individuals who are already fit.	Get in shape or stay in shape	Didn't achieve fitness goals

Figure 3.5. Dichotomy between consumer perceptions, attitudes, and behaviors

Figure 3.5 shows that the perceptions that consumers have about the health/fitness industry are mostly related to beliefs around the "people" in the business, such as the quality of the staff, the type of members using the club, and whether they will have fun if they become members of the club. When it comes time to join a club, the attitudes that consumers have regarding people-related issues impact their decision. On the other hand, their decisions concerning whether to purchase a club membership seem to be more driven by facility and program-related factors (women are an exception given that they have certain social expectations). Finally, when a member makes the decision to stay in or leave a club, their reasons are primarily relationship and connection driven, with the obvious exception of whether they achieved their personal fitness goals.

Given the aforementioned, it is logical to conclude that if a health/fitness club wants to create the most favorable environment for attracting and retaining members, they need to focus on the following factors:

When it comes time to join a club, the attitudes that consumers have regarding people-related issues impact their decision.

- Target their message to their market. A successful club should not create a generic marketing message, especially if it features young, fit people as role models. Rather, it should try to develop a message that speaks to a non-intimidating environment, where everyone is welcome and comfortable.

- Align the price with the experience. Clubs should try to avoid falling into the pricing game. Potential members see value as being a balance between the experience they have in a club and the price that the club charges for membership.

- Send a message that their club is clean.

- Make sure their club is seen as having staff who are not only credible and professional, but also warm and service-driven.

- Build programs that are entertaining, diverse, and motivating.

- Engage their members immediately and make sure that they introduce them to other members. They should think partnering.

- Have their employee team engage each new member; focus on helping them establish relationships at some level with every member.

- Find out exactly what prospects and new members want to achieve physically and emotionally, and then make sure that the club's professional staff is there to help guide, motivate, and support the achievement of each member's goals.

- Create activities in the club that are member-driven and in which members can take ownership.

- Recognize the achievements of the club's members.

- Make sure that the club has more equipment than the number of members expected to be in the facility at any given time.

- Make the club convenient; remove any barriers that might otherwise prevent the relatively easy use of the facility and don't make the members sacrifice their time or needs to use the club.

- Create a system so members can communicate with management about club-related issues that they perceive to be important and what their experiences are in the club.

- Make parts of the club non-intimidating, especially if attracting women is important to the club's business model.

Club operators should not sell their club on "closing techniques" and price. Instead, they should align the benefits that their club offers with the needs of the customer and create value for the members.

Club operators should not sell their club on "closing techniques" and price. Instead, they should align the benefits that their club offers with the needs of the customer and create value for the members.

MEMBERSHIP IN THE HEALTH/FITNESS CLUB INDUSTRY

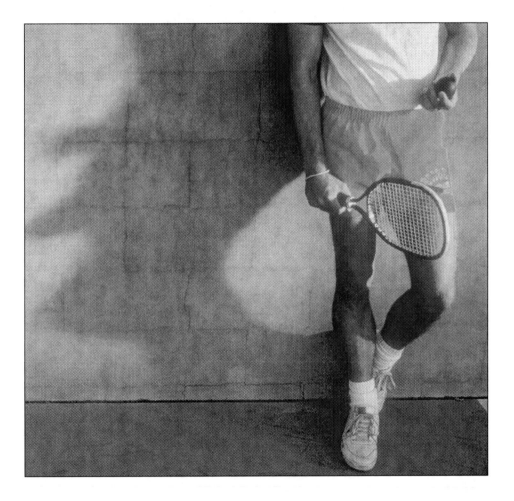

Part Two

4

Membership in the Health/Fitness Club Industry

Chapter Objectives

To a great degree, the financial success of the health/fitness club industry is dependant upon its ability to offer an experience that attracts and retains members. According to the report, *2004 IHRSA Profiles of Success*, over 70% of all health/fitness club revenues come from membership dues, making sustained membership growth the top priority of club operators. This chapter reviews the types of membership offerings currently offered by operators in the health/fitness club industry, and then discusses membership pricing and membership structures. Finally, the chapter examines what these membership policies and procedures mean to the club operator.

Defining the Differences between a Member and a Customer

The health/fitness club industry is unique in that to a great degree, its success depends upon selling and retaining memberships, whereas in most other hospitality and retail industries, success depends upon customer volume. With regard to the impact of membership on the level of success that a health/fitness club achieves, it is important to note that some very important differences exist between customers and members. In order for a health/fitness club to perform well financially, it must clearly understand that difference and create an experience that drives membership, not customer traffic. While the differences between a member and a customer are often subtle, they are nonetheless, very important.

A customer can be defined as an individual who uses a service, such as a health/fitness club visit, for a fee. A customer asks for no other privilege other than the right to use the service that they have paid for and understands that the fee is based upon the level of service provided or used. Customers are people who gain access based on a fee and have no commitment to the business they are accessing.

According to the report, *2004 IHRSA Profiles of Success*, over 70% of all health/fitness club revenues come from membership dues, making sustained membership growth the top priority of club operators.

A member, on the other hand, is someone who pays for the privilege and right to use a health/fitness club, as well as the privilege to associate with others of similar interests and backgrounds. Members establish an agreement with the business that they intend to honor. Members take a sense of ownership in the organization they join, connecting not to a service or facility, but to other people who are members of the same organization. A member expects certain privileges, which in most cases, extend far beyond just access to a service. Members pay not just for access, but for the unfettered privilege (schedule-wise) to access, with no restrictions placed on them when they access the service.

Types of Memberships in the Health/Fitness Club Industry

During the modern era of the health/fitness club industry, the membership offerings of clubs have varied, ranging from a customer-driven model of daily access for a fee to a model that is based on the payment of annual dues for the privilege of open-ended access year around. At the present time, the industry has three relatively standard types of membership offerings:

❑ *Membership Contract.* The membership contract was first introduced back in the 1940s and currently represents 44% of the industry's offering. Membership contracts are an agreement between the club operator and the member, which commits the member to a specified membership time period, usually one year to three years, for a specified amount of dues. In essence, the member is agreeing to pay the club operator a set fee (usually discounted) for the privilege of a long-term membership, whether they actually use the club or not.

At the present time, the health/fitness club industry has three relatively standard types of offerings.

In the past, many clubs offered lifetime contracts, but more recently, the length of a contract has been determined by laws that exist in most states. At the present time, most states limit a club membership contract to three years, and in many states, that limitation is set at one year in duration. A member perceives a value in the contract based on the opportunity to gain privileges for a reduced fee (a price-driven decision), while the operator sees value in the agreement arising out of the fact the club has received an agreed-upon amount of dues (resulting in a higher retention level of dues), that might otherwise not be available if a member chooses to leave before the year is out.

It is interesting to note that while this type of membership contract is offered by 44% of the industry, only 16% of members actually select this contractual option if given a choice. Many consumers who are looking to join a health/fitness club view membership contracts as legal agreements that require them to commit to a set length of membership and financial commitment, even though they are not sure that they will either want or need to use the club for the time commitment set forth in the contract. Membership contracts tend to be used most frequently by clubs that offer high-volume membership sales and high usage, while experiencing a high volume of member turnover (attrition).

❑ *Month-to-Month Membership.* This type of membership offering has been around the industry for years. Month-by-month memberships provide a member with club privileges for a period of one month, for which, in turn, the member commits to paying one month's dues in advance. This type of membership package is currently offered by 79% of all clubs and is selected by 45% of all health/fitness club members, making it the most popular offering in the industry. Many members and prospective members believe that the month-by-month membership is their more attractive option because it does not require them to make a commitment beyond a month's period of time. At the same time, owners tend to find this type of membership offering desirable because it presents less of an up-front barrier to joining their club based on price.

For the member, a month-by-month membership is easier to terminate and requires less of a commitment to using the club. For the club, a month-by-month membership tends to be associated with higher turnover than with a membership contract, and as a result, also offers slightly less financial security to the owner and operator of a club.

On the other hand, this type of membership offering also has some downsides for both the member and owner. For the member, a month-by-month membership is easier to terminate and requires less of a commitment to using the club. For the club, a month-by-month membership tends to be associated with higher turnover than with a membership contract, and as a result, also offers slightly less financial security to the owner and operator of a club.

Month-by-month memberships tend to be used more frequently by clubs that are focused on providing a higher degree of member service, as well as serving a more affluent population of members. These clubs tend to focus less on the volume of membership and more on the quality of the membership.

❑ *First-Year Membership Contract, with Monthly Membership.* This type of membership agreement is the most recent contractual offering of the industry. Years ago, the industry discovered that by offering a blended membership package, they were able to provide an offering that appealed to prospective members more than the standard contract. A blended package also gives a club more financial protection than a month-by-month membership.

A driving force behind the development of this type of membership offering was research showing that if a member was engaged for a full year, they would be far more likely to stay active in the club going forward. Owners believe that a blended-membership package presents a viable strategy to reduce the first-year attrition of a month-by-month membership, yet offer the member the ability to stay or leave as they choose after the first year.

This type of membership package is offered by 50% of the industry, a level that reflects a slightly higher percentage than full-contract offerings. This particular membership offering is the second most popular among members, given that 31% of members select this package when joining a club. This membership offering is equally popular among the high-volume and low-dollar health/fitness clubs as it is among the lower-volume, higher-dollar health/fitness clubs.

Membership Categories Typically Offered in the Health/Fitness Club Industry

As was detailed earlier in this chapter, health/fitness clubs have developed three basic types of membership offerings. To help differentiate these offerings, the industry has gone one step further and created special membership categories that allow the industry to further personalize their membership offerings to their prospects. In this regard, the categories most frequently offered by clubs include the following:

- *Individual Membership.* This type of membership bestows the privileges of membership on one designated individual for a specified dues rate. The most frequently selected type of membership, this particular membership category is most popular in urban settings.

- *Couples Membership.* This type of membership bestows membership privileges to two individuals for a specified membership dues rate. In some cases, clubs refer to couples as two people from the same family (i.e., married couple, parent and child), while in other markets, a couple might be defined as two individuals who live or work together. This basic category is most often employed in large metropolitan markets.

- *Family Membership.* This type of membership provides membership privileges to an entire family, usually defined as two adults and their offspring, for a specified membership dues rate. This particular category is popular in the suburban market. The greatest challenge with this category comes when a club has a large family using the membership, which can result in a club losing potential dues revenue that might otherwise be derived from selling separate memberships to several members of the same family.

- *Individual Membership with Family Add-on.* This type of membership offering grants membership privileges to an individual for a designated dues rate, but then allows that individual to add on additional individuals at lower price points. This category is designed to allow a family to determine how many of their offspring for whom they want to provide privileges or to be used by someone who joined the club as

The first-year membership contract, with a monthly membership-type of membership package is offered by 50% of the industry, a level that reflects a slightly higher percentage than full-contract offerings.

an individual and later has someone else who wants to become a member of the club with that person. This category of membership has become popular in both suburban and urban markets and provides the club operator and member greater flexibility and value. For members availing themselves of this type of membership, they only have to pay dues for those individuals who have privileges, which might not be the case with a family membership structure. For club operators offering this type of membership, they gain benefit by collecting membership dues from every family member with access to their facility.

While the four previously mentioned categories dominate the industry, there are some less frequently offered membership categories that clubs employ to target specific niche markets. The following categories provide a sampling of the growing trend in the industry to branch out to less typical membership offerings:

- *Singles Membership*. This category does not involve an individual membership, which could be purchased by a single or married person, rather it is a membership offered only to someone who is single. This category is popular in urban markets that have a large population of single professionals.

- *Junior Membership*. First offered in the country-club industry, junior memberships provide membership privileges to younger individuals, who might not yet have the earning potential and expendable income to purchase a standard full-privilege membership. The membership usually has an upper age limit for eligibility, such as being under the age of 21 or under 25.

- *Seniors Membership*. This category of membership is offered in markets that have a high concentration of seniors (usually defined in the industry as individuals who are over the age of 55). This category allows senior adults to have full club privileges at a reduced cost.

- *Corporate Membership*. This category is very popular among clubs that are located in settings surrounded by a high concentration of businesses. A corporate membership usually allows groups of individuals from a specific company to join a club at a reduced rate.

- *Executive Membership*. This category of membership is relatively new to the industry and is based on packaging special benefits with the membership, such that a member will pay additional dues for the perceived extra benefits included in the category.

- *Multiple Club Membership*. With the expansion of club chains, many club operators have found value in offering a membership option that gives members access to more than one club in a chain. Most of the regional club chains (e.g., Multiplex in Chicago, Healthworks in Boston, etc.) currently offer multiple-site memberships. Many national chains offer both regionally based and nationally based multiple-club

With the expansion of club chains, many club operators have found value in offering a membership option that gives members access to more than one club in a chain.

memberships as well. This type of membership offering has gained popularity with members because of the convenience factor, especially for those members who commute within a city or for those individuals who travel a lot. For the club operator, this category provides an avenue for up-selling and adding incremental dues dollars.

Packaging Membership Category Offerings

Up to this point, this chapter has reviewed how clubs package their memberships from the perspective of a particular category and contractually. In most cases, the industry sees differentiation of a membership being based on the length of the contract, category of membership, and the associated pricing. In essence, the industry, as a whole, has created multiple membership offerings, using a commodity and goods approach, where the difference in the offerings is based mostly on how the product is priced and wrapped.

> In recent years, several of the leading health/fitness club operators have created differentiation in their membership offerings not just on the basis of category and price, but also on what additional benefits they ultimately roll into the offering.

In recent years, several of the leading health/fitness club operators have created differentiation in their membership offerings not just on the basis of category and price, but also on what additional benefits they ultimately roll into the offering. This approach to membership differentiation follows a service or experience model, allows clubs to create greater separation from their competitors, and generates improved margins on their membership offerings. Examples of how clubs package their various membership offerings (categories and contracts) include:

- Package a specified number of complimentary personal training sessions with the membership

- Incorporate certain discounts to various club services, such as child care, dining, massage, etc.

- Include special privileges to certain areas of the club, such as executive locker rooms, Pilates room, private training area, etc.

- Include affiliated services with other service providers, such as restaurants, dry cleaning, car washes, etc.

- Incorporate charging privileges at the club

Pricing Strategies for Memberships

The health/fitness club industry has developed a replicable model for the pricing of its membership packages and categories. This pricing model is based on a fee associated with entry or access to the membership privileges and then another fee associated with the actual usage of that privilege. In that regard, the two types of club charges are initiation fees and dues:

❏ *Initiation Fee.* The initiation fee is the up-front fee a prospective member pays to a club for the privilege of becoming a member and associating with the individuals who belong to that club. The initiation fee is often used as a differentiating factor for clubs, with those clubs that charge a higher upfront fee often being seen as more exclusive and less crowded. Research conducted both by IHRSA in the United States and by the Fitness Industry Association (FIA) in England shows that members who pay a higher initiation fee tend to remain members for a longer period of time. As a result of this research, the initiation fee is also seen as a pricing strategy related to gaining a greater level of commitment from members and therefore enhancing the retention level of members.

Initiation fees range from a low of $0 to as high as $20,000 in the health/fitness club industry. The initiation fee often is classified under other names, such as enrollment fee, administrative fee, processing fee, etc. The tendency in the industry is for clubs that sell higher volumes of membership at lower dues points to refer to their initiation fees as administrative or processing fees, as a way of getting fees despite the fact that they proclaim that they have no initiation fees. Initiation fees are more common in clubs that sell month-to-month memberships. Clubs that sell membership contracts rarely charge initiation fees, instead offering low upfront processing fees.

In most cases, initiation fees are collected by the club at the time the new member enrolls for membership. The initiation fees are normally collected via a check or credit card. Since 2000, a new approach has arisen with regard to the pricing and collection of initiation fees. Taking the lead from the car industry, clubs are now offering installment initiation fees, which allow a member to put down

Research conducted both by IHRSA in the United States and by the Fitness Industry Association (FIA) in England shows that members who pay a higher initiation fee tend to remain members for a longer period of time.

Membership Category	Club Size in S.F.	Initiation Fee	Monthly Dues
Individual	Under 20k	Range: $50 - $150 Average: $100	Range: $39 - $53 Average: $48
	20K to 35k	Range: $66 – $150 Average: $100	Range: $42 - $56 Average: $49
	35K to 60k	Range: $96 - $234 Average: $112	Range: $45 – $59 Average: $50
	60K and greater	Range: $115 - $397 Average: $250	Range: $49 - $102 Average: $73
Family	Under 20k	Range: $75 - $250 Average: $105	Range: $60 - $109 Average: $85
	20K to 35k	Range: $89 - $169 Average: $100	Range: $70 - $105 Average: $90
	35K to 60k	Range: $96 - $284 Average: $187	Range: $70 - $133 Average: $90
	60K and greater	Range: $185 – $450 Average: $300	Range: $86 - $183 Average: $125

Figure 4.1. Initiation fee and dues ranges for clubs of various sizes*
*From pages 22-23 of *IHRSA's 2004 Profiles of Success*

By combining initiation fees with dues, clubs have the ability to differentiate their product offering and create multiple price points for the various markets they are attempting to target.

a percentage of the initiation fee upfront, and then over a period of time, pay off the balance of the initiation fee. In most cases, the initiation fee balance is included with the monthly billing of dues. In some cases, clubs are promoting initiation fees similar to car leases, in which they show the initiation fee as a monthly payment to be made over a designated time period. This strategy allows clubs to charge a higher initiation fee, but also enables the customer to have more flexibility to complete the payment.

❑ *Dues*. Dues are the fees charged to members for the ongoing privilege of being a member. Dues allow the member freedom to access the various privileges of the club, per the terms of the membership they have purchased. Dues, as presented earlier in this chapter, are billed either on a monthly basis, on an annual basis, or some combination of both. Clubs bill dues using various methods, including monthly statements from the club, billing through a designated charge card, or an electronic funds transfer, also known as EFT. The most popular form of billing dues is through EFT, with the second most popular being credit card billing. A few clubs exist, however, that have members pay their dues monthly, using a coupon that they forward in with their check. EFT is very popular because members are automatically charged their dues, and the club receives its dues income with limited liability for uncollected dues income. Dues for health/fitness club memberships range from a low of around $10 a month for an individual to as high as $300 a month for some family memberships.

By combining initiation fees with dues, clubs have the ability to differentiate their product offering and create multiple price points for the various markets they are attempting to target. Figure 4.1, based on data compiled in *IHRSA's 2004 Profiles of Success,* shows some of the variability that exists in the market when it comes to the pricing of both initiation fees and dues.

While the data in Figure 4.1 reflects industry averages when it comes to initiation and dues pricing, the industry has increasingly moved toward a dues-pricing strategy as a point of brand differentiation. Among the various dues-pricing strategies that are employed in the industry are the following:

• *Under $20 a month*. This strategy has grown in popularity over the past five years and is exemplified by club operators such as Planet Fitness in the Northeast. Clubs that take this approach to pricing are focused on delivering a "fitness box" that provides a workout facility with abundant equipment and no amenities (e.g., no towels, no locker room facilities, etc.), no programming, and limited staff, other than sales people. These clubs focus on high-volume membership sales to generate the revenue that they need to be profitable, normally looking at over 10,000 members per facility.

- *$20 to $49 a month.* This pricing strategy seems to be the most popular approach to membership pricing in the market, especially among the major multiple-club operators (e.g., LA Fitness, 24 Hour Fitness, Gold's, Bally's, Lifetime Fitness) and regional players, such as X-Sport Fitness in Chicago. Clubs that take this approach focus on providing a medium-to-large "fitness box" that is very well-equipped and offers the basic amenities. These clubs provide basic programming opportunities for members, especially in the area of group exercise. Due to their low pricing, these facilities focus more on their equipment offering and convenience, than on service. In most cases, these clubs have limited staffing and programming. These clubs focus on high-volume membership sales to generate the revenue they need to be profitable, normally looking at between 6,000 and 10,000 members per facility.

- *$50 to $74 a month.* This pricing strategy has grown in popularity over the past ten years. It is the strategy most often taken by independent clubs in smaller markets and local/regionally based multiple-club operators (e.g., Wisconsin Athletic Clubs, New York Sports Clubs, Lifestyle Family Fitness in Florida). Clubs that take this pricing approach are focused on delivering a service-driven experience for their members and provide a balance of more-than-adequate facilities, plentiful equipment, amenities, program options, and relatively high levels of staffing. These are the clubs that have shifted their focus from mostly on sales to achieving a balance of membership sales and member service. These clubs, depending upon their size, will normally have membership levels ranging from 2,000 to 5,000 members, with the exception of the clubs in smaller geographic areas.

- *$75 to $99 a month.* This pricing strategy reflects the high-service area of the club industry. This strategy is found among many regional club operators (e.g., Spectrum Clubs, Sport and Health, Club One), as well as in larger independent club operators in small- and medium-sized markets. Clubs that take this approach primarily focus on the goal of delivering high levels of member service. These clubs normally have higher levels of finished-out areas in their facilities, which are accompanied by a wide variety of equipment. These clubs offer considerable programming options, especially in the area of group exercise. These clubs also are focused on providing a reasonably high level of staff-to-members ratio. These clubs, depending upon their size, will normally have between 1,500 and 4,000 memberships.

- *$100 a month or more.* This pricing strategy is used by operators who are targeting an affluent market and are focused on delivering a high-end service experience that resembles a resort-type experience. This approach has been taken by several well-known independent club operators (e.g., Houstonian, Michigan Athletic Club), as well as some

The "$50 to $74 a month" pricing strategy is the strategy most often taken by independent clubs in smaller markets and local/regionally based multiple-club operators.

regional and national club operators (e.g., Western Athletic Clubs, Sports Club/LA, Equinox). These clubs provide luxurious physical environments that are supported by well-trained staff and extensive programming.

Key Points to Consider

Without question, decisions concerning membership pricing, procedures, and policies are some of the most important issues with which club operators will ever have to deal. In that regard, this chapter has addressed the following key points:

Without question, decisions concerning membership pricing, procedures, and policies are some of the most important issues with which club operators will ever have to deal.

- Membership is the heart of the health/fitness club industry, contributing over 70% of a club's overall revenue in most cases.

- Membership is about privileges and benefits, not just about access. Membership is about connecting with the club's people.

- Clubs have many options for packaging their membership offering. They can offer membership categories that are grouped by such factors as age group, size of group, family status, level of privileges, access to multiple sites, etc.

- Clubs can offer their membership packages on a month-by-month basis or through contracts of specified periods of time.

- When pricing membership, clubs can consider both initiation fees and dues as a means to differentiate themselves from their competitors. Research shows that higher fees usually lead to greater membership retention.

- Clubs should not fall prey to pricing as the main differentiation of their club membership offering from their competitors. Rather, they should consider the benefits and privileges that they bundle into the membership offering as a means to differentiate themselves.

5

Branding and Marketing of Health/Fitness Clubs

Branding and marketing are the processes by which a club develops a distinct position of the club's membership offerings in the public's mind and makes the public aware of its membership offerings, thus creating an enhanced opportunity to uncover leads and prospects for membership.

Chapter Objectives

As was discussed in the previous chapter, the health/fitness club industry has a unique product offering—membership. While the membership offerings of clubs can vary widely, a basic question arises concerning what is it that allows some clubs to achieve success with their membership offerings while others do not? With regard to that issue, one fundamental factor is how clubs market and sell their membership offerings. As such, this chapter focuses on how clubs brand and market their membership offerings. Branding and marketing are the processes by which a club develops a distinct position of the club's membership offerings in the public's mind and makes the public aware of its membership offerings, thus creating an enhanced opportunity to uncover leads and prospects for membership.

Branding in the Health/Fitness Club Industry

Branding involves the efforts of a club to create a distinct perception of what its membership offerings are in the mind of its audience. A club's brand is its membership promise; it is what a club is able to get its prospective members and the public at large to believe is the membership experience that the club has to offer. When a brand is developed for a club, the effort involves creating an image that the public and the facility's members will associate with the experience that will be provided by the club.

Branding is particularly important when the goal of a club is to differentiate its membership offerings in the mind of the public. The clubs that are successful at branding are those whom the public and members talk about and whom they associate with a specific message. Branding does not happen by accident, but rather through disciplined business practices. While many factors influence the ability of a health/fitness club to create and sustain a strong brand, there are a few business practices that tend to be critical in that regard, including:

A critical aspect of a club's branding efforts is to make sure its product (e.g., the experience the club delivers to the members) is consistent with the image its marketing portrays.

- *First to Market.* If a club is the first to market, it has a distinct advantage over its competition in creating a strong recognizable brand. For example, Nautilus, which was the first variable-resistance circuit line to the market, has benefited from that situation by continuing to hold one of the most recognizable brands in the fitness-equipment industry. Even today, 30 years after being introduced, many consumers still think that resistance equipment is called Nautilus. By the same token, StairMaster was the first company to develop and market a mechanical stairclimbing machine and, like Nautilus, has benefited immensely from being the first such machine available to the public. Accordingly, many consumers often call a stairclimber a StairMaster. Yet another example of being first to market in building a brand was Precor with its highly popular elliptical trainer. Not surprisingly, most consumers think Precor when they stop to consider an elliptical machine. In turn, the strong brand recognition for the aforementioned equipment impacts the operators of health/fitness clubs, as they are often confronted by consumers asking for those specific brands. In the health/fitness club industry, Bally's has benefited by being one of the first national club chains to market, as has Lifetime Fitness in the family fitness and recreation market.

- *Marketing an Image.* Successful brands are built and sustained through a concerted marketing effort that typically includes a recognizable logo and image. By creating an appealing look and image, a health/fitness club can develop a brand image that will occupy a position in the consumer's mind. Crunch Fitness, founded by Doug Levine, has built one of the most recognizable brands in the health/fitness industry through a well-coordinated marketing and merchandising effort that puts their logo and image on clothes, videos, advertisements, and more. Gold's Gym is another example of an organization whose brand has achieved an exceptional level of consumer recognition through the marketing of an image. In addition to Crunch and Gold's, Lifetime Fitness has also been able to establish a strong national brand through marketing.

- *Delivering an Experience that Aligns with an Image.* A critical aspect of a club's branding efforts is to make sure its product (e.g., the experience the club delivers to the members) is consistent with the image its marketing portrays. An excellent example of this practice is Crunch Fitness. Crunch has a product that aligns very well with its marketing message. The facility design, the staff attire, the programs, and even the way Crunch personnel communicates to its members all support and build on the brand image created by Crunch through its marketing.

The following seven companies have some of the more successful brands in the health/fitness club industry:

❏ *Bally's.* The Bally's brand is one of the top nationally recognized brands in the health/fitness club industry. When the public sees the Bally's name, as a rule, they know it's a health club chain that features low prices, high energy, younger people, an environment geared towards singles, and popular culture. Bally's created this brand by being first to market, by supporting the brand image through extensive advertising efforts based on popular culture, and, to some degree, by delivering a product that has matched the image it created through advertising.

❏ *Gold's Gym.* The Gold's brand is widely considered as one of the top national brands in the health/fitness club industry. When the public sees the Gold's name and logo, the image of a facility catering to weightlifters and bodybuilders comes to mind. If average citizens were asked what they initially think about when they hear someone refer to Gold's Gym, most individuals would probably respond that it's a club for serious fitness people. This brand image is built partially by being one of the first gyms to receive substantial publicity (e.g., from the movie *Pumping Iron*), by extensively merchandising its logo, and by the visibility offered of its first spokesperson, Arnold Schwarzenegger. It is interesting to note that the Gold's Gym name, through its franchising efforts, has come to be much more than what its brand is perceived to be.

❏ *Crunch.* The Crunch brand is one of the most recognizable regional and national club brands in the United States. When the public hears the name Crunch or sees its distinct logo, it is likely to think of a facility that is out of the box, an environment that is particularly appropriate for young creative people, and a club for people of all walks and lifestyles. Crunch has a public persona of a club for those individuals who want an unusual and entertaining experience—one where no judgments are made. Crunch has developed its image through a combination of uniquely designed facilities, creative marketing, creative merchandising, and creative programming.

When the public sees the 24 Hour Fitness brand, they tend to think about a facility that is characterized by such attributes as convenience, all-day access, plenty of equipment, and affordability.

❏ *24 Hour Fitness.* The 24 Hour Fitness brand is one of the more visible brands nationally. When the public sees the 24 Hour Fitness brand, they tend to think about a facility that is characterized by such attributes as convenience, all-day access, plenty of equipment, and affordability. 24 Hour Fitness has built its brand image through a combination of mass-media promotions, building and locating clubs in large numbers in major markets, and keeping its clubs open 24 hours a day. Recently, 24 Hour Fitness has aligned themselves with several celebrity sports stars (e.g., Andre Agassi, Magic Johnson, Lance Armstrong, Jackie Chan, etc.) in an attempt to create an even more recognizable brand.

❑ *Healthworks.* Healthworks is a women's-only group of clubs in the Boston area that is one of the most familiar regional brands in the Northeast market. Healthworks has built its brand recognition by being the first quality women's-only club to market, by delivering an experience women respect and enjoy, and by marketing that image in the community. Healthwork's marketing, in large part, has been developed through its community involvement and charitable work for women and families in need, both of which play a significant role in the strength of its brand.

❑ *East Bank Club.* The East Bank Club is a 450,000 square-foot club that is located along the river in Chicago. It could be argued that everyone in Chicago knows of the East Bank Club. East Bank's reputation as a premier club, providing every imaginable service to its members, has been built through each of the three key steps to branding. East Bank was the first mega high-end club to market, it continues to deliver an extraordinary service with incredible facilities, and its members seem to willingly serve as promoters of the club's numerous positive features. Over the past 25 years, many high-end mega clubs have been built in Chicago, but every one of them finds itself measured against East Bank as the top brand in the market.

❑ *Red's.* Red's is located in Lafayette, Louisiana. Red's was founded in the early 1960s as a small 3,000 square-foot club and has expanded over the years to become a 180,000 square-foot facility. As of 2004, Red's club had approximately 15% of the total city population as members, even though they had over a dozen competitors. A local landmark, Red's is an exceptional brand. The Red's brand was first to market, but more importantly, it has built a strong reputation as a result of having a great product and being extensively involved in the community.

A number of other brands exist on a national, regional, and local level that are excellent examples of well-established brands, including the New York Sports Clubs (regional), Sports Club/LA (regional), Fitcorp (local), Houstonian (local), Cooper Activity Center (local), Curves (national and international), and Lifetime Fitness (national).

> Over the past 25 years, many high-end mega clubs have been built in Chicago, but every one of them finds itself measured against East Bank as the top brand in the market.

Marketing in the Health/Fitness Club Industry

As was discussed in the previous section, marketing is one of the critical steps in branding. Marketing, however, involves much more than just creating a brand image. Not only does marketing help create awareness of the club in the mind of the public and help establish a reason for the public to visit the club, in essence, it also assists in bringing leads to the club. Marketing is not selling, however, since marketing never closes a membership sale. Instead, marketing enables a club to instill an image in the public's mind and then provides a compelling reason for the public to consider the club to pursue their exercise and recreation needs. Too many individuals in the health/fitness club industry, however, equate marketing with engaging in advertising and generating lead boxes. In reality, marketing can take many forms, each with the ability to create an image and provide the public with a compelling reason to visit the club.

Proven Marketing Approaches in the Health/Fitness Club Industry

❑ *Advertising.* Advertising represents a very broad-stroke approach to marketing in the health/fitness club industry. As a rule, advertising is not a targeted approach to marketing, but rather a method for hitting a larger, less-targeted audience. Advertising can take many forms, including:

- *Print Media.* Print media advertising includes placing advertisements in such venues as newspapers, magazines, company newsletters, etc. Print media varies in its effectiveness. If a club is in a small market with a relatively small local paper, then print advertising can be an effective approach. On the other hand, if a club is located in a large market, such as New York, print advertising is not a good strategy, all factors considered. At the least, print advertising can be very expensive. Not only must a club pay for the production of the advertisement, it is also responsible for the cost of its placement as well. In some cases, the cost of producing a quality print media ad can run thousands of dollars, while the cost to place it can run over $25,000 for a full-page advertisement in some large papers. Clubs that chose to use print media may want to consider using other print media, such as local community circulars, or flyers, which are less expensive and can be more easily targeted to your audience.

- *Radio.* Advertisements on radio can be placed on stations that have a demographic audience similar to demographics the club wishes to target. In fact, every radio station has detailed information on the demographics of its audience, which can help a club determine with which stations it should place its advertising dollars. Furthermore, most radio stations, for an extra cost, will also agree to broadcast live from a club, which can really add some visibility to the facility's marketing efforts. Radio advertising is not inexpensive, but if a club is relatively selective in how and where it advertises, such an approach can be effective.

Not only does marketing help create awareness of the club in the mind of the public and help establish a reason for the public to visit the club, in essence, it also assists in bringing leads to the club.

Direct mail marketing is far more likely than advertising to bring potential members to the club's doors.

- *Local and Regional Cable Television.* Using cable television to communicate the club's desired message can be a very effective approach to advertising, especially if a club does it on a regional or local level. On the other hand, it is important for a club to keep the cost of production and placement of an ad on cable television in mind when deciding whether this is an appropriate way for it to advertise.

- *Billboards.* Billboard advertising is an excellent alternative for advertising, especially in large, urban markets such as Dallas, Houston, and Los Angeles, where people spend considerable time in their cars. Billboards, if placed along the proper thoroughfare, can bring considerable attention to the club. Like most advertising efforts, billboard advertising involves both production and placement costs. With billboard advertising, similar to the other media, the club can pay for the space it chooses to use for a given period of time.

- *Internet.* Over the last few years, internet advertising has become very popular. Club operators, however, should be aware of the fact that internet advertising is not always targeted. With the increase in software that stops pop-ups, the value of internet advertising to a club might not be as high as the other available forms of advertising.

- *Yellow Pages.* The *Yellow Pages* are still a main source of information for much of the public. Accordingly, given a choice of the various types of advertising media, club operators should look at utilizing the *Yellow Pages*.

When looking at advertising, club operators should be aware that there are two basic types of advertising—image advertising and call-to-action advertising. With image advertising, a club is sending a message about the image of its brand. Image advertising involves efforts by a club to create awareness of its brand and establish exposure of its business in the marketplace. Call-to-action advertising, on the other hand, focuses on providing a compelling reason for the club's audience to take action (e.g., join the club, sign up for a product or service, etc.). Call-to-action advertisements usually offer some inducement for the public to visit the club, such as discounts, a free week's membership, raffle for a free membership, etc.

❑ *Direct Mail Marketing and E-Mail Blasts.* Direct mail marketing is a far more targeted approach for a club to send its message to the public. Direct mail allows a club to select its audience. The effort can be as small or as large as the club likes. Direct mail marketing is far more likely than advertising to bring potential members to the club's doors. On average, most direct-mail efforts will generate a response rate that varies from .5% to three percent. The more targeted a club's initial audience, the higher its percentage of responses will be. Direct mail can be accomplished either through actual mailings or, in recent years, by using e-mail. Among the ways that clubs can enhance their direct-mail marketing efforts are the following:

- *Keep the message simple.* A direct-mail message needs to be direct and simple, otherwise consumers will not spend much time reading it.

- *Make the message different and appealing.* Consumers get hit all the time, so if a direct-mail piece does not "knock their socks off" at first glance, then the consumer's attention has probably been lost. Some of the best direct-mail pieces feature unique pictures, special offers, and a look and feel that is different. The best examples of these are what are termed 3D direct-mail pieces. A 3D piece could be a box that when opened has a barbell paperweight or it could be a tennis-ball container that when opened has a ball with a gift certificate attached to it.

- *Personalize the mailing.* If a club employs pre-printed labels in its direct mailings, they don't separate themselves from the crowd. Research has shown that handwritten cards and envelopes get far more attention when they arrive in the mail.

- *Make an offer.* A direct-mail piece needs to provide a reason for the consumer to visit your club. For example, the piece could include/feature an eye-catching enticement such as a guest pass, a gift certificate, or a discount coupon.

- *Obtain good mailing lists. The club's best source for names to contact is* names provided by its members. As a rule, the next best avenue for securing names is from a direct mail house that provides mailing lists (for a fee). These lists can be sorted (organized) by a number of critical factors, including zip code, age, gender, household income, etc. The better job a club does in identifying the desired parameters, the better its mailing list will be.

A more modern form of direct mailing is the e-mail blast. Research indicates that the response rate to an e-mail blast can range from seven percent to as high as 15%. Successful e-mail blasts generally involve the same approach to direct mailing as traditional direct mail, with the exception that a club can't personalize its message quite as well. E-mail blasts can be enhanced by including video segments, photos, coupons, or whatever the club chooses.

- ❑ *Reputation Management.* Reputation management is another way of expressing involvement in community and public relations. Reputation management is about a club creating and sustaining its brand image through relationships in the community. Reputation management can be one of the most powerful marketing avenues a club can employ. Examples of reputation management include:

  - *Serving on community boards and committees.* A club can have members of its staff get involved in the community by serving on local boards or groups, such as the chamber of commerce, rotary, local hospital board, school board, PTA, or other locally active organization serving the public.

Research indicates that the response rate to an e-mail blast can range from seven percent to as high as 15%.

> **Clubs need to develop marketing materials that they can provide to leads and prospects that will articulate the "story" of their club.**

- *Sponsoring community activities.* A club can get involved with community activities by serving as a sponsor for a local community event, such as a rotary function, school PTA function, special charity event, etc. If a club is particularly sensitive to the value of such an approach, it will go one step further and actually agree to host community events and meetings. For example, a club could host the parent meetings of the local Little League.

- *Creating a press kit and sending out press releases.* Every club should create an attractive and compelling press kit. Such a press kit should include a background statement about the club, a fact sheet, some biographies of key staff, etc. The press kit should then be forwarded to the local media, along with a human-interest story. The club should consider inviting the press to special events conducted at the club (e.g., grand opening, special activities, community-interest events, etc.) and get the media actively involved in promoting the occasion. Finally, the club should make sure to send stories to its media contacts on a regular basis. The press is almost always looking for great human-interest stories, and almost every club has members or staff that have compelling stories.

- *Becoming a health and fitness resource for the community.* A club could contact the local press and see if it can write a question-and-answer column for the paper. A club could also take this approach with a local radio or television station. For example, in Dallas, Texas, Larry North, owner of the Larry North Fitness clubs, is frequently featured as an expert on health and fitness matters on local radio.

- *Developing a charity event or foundation.* A number of clubs in the United States have created actual charity foundations that involve their members and staff in providing support and funds to a specified charity. The charitable activities of Healthworks in the Boston area are a perfect example of a club taking this approach.

❑ *Club Marketing Materials and Literature.* Clubs need to develop marketing materials that they can provide to leads and prospects that will articulate the "story" of their club. These marketing materials can be used as handouts, both when they're utilized outside the club, and when potential leads are visiting at the club. Examples of some of the most effective marketing literature and media used by clubs include:

- *Print brochures.* Every club should have a print brochure. The brochure should represent the image of the club and tell the story of the club. An effective brochure, in this instance, should feature a number of items, including pictures, testimonies by members, bullet points on the attributes and benefits of the club, a map with the location of the club, and information on how to contact the club (including e-mail and web site addresses). Sample brochures are included in the appendices of this book. Cost-wise, a wide variety of print options are typically available. It is money well-spent, however. A quality color brochure might run as high as one to two dollars a brochure when the club prints 500 or more at a time.

- *CD/DVD Brochure.* One of the most recently developed tools that a club uses to market and promote itself is an actual CD or DVD brochure. At a minimum, the DVD/CD should contain a virtual tour of the club, clips of member testimonies, information about the club in story format, and a direct link to the club's website. CDs and DVDs are a relatively inexpensive item to produce (generally ranging from fifty cents to one dollar to replicate). It should be noted that this cost is the same or less than for a printed brochure. Clubs, such as The Athletic and Swim Club in New York, ACAC in Charlottesville, Virginia, and LeClub in Wisconsin, are excellent examples of facilities that successfully employ this approach.

- *Website brochure.* No club should be without a web-based brochure. This method can enable a club to use streaming video, photos, samples of club schedules, and other relevant information from the facility. Furthermore, a club can link its site to the web-based *Yellow Pages* and to IHRSA's healthclubs.com.

❏ *Strategic Alliances.* Another effective marketing approach that can benefit a club is to develop strategic alliances or cross-marketing relationships. A strategic alliance or cross-marketing relationship involves a situation where a club establishes a working relationship with another organization that allows each of the respective organizations to benefit from the relationship, for example, in attracting new customers. Among the types of strategic alliances that a health/fitness club might consider are the following:

- *Alliance with local restaurants.* Clubs can approach restaurants whose clientele have the same demographics and establish a relationship in which both organizations are marketing the others to its clients. This approach can be as simple as employing table-top advertising, or could involve special coupons that members and customers receive when they use the club or restaurant.

- *Alliance with local healthcare organizations.* By establishing an informal relationship with other healthcare organizations, a club could gain valuable leads.

- *Alliance with local homeowner associations.* The club could establish a relationship in which new homeowners obtain, as part of their homeowner membership, a coupon that enables them to join the club at a discounted price or even a one-month, complimentary membership.

A strategic alliance or cross-marketing relationship involves a situation where a club establishes a working relationship with another organization that allows each of the respective organizations to benefit from the relationship, for example, in attracting new customers.

- *Alliance with local realtors.* Clubs can work with local realtors to create special welcome gifts. These gifts could be included with all new home purchases or could be positioned as a special-benefit package if individuals satisfy some set of predetermined criteria set by the local realtor. In an urban market, a club might want to work with local apartment/condominium landlords to create the same type of package.

❑ *Community and Corporate Health Fairs.* Clubs can build their reputation as a member of the healthcare network by sponsoring local health fairs. If the club is in an urban market or an area heavily populated by corporations, the club should contact the various companies and offer to sponsor a health fair for the company. These health fairs can include both club-related services and demonstrations, but also involve bringing in outside healthcare providers, such as physical therapists, opticians, etc. In some urban settings, building landlords are often receptive to activities such as these to offer as a benefit to their tenants. If a club is in a suburban or residential market, contact should be made with local city leaders or local associations to gage their possible interest in having the club sponsor a community-based health fair.

❑ *Member Referral and Sponsor Programs.* Research has shown that the single best source of new members is the club's existing members. Clubs who understand the value of leveraging existing member involvement in their club as a marketing tool usually achieve the greatest success. Every club should have an ongoing member referral program that provides a process and incentive for existing members to share the club's story with friends and associates. Over the years, club companies such as ClubCorp in Dallas and Western Athletic Clubs based in California, have done an excellent job with their referral programs. Among the factors that referral programs focus on are the following:

- *Providing a means for members to submit and refer the names of friends and associates.* This process could be as simple as having referral cards and a box, a special web address, or encouraging members to contact the membership sales department.

- *Providing recognition for the members who provide referrals.* This policy can vary from providing special awards for club services to special grand prizes.

- *Resisting the tendency to overextend the welcome.* A good member referral program is not promoted too blatantly; rather, it is incorporated into the overall fabric of the club's membership and marketing process.

> **Research has shown that the single best source of new members is the club's existing members.**

❑ *Lead Boxes*. Lead boxes were among the first marketing tools employed by health/fitness clubs. Lead boxes involve placing a special box, accompanied by a promotional offer and a special information card, at specific locations throughout a particular market. As a rule, a club will place the lead boxes in various retail locations, where the demographics of the retail customers match the profile of the club's membership. A lead box is normally accompanied by a flyer or poster that extends the to public a chance to win a membership or other service just by filling out a card and placing it in the box. Clubs subsequently check their lead boxes on a regular basis and collect the names of those individuals who want a chance to win whatever prize has been promoted. A prize is always awarded. At the same time, however, the club has also collected the names of people who are potential prospects and future members.

Membership sales staff cannot sell memberships if they do not have a sufficient number of leads and prospects.

Key Points to Consider

Branding and marketing are critical undertakings for clubs that are interested in building and sustaining a vibrant membership. Branding helps establish the image and the story of the club in the mind of both the public and the members. Such an image can help create a greater level of awareness of the club in the market and help attract the public to its front door. Marketing involves the steps undertaken to help build the brand image of the business and generate interest in the club's membership offering. Marketing is critical to generating both membership leads and membership prospects. Membership sales staff cannot sell memberships if they do not have a sufficient number of leads and prospects. Accordingly, marketing should be a significant part of the prospecting strategy utilized by a club's membership sales staff.

6

Selling Club Memberships

Chapter Objectives

In the previous two chapters, the principles of membership and the art of marketing were reviewed. This chapter logically extends that line of discussion by examining the process of selling memberships. To many individuals in the health/fitness club industry, the word "sales" elicits negative perceptions. In reality, however, sales essentially involves nothing more than providing a worthwhile product for which a market exists, a needed service, or an exceptional experience that fulfills a prospect's wishes. This chapter initially presents an overview of the sales process, and then discusses several actual practices, such as the club tour, corporate sales, and sales management, which can assist club operators in driving their membership sales.

Understanding the Mathematics of Selling Memberships

As was discussed earlier, a thriving membership is at the heart of every successful club. The challenge of sales is to make sure that the club's membership level continues to grow, thus ensuring the overall profitability and vitality of the club. According to *IHRSA's 2004 Profiles of Success*, a profile of the health/fitness club industry, overall in 2004, IHRSA health/fitness clubs had net membership growth, ranging from 3% to 6%. This profile also indicates that most mature club operations had membership growth closer to 3%. Figures 6.1 and 6.2 show that most clubs have to sell between 800 and 1,300 memberships on an annual basis to succeed, with some of the larger club operators having to sell as many as 5,000 memberships annually.

What is most evident from the aforementioned figures is the fact that for most clubs, whether small or large, is that on an annual basis, they are generating new sales at a rate ranging from 28% to 54% of their base membership. The point is that when it comes to membership sales,

> The challenge of sales is to make sure that the club's membership level continues to grow, thus ensuring the overall profitability and vitality of the club.

	Mean	Lower 25%	Median	Upper 25%
Accounts Added	1,011	508	730	1,124
Accounts Dropped	870	414	662	1,947
Net Accounts	141	94	68	177
Total Members	1,871	1,298	1,640	2,127
Sales %	54%	39%	45%	53%

Figure 6.1. Annual membership sales for health/fitness clubs 20,000 to 35,000 square feet in size*

	Mean	Lower 25%	Median	Upper 25%
Accounts Added	1,557	675	1,000	1,459
Accounts Dropped	970	448	965	1,415
Net Accounts	587	227	35	44
Total Memberships	4,654	2,040	3,277	5,288
Sales %	33%	33%	31%	28%

Figure 6.2. Annual membership sales for health/fitness clubs over 60,000 square feet in size*

It is important to understand that a high performing sales person will, on average, make approximately 10 membership sales a week.

health/fitness clubs have established a historical pattern requiring a high rate of membership sales. If for example, the mean number of total sales for clubs over 60,000 S.F., which is 1,557 memberships, is used as a basis for identifying the extent of the need to sell club memberships and that number is converted to a weekly sales rate, a club ends up having to sell 20 memberships a week. If the annual sales ranges indicated in Figures 6.1 and 6.2 are examined, the average sales required on a weekly basis for the majority of clubs would range from a low of 10 sales a week to a high of 30 sales a week. It is interesting to note that clubs such as Lifetime Fitness, 24 Hour Fitness, and Bally's often have to sell an average of 100 memberships a week. It is important to understand that a high performing sales person will, on average, make approximately 10 membership sales a week. In other words, most clubs will need to have at least two full-time membership sales people.

*Taken from IHRSA's 2004 Profiles of Success

While the percentages tend to vary from market to market and club to club, the average club can expect to convert 20% to 50% of its leads to prospects and 20% to 80% of its prospects to actual members.

In fact, high sales volume clubs, such as Lifetime Fitness or Bally's, will often need as many as 10 membership sales people. Obviously, sales are most definitely a numbers game.

Understanding the Membership Sales Continuum

Membership sales involve three distinct stages: identifying leads, qualifying prospects, and closing the sale. Each of the sales stages is like a filtering screen, with the number of people at each stage being screened until it becomes a smaller population with better qualifications for membership. As Figure 6.3 indicates, the sales process can begin with 100 leads, that then develop into 30 prospects, and finally result in 15 sales.

Using the aforementioned example as a reference, a club that requires 20 new memberships a week would need to generate a total of 40 prospects and 130 leads weekly. When examined in this perspective, the sales process requires a club to create a large reservoir of leads in order to produce the required level of membership sales. While the percentages tend to vary from market to market and club to club, the average club can expect to convert 20% to 50% of its leads to prospects and 20% to 80% of its prospects to actual members.

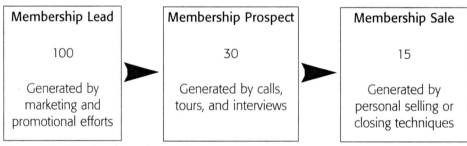

Figure 6.3. Membership sales continuum

Membership Sales Stages Up Close and Personal

❑ *Identify Leads.* A lead is defined as an individual whose demographics (personal characteristics and behaviors) align with the demographics of a club's membership and whom has given an indication that they might be interested in a club's membership offering. Examples of leads include individuals who complete a lead card, individuals who have responded to an advertisement, and individuals who have called the club, based on a direct-mail piece that they received. Leads are just that, individuals who, when exposed to the features and benefits of the club, may become more interested and eventually decide to join the club.

The process of generating leads should be considered the top priority of a membership sales team and the marketing department. By generating a sufficient reservoir of leads, a club can be assured of generating a sufficient number of membership sales. The lead generation process involves two distinct phases. The first is marketing, which is designed to generate consumer interest and awareness of the club, while the second is lead tracking or database mining, which enables a club to place a name with a lead. Because marketing was reviewed in the previous chapter, this chapter does not reexamine this aspect of lead generation. Instead, this section details some of the key aspects of database mining (name recording), including:

- Every time a club gets a phone call or inquiry, an effort should be made to get the caller's address, phone number, and e-mail address.

- Clubs should make sure that their lead cards provide space for the name, address, phone number, and e-mail address. An incentive should be offered to the lead to provide this information.

- For any marketing piece that gives an individual an opportunity to respond to the marketing offer, the response form should require the lead to provide the appropriate contact information.

- If a club is engaged in a health fair or community event, contact information should be collected on every individual with whom the club comes into contact.

- A club should make it a habit for its sales staff to collect the required contact information on every individual with whom they come in contact.

- If a club utilizes guest passes as a marketing strategy, the guest pass should include space for the contact information.

As the aforementioned points indicate, generating leads is a full-scale effort that ties marketing to information collection.

❏ *Qualifying Prospects.* A prospect is a lead who has expressed a need for or an interest in the club. A prospect differs from a lead in that that person has been identified as having a desire, need, or want that can be filled by the services offered by the club. Accordingly, a prospect is more likely to become a member than someone who is a lead. Turning leads into prospects and qualifying people as prospects occur in many ways. The most critical factor in qualifying prospects is to talk with the lead/individual and identify that person's desires, needs, and wants and then get that individual to express it to the sales person. Several core marketing strategies exist that are relatively likely to be successful at generating prospects, including member referrals, guest visits from distributed guest passes, and referrals from corporate accounts. In the end, to turn a lead into a prospect requires that a conversation take place between the membership sales person and the individual who is a prospective club

The process of generating leads should be considered the top priority of a membership sales team and the marketing department.

When a sales person determines that a lead has become a prospect, it is that person's responsibility to move forward with the final process of closing the sale.

member, during which the membership sales person picks up an indication that qualifies the lead as a prospect. Among the more common indications that a lead is now a prospect are the following:

- An individual indicates verbally or non-verbally that the club offers them an opportunity to fulfill a specific need.

- The individual has been a member of another health/fitness facility in the past.

- The individual has a history of being physically active and is looking to resume exercising.

- The individual is looking for a way to achieve a personal fitness or weight-loss goal.

- The individual contacted the club, based on the recommendation of a current club member.

- The individual has taken a tour of the club or has utilized a guest pass they received and has actually used the club.

When a sales person determines that a lead has become a prospect, it is that person's responsibility to move forward with the final process of closing the sale.

❏ *Closing the Sale.* The process of closing a sale refers to the process of moving a prospect to the point where that person decides to become a member of the club. The process of moving a prospect to membership usually takes place in one of two ways. The first way is what is referred to as relationship selling, where prospects choose to become members because the club has demonstrated to them that the club can fulfill an expressed need. The second method is often referred to as "high-pressure sales," a practice in which the membership sales representative applies pressure for the prospect to join using certain "closing" techniques. While the relationship approach is likely to generate the highest closing percentage (i.e., the percentage of prospects who become members) and the highest quality member, while "high-pressure" closing techniques usually produce high closing percentages, but low-quality members. The primary differences between the two basic methods of closing are highlighted in the following points:

- *Relationship Selling.* This approach to selling is preferred by those clubs that are interested in bringing in members who will remain members. This approach to turning a prospect into a member involves an in-depth process of uncovering a prospect's needs and then connecting the club's services to the expressed needs of the prospect. The process involves creating a series of benefit statements that enable the prospect to see how the club can fulfill their expressed needs. This process does not intimidate the prospect, and it does not employ discounting or other rehearsed processes to move the prospect to membership. The relationship sale involves the following simple steps:

✓ Asking questions of the prospect so that person's needs can be determined. Normally, at least two expressed needs must be identified. The questions usually start as open-ended probes (no definitive answer) and then move into closed probes (yes- or no-type questions).

✓ When a need is uncovered, the sales person will reiterate what has been said and then create a benefit statement that connects a particular service to the expressed need of the prospect.

✓ When a prospect confirms (verbally or non-verbally) that the benefit exists, then the membership sales person will confirm the benefit.

✓ After confirming the benefit agreed to by the prospect, the membership sales person will repeat the process to inject yet a second confirmed benefit into the process.

✓ Once the prospect has confirmed that the club benefits them in at least two ways, the membership sales person will ask for the sale in a non-intimidating way.

Relationship selling is far more effective in generating quality membership sales than high-pressure selling and typically will lead to a very high closing ratio.

❑ *High Pressure Closing.* Clubs and membership sales people who use this process start by asking questions that uncover a prospect's needs and vulnerabilities. While uncovering the prospect's needs is an important facet of this process, what is more important is identifying the prospect's vulnerabilities, such as time, cost, support of a significant other, self-confidence, etc. When the membership sales person identifies the vulnerability, the next step involves having the sales person use rehearsed closing lines that have a proven record of intimidating and pressuring the prospect to sign up for membership.

The following case study can help illustrate the process. For example, a membership sales person has uncovered the fact that the prospect has low self -esteem and does not perceive that he has sufficient funds to join the club. A possible high-pressure closing technique that this membership sales person might use is to say, "You don't want to continue feeling so bad about yourself, so why don't you join now and get started with changing your image! I know you don't think you have the necessary funds for joining, so the club is prepared to offer you a $0 initiation fee and reduced membership dues of $39 a month if you sign up for a two-year contract."

Membership sales representatives who use this approach to attempt to turn a prospect into a member tend to discount the price of the memberships that they are selling and present multiple closing lines, before allowing the prospect to leave. In many cases, the membership sales representative will tag team with another membership representative

Relationship selling is far more effective in generating quality membership sales than high-pressure selling and typically will lead to a very high closing ratio.

to further intimidate the prospect. While this approach to closing is considered inappropriate by much of the industry, consumers are likely to face such strategies from clubs who depend on high-volume sales.

Staging the Membership Tour

Earlier in this chapter, the various strategies for moving a lead to a prospect and then turning that prospect into a member were discussed. Among the many approaches employed in the health/fitness club industry in this regard, the club tour is the strategy that has been shown to produce the highest percentage of prospects from leads and also the highest percentage of memberships from prospects. A membership sales person who has mastered the art of the club tour can be assured of generating quality prospects and membership sales. Staging the winning club tour involves the following steps:

❑ *Begin the tour with a relaxed Q-and-A session.* When sales people first meet prospects, they should sit down in an open, non-intimidating setting. The sales person should offer the prospect a beverage or water and then proceed to uncover the following key pieces of information:

> The club tour is the strategy that has been shown to produce the highest percentage of prospects from leads and also the highest percentage of memberships from prospects.

- Are they currently a member of a sports or health club, and if so, what activities do they currently pursue?

- If they are currently a health/fitness club member, why are they considering another club?

- Do they currently exercise? If yes, what kind of exercise do they currently perform? If not, what factors do they feel will help them be more likely to engage in a regular exercise program?

- What is it they would like to accomplish as the result of joining the club? Do they have any specific goals that they have established?

- Are there any activities that are of particular interest to them, such as group exercise, yoga, running, weights, etc.?

- Do they have a friend or associate who currently uses the club?

- Do they prefer a competitive or social atmosphere or are they more inclined to prefer a relaxed, private atmosphere?

- How much time do they have available at the moment to learn about the club and the benefits it can offer?

The aforementioned inquires are the most critical questions that should be asked. Obtaining answers to these questions will not only increase the chances of the membership sale being closed, but the information can prove invaluable in setting up for the prospect's first visit to the club. This information can also be used by a club's fitness department to help identify those members who may be at a heightened risk for attrition. The information obtained by this process can also help the entire club to focus on improving membership growth and retention.

❑ *Start the Tour at the Prospect's Hot Spot*. It is critical that the club tour begins in the area the prospect indicates as having the highest importance to them. It is important to keep in mind that the "club shoppers" of today are very knowledgeable about clubs and to give them a "canned" tour is one of the worst things a club can do. It can turn them off and detract from the club staff's level of professionalism. The tour should be personalized for each prospect, based upon the areas that the prospects indicated were their priorities in the Q-and-A session. A sales person should not waste time taking the prospect through the entire club, unless the sales person asks the prospect first.

❑ *Introduce the Prospect to the Experts*. It is critical during the tour that the sales person introduces the prospect to the club's experts in the prospect's indicated areas of interest. If the tour has been scheduled, arrangements should be made for the experts to be present. For example, if the prospect is interested in group exercise, then the group-exercise coordinator or instructor should be made available. If the prospect is interested in free weights, then the fitness director or a personal trainer should be present to answer the prospect's questions. If the tour is unscheduled and an expert is not available, an effort should be made to get the fitness director or an assistant to show the prospect around the fitness area.

A sales person should never lead off a tour of the fitness area by saying, "this is our cardiovascular room," or "we have Nautilus equipment." These are obvious statements, and to the club shopper, who has probably been a member of other clubs, these statements indicate a lack of professionalism and understanding of the prospect's specific needs by the individual leading the tour. The sales person should focus on what sets the club apart from all the other clubs. The sales person should address what the key differences mean to the prospect and why the individual should join the club. This is the time the sales person should focus on the staff, service, members, programming, etc.—not the equipment.

❑ *Extend the Invitation to Try the Club That Day*. The sales person should make sure that they give the prospect is given the opportunity to use the club that day if the prospect desires. Better yet, the prospect should be connected with another member or a staff person who can provide any needed assistance.

❑ *Introduce the Prospect to a Member*. From a sales perspective, nothing is stronger than the testimony of a member in showing a prospect the value of a club. The introduction between a prospect and a member should be short and brief. The club should always keep in mind that a satisfied member can be their best sales person.

From a sales perspective, nothing is stronger than the testimony of a member in showing a prospect the value of a club.

❑ *Provide a Brochure/Club Information Package.* Every prospect should be provided with the club's brochure. Doing this enables certain parts of the information presented in the brochure to be referenced during the tour.

❑ *Use the Club's Program/Events Calendar.* The tour should include a brief review of the club's program and/or events calendar. It is important that the prospect gets a feel for the various activities that the club sponsors, along with a sense of the traditions of the club. This situation also represents a great opportunity to allow prospects to ask any questions that they may have and it gives the sales person an excellent chance to elaborate on the level of activity in the club.

❑ *Ask for the Sale.* After the tour is completed, the sales person should sit down with the prospect in a non-intimidating setting and ask if tthe prospect has any further questions. After answering the prospect's questions, the sales person should ask for the sale. If the tour went as planned, the sale will be made. If the sale doesn't occur, the sales person should make sure that the prospect is given a guest pass and then follow-up with the prospect at a later date to see how the individual's visit to the club went.

The Corporate Membership Sale

In urban markets and suburban markets with a high concentration of businesses, corporate membership sales present an unparalleled opportunity for clubs to develop large reservoirs of leads and prospects, which often result in high closing rates.

The corporate membership sale involves a unique process and situation in the health/fitness club industry. In urban markets and suburban markets with a high concentration of businesses, corporate membership sales present an unparalleled opportunity for clubs to develop large reservoirs of leads and prospects, which often result in high closing rates. For many health/fitness clubs, the corporate market represents a majority of their membership growth opportunity. Since the process of generating corporate leads and prospects, along with the process of closing those leads, is different than the typical sales process, this section of the chapter reviews the most effective approaches for selling to the corporate market, including:

❑ *Learn and Understand the Corporate Mindset towards Club Memberships.* The club's first step should be to learn about the corporate fitness arena and what corporations are seeking when they purchase corporate memberships. In this regard, the University of Michigan's Health Management Research Center produces an annual report detailing the current research on the benefits and costs associated with worksite wellness. This report offers a useful overview of the cost benefit data that corporations typically consider when they evaluate the need for a corporate membership program. Another excellent resource is the 1998 IHRSA publication, *The Corporate Market; How to Capture and Keep Corporate Memberships.* In general, most corporations purchase corporate memberships for one of the following reasons:

- Use it as a tool for recruiting high-caliber talent. Many corporations indicate that fitness memberships are a benefit frequently sought by new employees.

- See it as a means to help improve employee morale and productivity.

- See it as a means to reduce healthcare-related costs for the company (current research validates the fact that low-risk employees cost companies less).

- See it as means of improving the image of the company.

- See it as a means to reduce worker's compensation costs, absenteeism, and work-related disability.

While most companies pursue a fitness membership program for their employees based on one or more of the aforementioned factors, they also evaluate a corporate fitness membership program based on a club being able to provide one or more of the following services:

- Corporations look for health/fitness programs that include fitness, nutrition, health education, health screening, and behavioral change.

- Corporations look for membership packages that offer more than just memberships, but also allow access to specific programs, such as back care, weight loss, stress management, health fairs, health-risk screening, etc.

- Corporations look for clubs to provide them with reports on employee usage of both the club in general and particular programs specifically. These reports should provide the corporation with detailed insight into how much use their employees are getting out of the membership.

- Corporations prefer a situation where clubs offer a variety of options for billing, including the options of dues sharing with employees, payroll deduction, discounted fees, etc.

Corporations prefer a situation where clubs offer a variety of options for billing, including the options of dues sharing with employees, payroll deduction, discounted fees, etc.

❑ *Identify the Club's Corporate Market.* Once a club gains an understanding of the corporate market, its next step should be to develop a list of the most appropriate corporations to pursue. Among the most effective means for accomplishing this task are the following:

- *Identify which corporations are represented by the club's current membership.* This step can be done by doing a search of the club's membership roster and identifying the corporations listed on the membership applications. If the club has a good relationship with its members, it might also consider having discussions with those members of the club who are known to be affiliated with local companies. Clubs should always keep in mind that its members are the best source of information in this arena.

- *Compile a list of companies that fall within the club's market area.* While not as effective as utilizing the club's membership roster, this strategy is a good alternative. Clubs should focus primarily on those companies that are located within a few miles of the club.

- *Find out who the decision-makers are at the corporations.* In most cases, either the human resources department or the medical department is involved in the process of deciding whether to purchase health/fitness club memberships for their company's employees. In smaller companies, it might be the manager or president of the company. Of course, if a club has a good relationship with its members, it may be able to find out from them who the key decision-makers are at the companies at which they work.

- *Learn about the company's values and needs.* As part of the process, clubs should make an effort to learn as much about a company as it can. The club can start the effort by searching the company's web site. The best approach in this regard, however, is for a club to talk to its members who are employed by the company. The club should learn as much as it can from these discussions with its employees.

❑ *Develop a Corporate Presentation Package.* Most companies, both small and large, expect the sales process to feature professionally presented materials. As a result, a club needs to prepare a professional presentation about the club and the value of corporate memberships. Among the key elements that such a presentation package might include are the following:

- *Develop a PowerPoint or DVD presentation.* A powerpoint or DVD presentation should be developed that not only tells the story of the club, but also integrates information on the benefits of fitness and wellness for the corporation.

> **Most companies, both small and large, expect the sales process to feature professionally presented materials.**

- *Make the presentation company relevant.* The materials should be customized to the respective company with which the club is dealing.

- *Have a printed presentation package or DVD/CD package.* The club should leave a professionally done package with the company after its presentation is completed. In this regard, the most recent trend is for a club to use CDs or DVDs that also link to the club's web site.

- *Get away from a standard corporate discount package.* The club should avoid making its presentation a discount presentation. The club's primary goal during a presentation should be to increase the perceived value of what it has to offer the company.

❑ *Get an Audience at the Corporation.* This step is often the most challenging aspect of corporate sales. Similar to the typical membership sale, when converting a lead into a prospect can be a demanding task, getting an opportunity to meet with the corporation can be a long tedious process. Clubs experienced in corporate sales have found the following approaches to be effective in getting the club's foot in the door:

- *Member referral*. The best approach for getting an audience at a corporation is for a club to have one of its existing members introduce a designated person from the club to the company decision maker by setting up an appointment for them. If members cannot set up an appointment for that person, then the member should be asked to at least provide an introduction for the sales person.

- *Building relationships in the community*. If possible, appropriate staff members from the club should join the local chamber or business-networking group. They should establish relationships that they can later use to help get them an audience at the targeted company.

- *Forward a personalized invitation*. If the company contact is known, the club should forward an invitation inviting them to the club for a special presentation. The invitation should be compelling and eye-catching. The more professional and out-of-the-ordinary it is, the more likely it is to get the company's attention.

- *Always confirm an appointment with a follow-up call*. Whether the club's appointment is obtained by an invitation or a personal introduction, the club should be sure to follow-up by phone and/or e-mail to confirm the appointment.

❑ *Make the First Appointment a Learning Experience*. In corporate sales, the first appointment is not designed to close the sale, but rather as a means to learn about the company's needs and wants (sound familiar?) and to present general information on the benefits the club can offer. At this meeting, typically more time is spent learning about the company than presenting information on the club. The basic goal of this first meeting should be to have the company agree to have the club forward a proposal specific to the company.

❑ *Forward a Customized Presentation*. Upon completion of the initial meeting, the club should prepare a customized proposal on membership for the company. The proposal should be relevant to what the club has learned about the company. The proposal might include an invitation for the contact to use the club or possibly an invitation that allows the company to send its employees to the club for a week's complimentary usage. Some clubs have developed special activities at the club, such as featured evenings for the targeted companies. In any event, the club should make sure to follow-up its proposal with a call to confirm that its proposal has been received. The call should include an inquiry about when a good time to follow-up might be.

In corporate sales, the first appointment is not designed to close the sale, but rather as a means to learn about the company's needs and wants (sound familiar?) and to present general information on the benefits the club can offer.

❑ *Maintain Contact*. Once its proposal has been forwarded to the company, the club should be vigilant with following up. The club will often find that it may take a few months between the time it forwarded its initial proposal and the next meeting it has with the company.

The clubs who constantly achieve membership sales success are fully aware of the fact that membership sales must become part of the club culture.

❑ *Be prepared for Additional Meetings and Counterproposals*. When pursuing corporate sales, the club needs to be prepared for the fact that it will typically have to deal with additional meetings and revised proposals. It is a rare event that a club's first proposal becomes the one the company accepts.

❑ *When Closing the Sale, the Club should Throw a Party for the Company*. Once the company agrees to the club's proposal, then a special function should be held at the club in honor of the company, welcoming the company to the club.

❑ *Make sure to Assign a Corporate Representative*. Over the years, clubs have found that it is essential for them to assign a staff person to represent the account and maintain an ongoing contact with the company representative once the contract has been signed. More often than not, corporations need hand holding. Accordingly, clubs should make sure that they have a staff person meet with the designated corporate representative on a regular basis. These meetings should include providing information about the usage of the club by company employees and other relevant data to the company representative. Maintaining regular contact with the company can help assure ongoing support from the corporation.

It is important to understand that corporate membership sales are a high-reward and high-risk approach to membership sales. While corporate sales can lead to a relatively large number of sales, they can also often lead to high level of turnover.

Sales Management: Creating a Culture of Sales Success

The clubs who constantly achieve membership sales success are fully aware of the fact that membership sales must become part of the club culture. The most critical part of creating a sales culture is to establish disciplined sales-management practices. In the health/fitness club industry, a disciplined sales management approach would encompass several activities, including:

❑ *Identify and Appoint a Sales Manager*. It is extremely important that a staff person be accountable for the club's overall sales performance. The sales manager should be the individual who helps set sales goals, leads sales meetings, provides coaching and instruction for the sales staff, and otherwise supports the efforts of the sales staff.

❏ *Establish Sales Goals for the Team and Individuals.* The sales manager, working with ownership, needs to establish annual, monthly, weekly, and even daily sales goals for the team and individual sales staff. Many clubs set goals based on the number of membership units sold, but the wise sales manager focuses on sales goals founded in dollar volume. The individual and team sales goals that are established should be somewhat of a stretch, so that if they're achieved, the club exceeds its baseline membership parameters for being successful.

❏ *Monitor and Track Sales Performance.* The sales manager should implement a system that allows the club's sales-performance level to be tracked on a daily, weekly, monthly, and annual basis. The system should enable the sales manager and sales staff to identify positive and negative sales trends.

❏ *Conduct Weekly Team and Individual Sales Meetings.* The sales manager needs to have weekly sales meetings with the team that focus on results, challenges, and solutions. Concurrently, the sales manager needs to meet individually with their sales team members to provide support, coaching, and education.

The individual and team sales goals that are established should be somewhat of a stretch, so that if they're achieved, the club exceeds its baseline membership parameters for being successful.

❏ *Create Special Incentives.* Sales are filled with highs and lows. Sales managers need to create incentives that reward great performance and also help drive performance during down times. While these incentives can be ongoing, in many cases, they should be designed to be employed during specific periods of time.

❏ *Recognize Success.* Sales managers need to realize how important recognition is to sales people. Accordingly, a means to recognize individuals who perform well should be designed and implemented. Such an undertaking can produce great results.

❏ *Compensate the Sales Staff Based on Performance.* Sales people need to be compensated based on how well they achieved their individual and team sales goals.

❏ *Integrate the Sales Team with the Operations Team.* Club managers and sales managers both need to realize that the greatest membership sales

An effective sales manager will realize that the entire club staff can contribute to the success of the sales department and will work hard to integrate the two.

success comes when the operations team and sales team work together. Unfortunately, some clubs forget this precept and create silos (individual pockets of focus) where membership sales are not connected to the other areas of the club. An effective sales manager will realize that the entire club staff can contribute to the success of the sales department and will work hard to integrate the two.

❑ *Hold the Sales Team Collectively Accountable.* The club manager needs to hold the sales manager accountable for the club's sales performance against the predetermined plan. By the same token, the sales manager should hold the sales staff accountable for their individual and team performance.

Key Points to Consider

As illustrated by the information presented in this chapter, membership sales are a continuation of a club's membership and marketing efforts. More importantly, membership sales are a by-product of very disciplined business practices that require a detailed system of checks and balances.

MEMBERSHIP RETENTION IN THE HEALTH/FITNESS CLUB INDUSTRY

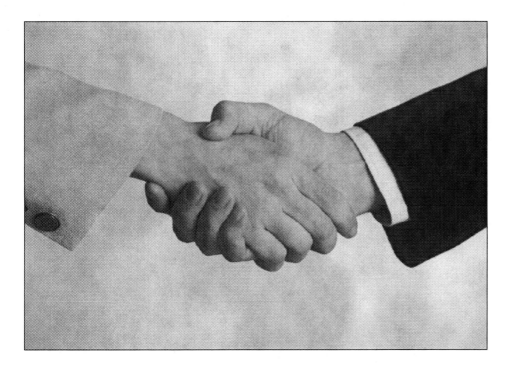

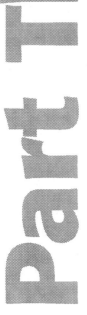

7

Member Retention and the Value of a Member

Chapter Objectives

Members are the heart of every club. Without them, health/fitness clubs would cease to exist. It is a widely held belief in the industry that membership is all about sales. In reality, however, membership is a balance between the process of selling and retaining memberships. Membership retention is about engaging members in the club experience so that they continue to stay a member. The more members stay, the fewer the number of memberships a club has to sell. In other words, membership retention involves the process of keeping members after the sale. This chapter begins by providing an overview of membership-retention data in the health/fitness club industry, and then discusses the value of a member. Finally, the chapter details several of the variables known to influence a club's membership retention level and some of the steps that clubs can take to affect those retention variables.

> It is a widely held belief in the industry that membership is all about sales. In reality, however, membership is a balance between the process of selling and retaining memberships.

The Industry's Experiences with Membership Retention

For a long time, membership retention has been a hurdle for the industry. In the late 1980s and early 1990s, membership retention levels in the health/fitness industry ran around 60% to 65%. In other words, on an annual basis, 60% to 65% of existing memberships would remain, and 35% to 40% of a club's members would depart. From a sales and retention perspective, that

	All Clubs		Multipurpose		Fitness-Only		Multi-Club		Independent	
	2002	2003	2002	2003	2002	2003	2002	2003	2002	2003
Retention	65%	66.5%	69%	67.5%	59.2%	62.2%	64.7%	61.9%	65.3%	68%
Net Member Growth	3.9%		3.0%		6.1%		3.6%		4.4%	

Figure 7.1. Industry retention data from IHRSA's *2003 Profiles of Success*

means that two out of every five sales would be lost before the year was out. Figure 7.1 summarizes the retention data for the industry in 2002 and 2003.

As Figure 7.1 shows, irregardless of the type of club—fitness only, multipurpose, part of a chain of clubs, or independently owned—the retention percentages were approximately the same, around 66%. In other words, most clubs have over one-third of their members choose to leave each year. This statistic is alarming, since the long-term growth of any business cannot be sustained if it has to continually attract such a high percentage of new customers.

Most clubs have over one-third of their members choose to leave each year. This statistic is alarming, since the long-term growth of any business cannot be sustained if it has to continually attract such a high percentage of new customers.

Membership attrition =	Aggregate of dropped memberships for the year divided by the twelve-month average beginning membership level	
Membership retention =	100% minus the membership attrition percentage	

Month	Beginning Membership Level	Dropped Memberships
January	2,000	50
February	2,040	55
March	2,090	55
April	2,120	60
May	2,120	60
June	2,110	70
July	2,090	70
August	2,085	75
September	2,090	65
October	2,100	50
Novemeber	2,105	55
December	2,100	60
Total	25,050	725
Average	2087.5	
Attrition Rate	34.7%	
Retention Rate	65.3%	

Figure 7.2. Example of average membership attrition and retention rates on a hypothetical health/fitness club.

The retention data presented in Figure 7.1 is reflective of the sample of clubs that were surveyed by IHRSA. In reality, there are clubs in the industry who report retention rates closer to 50%, while there are also others who report retention rates that average between 80% and 90%. According to IHRSA's research, the larger clubs (over 60,000 S.F.) and those clubs generating over five million dollars in annual revenues have retention percentages in the 70%-to-75% range. In fact, clubs, such as the Houstonian in Houston, LeClub in Wisconsin, Cooper Activity Center in Dallas, and East Bank Club in Chicago report that they are able to keep their retention rate at 80% or more on an annual basis.

In other words, if the average club were to focus more attention on retaining its members and improve its rate of retention by just five percentage points, it could bring another $200,000 to $800,000 in revenues to the club!

The Value of a Membership and the Value of Retention

To understand the importance of membership retention, it is important to understand the value of a membership. Many club operators don't really understand the dollar value of a member and thus don't devote as much energy and resources into retaining members as they should. Based on data found in the *2004 IHRSA Profiles of Success,* the dollar value of a single membership can be substantial (refer to Figure 7.3).

As Figure 7.3 indicates, the value of one membership ranges from $1,998 to $5,364 (amounts calculated before factoring in the value of new members referred by that member). The impact of these numbers is even more meaningful when they are considered in a wider context. For example, if clubs extrapolated their data based on their average annual retention percentage, the average value of dollars lost pr club would be very substantial (refer to Figure 7.3).

According to Figure 7.4, the average IHRSA club loses between $923,187 and $7,713,202 each year from memberships that leave. It is hard to imagine another commercial venture that allows that much business to escape, thereby creating a situation where it has to try to sell constantly to avoid the irreparable erosion of itself. If the average IHRSA club were to increase its retention percentage by just five points, it would save between $200,000 and $800,000 each year. In other words, if the average club were to focus more attention on retaining its members and improve its rate of retention by just five percentage points, it could bring another $200,000 to $800,000 in revenues to the club! Based on the average earnings percentage for the industry, those increased revenue totals translate into another $50,000 to $200,000 in the bank. Obviously, members have considerable worth. As such, if a club retains just one more member, it is adding to its bottom line.

Variables Known to Influence Attrition and Retention

In 1998, IHRSA funded research into uncovering the reasons why members leave clubs, with the intent of gaining a greater understanding of what factors

Club Size	Under 20,000 S.F.	20,000 to 34,999 S.F.	35,000 to 59,999 S.F.	Over 65,000 S.F.
Average # of memberships	1,1114	1,871	2,407	4,654
Average IF Collected per Membership in $	$100	$100	$112.50	$249
Average Annual Dues per Membership in $	$576	$588	$600	$882
Average Non - Dues Revenue per Membership Annually	$156.60	$137.26	$328.91	$545.20
Total Annual Revenue per Member in $	$832.60	$825.26	$1,041.41	$1,676.20
Average Length of Membership in Years	2.4	2.4	3.4	3.2
Total Value of a Membership	$1,998.24	$1,980.62	$3,540.79	$5,363.84

Figure 7.3. Dollar value of a membership in the health/fitness membership

might influence the individuals to stay. In 2000, IHRSA sponsored additional research that looked at these factors that correlated to individuals remaining as a member of a club, in an attempt to identify which of those variables might be alterable. Finally, in 2001, the Fitness Industry Association of England undertook research into membership retention. Cumulatively, the results of those three separate research endeavors provide considerable insight into why individuals forego their memberships in health/fitness clubs.

Club Size	Under 20,000 S.F.	20,000 to 34,999 S.F.	35,000 to 59,999 S.F.	Over 60,000 S.F.
Total Membership	1,1114	1,871	2,407	4,654
Retention Percentage	58.50%	57.90%	70.90%	69.10%
Lost Members	462	788	700	1,438
Dollars Lost	$923,187	$1,560,732	$2,478,566	$7,713,202

Figure 7.4. Average cost per club of lost memberships

Did not make enough use of the membership	43%
Lost interest or motivation	17%
Switched to outdoor exercise	15%
Did not have a partner	13%
Switched to home exercise	13%

Figure 7.5. Top five personal reasons people report for leaving

Overcrowded	27%
Dissatisfied with the staff	13%
Lack of personal attention from the staff	13%
Dissatisfied with programs and activities	8%
Unresponsive management	6%

Figure 7.6. Top five club-related reasons for leaving

The decision a member makes to remain a club member or leave the club is impacted to a significant degree by personal and relationship factors.

Did not have an exercise partner	81%
Favorite staff person left	81%
Switched to home exercise	77%
Lost interest or motivation	75%
Did not fit in	75%

Figure 7.7. Correlation between reasons for not renewing and the decision not to join a club during the coming year

As Figures 7.5 to 7.7 demonstrate, the decision a member makes to remain a club member or leave the club is impacted to a significant degree by personal and relationship factors. It seems that such a decision is most often influenced by not having an exercise partner, not fitting in, losing motivation, lack of attention from the staff, and dissatisfaction with the programs and activities of the club. Each of these variables involves an individual's social connection to the club—to the club's staff, the other members, and the activities of the club. These factors are also affected by how well the club gets each new member "engaged" with their new purchase.

In addition to the aforementioned data, research has also identified the following factors as critical determinants influencing membership retention:

- Members who feel the staff helped them to achieve their personal fitness goals were far more likely to remain a member.

- Members who felt that the staff was professional and took a personal interest in them were far more likely to remain a member.

- Members who made friends quickly and developed a sense of belonging or fitting in were far more likely to remain a member.

- Members who used the club most frequently during their first month reported they had a better relationship with the staff.

- Members who rated their satisfaction with the club as the highest were also the most likely to have a great relationship with the staff and were the most likely to remain a member.

- The percentage of members who remain in a club falls proportionally over the first 12 months. According to the FIA, at 12 weeks, retention is around 93%. It then drops to 78% by 24 weeks, and by 36 weeks, falls to just less than 70%.

- Older adults have a higher retention rate than younger adults, with those over 45 having the highest retention percentage of any age group.

- Those members who pay a higher initiation fee have a higher retention rate. According to FIA research, the retention rate for those paying an initiation fee is 21% greater than for those who don't pay a fee.

- Members who pay annually have higher retention rates than those who pay on a month-by-month basis. After one year, the difference between the two retention rates is negligible.

- A dose-response rate exists between use of the club and membership retention. In other words, the more engaged a member is in using the club, the more likely that person is to remain a member.

- The first month is the most critical period for the retention rate process. Those individuals who use the club less than four times in the first month have a significantly higher attrition rate.

- Those new members with a higher level of education and a higher level of income are more likely to remain members.

- Smokers and those individuals who are overweight are more likely to drop their membership.

As can be seen, a host of reasons exist why people decide to either remain a member or chose to leave. The aforementioned factors are similar in many respects to the data presented in the earlier figures. These factors lend further support to the contention that club members need to be engaged and connected with their clubs as soon as possible in order for them to continue with their membership. This step entails facilitating a connection between the individual member and both the staff and the other members. This undertaking also involves helping members achieve their personal goals and providing an entertaining and motivating environment for club members. Accordingly, club operators, with regard to membership retention, need to identify and focus on those factors that can have the greatest impact on their club's retention level and bottom line.

Proven Strategies for Improving Retention

The process of retaining members ultimately revolves around the club's ability to deliver experiences that are personally relevant and are facilitated by exceptional service. This section reviews several proven approaches for not only increasing the level of member connection, but also driving member retention. In the next two chapters, some of the key elements involved in creating positive experiences and establishing a service culture and a service-oriented level of programming will be addressed.

Among research-based strategies for enhancing the membership-retention level are the following:

- *Don't sell the club membership short.* Retention begins at the time of joining. Research shows that members who pay an enrollment fee stay longer than those who don't. Furthermore, the higher the fee, the higher the retention level. The key point is that the club operator should assign a real value to the club's membership experience. If membership is given away, all factors being equal, members will feel their membership is not worth very much.

- *Identify the members' fitness needs and focus on getting them to the goal.* The data is clear that with regard to membership retention, it is crucial that members achieve their fitness goals. This process not only involves identifying what those goals are, but also developing a program that provides a realistic avenue for them to be achieved. Finally, all clubs should provide monitoring, support, and encouragement to their members so their members' goals can be achieved.

- *Connect the new member to other members.* Most members express a strong desire to have a partner or to feel a sense of belonging. Satisfying this desire requires getting the members to meet other members and establish friendships. Clubs can accomplish this goal by having the staff introduce new members to other members. They can also achieve this objective by organizing and implementing such undertakings as welcoming parties, new member/existing member activities, member chat spaces, partner programs, etc.

The process of retaining members ultimately revolves around the club's ability to deliver experiences that are personally relevant and are facilitated by exceptional service.

- *Staff and members need to connect.* Clubs need to establish a service culture that is passionate about caring for the members. The staff should be encouraged to meet with members, learn about them, and respond to their needs and feedback. Responsive and friendly are two key attributes of a caring-oriented staff.

- *Get the members active.* The research is very clear about the "use-it-or-lose-it" aspect of membership. Members who are more active, especially in the initial stages of their membership, are far more likely to remain members. Clubs need to establish systems that introduce new members to club-based activities in a non-intimidating way and then track their activity-involvement levels so they can monitor and help reinforce each member's efforts to be physically active. Clubs might even consider offering incentive programs tied to activity during an individual's first three months of membership.

- *Be attentive to the members' comments and interests.* Club management needs to establish a system for maintaining an open dialogue with its members. This process should involve the use of such factors as a feedback system, service recovery system, focus groups, surveys, and even member committees. The members need to perceive management as being interested in and responsive to their experiences.

- *Keep the club clean and well-maintained.* While not a primary reason given by members for quitting, research shows that whether the club was kept clean and whether the club kept its equipment and facilities updated had an impact on the desire of individuals to maintain their club membership. Members want to feel that the dues they are paying are going back into the club. Clubs need to keep this factor in mind and let members know when the club is doing something to upgrade its facilities or equipment.

All employees, from the membership sales staff to the manager to the housecleaning staff, must view helping retain members as an integral part of their job.

- *Make retention a part of everyone's job description.* All employees, from the membership sales staff to the manager to the housecleaning staff, must view helping retain members as an integral part of their job. Sales people help retention by not selling the club short and by helping connect members at the time of joining. The fitness staff drives retention by helping members achieve their fitness goals and helping connect the members to other members. The front desk staff can have a positive impact on retention by making members feel welcome and responding to member comments. The house maintenance staff affects retention in a positive manner by keeping the club clean and by looking for ways to respond to member needs.

As club operators attempt to identify strategies that can help them retain members, they should remember that retention begins with a culture within the club that focuses on connecting people, creates memorable experiences, and always puts the member first. The next two chapters take a more in-depth look at member satisfaction and the need for a club to create exceptional experiences and service-oriented programs that will satisfy the needs and expectations of its members.

Retention begins with a culture within the club that focuses on connecting people, creates memorable experiences, and always puts the member first.

8

Creating Memorable Member Experiences

Chapter Objectives

In the previous chapter, the value of a membership and the importance of retaining members in driving the profitability and vibrancy of a club were addressed. As research indicates, members either stay or leave a club based on whether their experience at the club meets or does not meet their expectations and needs. Research also shows that in the majority of instances, the situations in which member expectations were not met revolved around the connection of members to members, members to the staff, and members to the club's activities. This chapter explores the importance of the fact that clubs should create a culture that drives memorable experiences that meet and exceed the expectations of their members. The chapter examines how individuals who belong to clubs respond to experiences that they encounter as members of a club and the impact that these experiences have on their level of retention. The chapter then reviews the importance of creating memorable experiences. Finally, the chapter details the process of creating the experiences that drive member retention.

> Members either stay or leave a club based on whether their experience at the club meets or does not meet their expectations and needs.

How Members Respond to the Service Delivery and the Experience Provided by the Club

When individuals decide to become members of a club, they join with certain preconceptions and expectations. For some, those factors may involve achieving a certain fitness goal, while the objective of other individuals may be to meet other people within the club setting. Irregardless of whether one or more of these factors is the primary reason driving their joining a club, each of these variables affects whether they remain a member. In this regard, these factors may include such diverse matters as personal attention from staff, facility cleanliness, program variety, program convenience, meeting other members, and a host of other reasons. In reality, because club operators cannot always identify these expectations, they must be prepared to create and deliver experiences that can meet or exceed expectations of which they may not even be aware.

A club's first indication of how members have accepted or perceived the delivery of the club experience is by the response they make (both verbally and non-verbally). Collectively, the members' responses then become an important factor in how club operators and their staff adjust the services and experiences they provide.

Research conducted on how individuals respond to their experiences indicates that four basic responses exist—one of which is good, one of which is outstanding, and all of which can be used to drive a club's ability to retain members. The impact of these responses on a club varies from factor to factor:

❑ *Outrage*. Outrage is an emotional response that members have when their experience has fallen well short of their expectations. Members who exhibit outrage feel great emotional displeasure and a sense of betrayal. When clubs do not deal immediately with member outrage, they are contributing to the formation of what can be called, "business terrorists," people who go out of their way to harm the business. Many of the individuals in the health/fitness club business are familiar with this response. Most clubs tend to ignore members who respond with outrage, not realizing that they are creating terrorists. When the club actually overcomes the outrage (not an easy thing to do), it is building a strong bridge to retaining a member.

❑ *Dissatisfaction*. Dissatisfaction is an unemotional response that members have when they do not receive the service or experience they expect. This response often occurs when a club makes its members "sacrifice" something of importance, the absence of which then becomes an inconvenience. Dissatisfied members normally don't tell the club about their sense of dissatisfaction. Rather, they might grumble to other members of the club or show up less often at the club. An example of a circumstance that could result in a degree of member dissatisfaction could be something as simple and basic as a trainer arriving five minutes late for an appointment with the member or the sauna not working. Eventually, dissatisfied members will leave the club if they are not identified. On the other hand, they are easily taken care of if the source of their dissatisfaction is addressed by the club.

❑ *Satisfaction*. To many individuals in the health/fitness club business, member satisfaction is considered the end point, the response of choice. A satisfied individual means that the club has been able to meet the member's expectations. A satisfied member is not necessarily a happy

Research conducted on how individuals respond to their experiences indicates that four basic responses exist—one of which is good, one of which is outstanding, and all of which can be used to drive a club's ability to retain members.

member, rather an individual who, for now, will continue as a member. Satisfied members are often the first to leave when a new club opens elsewhere, because although they are satisfied, they have not developed a sufficient sense of loyalty to the club. Far too often, satisfied members are relatively unknown to the club, because they haven't expressed their true feelings to the club.

❑ *Delight.* Delight occurs when the club exceeds a member's expectations. In other words, the club has provided an experience that was both memorable and beyond the member's perceptions or expectations. Delight is an indication of an emotional buy-in or personal ownership. Delighted members are often referred to as "business apostles"— individuals who "tell and sell" the club's story to others. Typically, club operators know who these individuals are, because they are often the most active and outgoing members of the club.

> **Delight occurs when the club exceeds a member's expectations. In other words, the club has provided an experience that was both memorable and beyond the member's perceptions or expectations.**

In the late 1990s and early 2000s, ClubCorp sponsored research that was designed to identify how the various aforementioned member responses impacted retention and profitability. In particular, ClubCorp wanted to better understand how these responses affected the members' desire to remain a member and their willingness to refer others for membership. This research found that delighted members were twice as likely to remain a member as a satisfied member and one tenth as likely to leave. Furthermore, a delighted

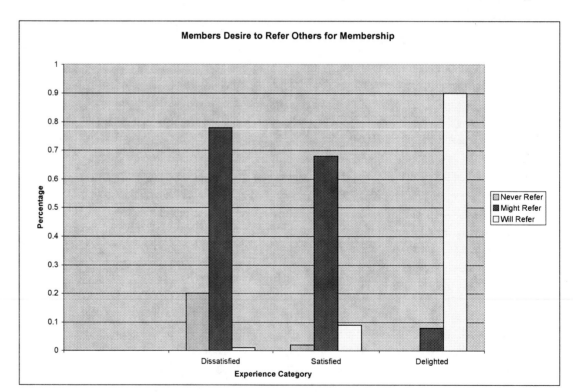

Figure 8.1. The members' desire to refer others for membership

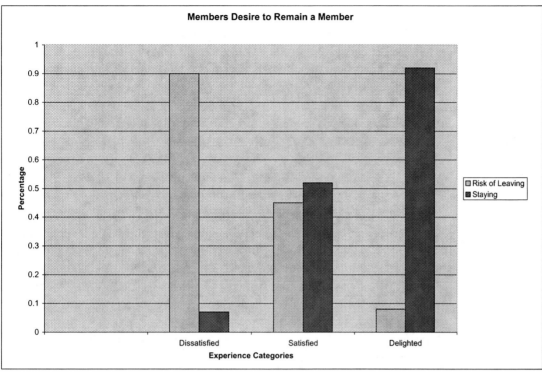

Figure 8.2. The members' desire to remain a member

member was nearly 10 times as likely as a satisfied member to refer someone for membership. The conclusion, which paralleled research results in other customer-service environments, was that a delighted member is the most valuable member a club has. These findings support the contention that a club should create a service and experience culture that is focused on driving member delight. Figure 8.1 and 8.2 illustrate the findings of the ClubCorp investigations.

When the membership retention and membership sales implications of these figures are considered, it is very clear that clubs can benefit by creating a culture that is focused on delivering the service necessary to create experiences that drive a member's sense of delight.

Defining a Positive Club Experience

As the previous section discussed, if a club wants to have an impact on member retention, it needs to have a service culture that is focused on creating and sustaining experiences that exceed the expectations of members. In that regard, two critical issues arise: what is meant by the term "an experience" and what role does service culture have in driving these experiences. In order to address those issues, the first step is to understand the relationship between service and experience. Both factors are defined as follows:

Clubs can benefit by creating a culture that is focused on delivering the service necessary to create experiences that drive a member's sense of delight.

> Service requires people and systems that can repeatedly deliver the club's product, with minimal sacrifice on the member's part.

❑ *Service*. Service is the process by which a club's people and systems are able to deliver the club's facilities, programs, and other amenities to the member. Service is the process that the club employs to deliver its product. Service requires people and systems that can repeatedly deliver the club's product, with minimal sacrifice on the member's part. The following example can help illustrate the differences between service and experience. A club offers yoga classes for novices, beginners, and advanced members. The classes are the club's product. The manner in which the club's instructors teach those classes and interact with the members is the service the club provides. If the service provided by the club enables members to participate freely, with minimal inconvenience, and enjoy the class, then the club is servicing the members with minimal sacrifice by the members. If instead, the yoga class instructors require members to say a pledge, ask beginners to perform advanced work, and never smile, the club's service in this instance would be requiring the members to make some degree of sacrifice to participate. In other words, in the context of service, the club should think of it as the delivery mechanism for all of the experiences it provides to members. Great service occurs when members sacrifice the least, and poor service exists when the club makes its members exert a considerable sacrifice.

❑ *Experience*. An experience involves the interplay of a club's product, the service process, the expectations and needs of the member, and finally, the club's ability to create the desired circumstances around a theme. In essence, an experience is what members receive or perceive they receive based on how the club themes the service it provides and how it impacts the members' expectations. It should be noted that experiences can be good or bad. Accordingly, the goal of the club should be to create experiences that require minimal sacrifice on the part of the member and enhance the member's sense of member delight.

One positive example of creating a desired experience is a class offered by one of the various Crunch clubs in New York City. This particular Crunch club offers an aerobic class called cardio striptease. The theme of the class is, of course, striptease. The club's product is an aerobic class. The service is the manner in which the instructor delivers the class, hopefully with passion, dressed in full striptease attire, and encouraging the members to do the same. While the foregoing is an extreme example, other programming efforts, such as Fireman's Aerobics, Hell Week, etc., also illustrate how clubs can create an experience at the micro level.

Creating Club-Based Experiences

Clubs can achieve noteworthy success with their members by creating a service culture that is focused on delivering unique experiences that not only exceed member expectations, but also help facilitate member delight. Among the relatively simple steps that a club can take to become more experience-oriented are the following:

❑ *Establish a theme.* The first step in creating a unique and differentiating membership experience is to identify a unifying theme. By establishing a theme for the experience that the club intends to provide, it can focus each aspect of its business toward the fulfillment of that particular theme. For example, Western Athletic Clubs, based in San Francisco, California, have a theme built around being a "sports resort." Each aspect of their design, product mix, and service culture is focused on creating a resort experience. Another example of theme building is Crunch Fitness, based out of New York, which has developed a theme that is designed to deliver out-of-the-box, non-judgmental experiences. When an individual enters a Crunch club, that person can easily see that the design of the club, the attire of the staff, the names of the classes and programs, and the service approach of their staff all align with the club's basic theme. Another club that is built around a theme is the Marsh, which is located outside Minneapolis, Minnesota. The Marsh's theme is focused on mind and body, in essence, attempting to make it an out-of-body retreat. The Marsh's facilities, programs, and service culture all center on creating experiences based on that particular theme. At a more micro level, numerous clubs have developed classes and programs around a highly recognizable theme, such as Boot Camp, Fireman's Aerobics, SWAT Classes, etc.

❑ *Add the "ING."* According to Gilmore and Pine in their insightful book, *The Experience Economy*, when a club takes a particular product and service and thinks of that item in the context of adding an "ING," then the club is more likely to generate the desired experiences. An excellent example of this concept in practice occurred when Johnny G. created Spinning. What was once just riding a stationary bike became a hot experience. By creating Spinning, he made the class more appealing as an experience. The key point for clubs to consider in this regard is for the club to think about the action-oriented aspects of its products and services.

When a club takes a particular product and service and thinks of that item in the context of adding an "ING," then the club is more likely to generate the desired experiences.

❑ *Build the proper stage.* Creating experiences is like putting on a play. In the first act, the club needs to construct the proper stage or set design. Clubs who want to create positive experiences have to first develop an appropriate theme and then make sure the stage for acting out that experience has been established. For example, Western Athletic Clubs (as was previously noted) have a theme based on a resort experience. As a result, their club facilities are designed to look and feel like a resort destination. From the beautiful exterior landscape, to the design of each room, each Western Athletic Club member gets the feeling they are in a resort. Another industry group that focuses on building the proper setting are Crunch clubs, which feature a theme that is non-judgmental and out-of-the-box. When an individual enters the Crunch club in West Hollywood, for example, they will notice that as they walk to the locker rooms, they can see the profiles of people in the showers or that when members are on the exercise floor, that all the mirrors are round and on stands. Crunch also places signs throughout their club with off-the-wall expressions that support their theme. As intended, the members of Crunch clubs definitely get the sense they are immersed in an unusual experience.

❏ *Have the right props.* Just as a stage is normally needed to put on a play, clubs also need the right props. From a club perspective, the props are the equipment, the signage, the physical amenities, the classes and programs, and even the staff attire. It is critical that the club's props align with the designated theme of the facility. At Crunch clubs, for example, several outrageous signs are posted throughout the club. Most members stop and read the signs and have a laugh—a process that is part of the intended experience. The Crunch staff can be found wearing cut-offs, earrings, and other unusual items, all of which reinforce the predetermined theme of Crunch clubs. Each Crunch club also offers classes such as cardio striptease and cardio funk, both of which align with their theme. At the Marsh in Minnesota, its theme of a mind/body retreat is reinforced by props such as curtains, chairs, candles, and other items that make the members feel as if they are escaping from the world.

Just as a stage is normally needed to put on a play, clubs also need the right props.

❏ *The club's staff must see their job as acting.* Actors are adept at stepping into a character and creating the feeling desired by the director. For a club's staff, they too need to know the club's theme and then be able to "act" in a manner that reinforces that theme. For example, at Western Athletic Clubs, which have a theme built around providing a resort experience, the staff welcomes and communicates with members in a fashion that is reminiscent of a well-run resort. At Crunch, members can definitely expect the unexpected from the staff, but always within the context of taking care of the member. Again, this approach is consistent with the theme at Crunch. The art of acting by the club staff is an essential aspect of what could be considered the club's "service culture."

❏ *The staff should be focused on creating transformations.* Not only must a club's staff members be focused on acting, they should also be prepared to deal with each individual member in a manner that allows them to personalize the experience for the member. Transformations occur when an experience takes on a high degree of personal relevance. In essence, a club's staff needs to find ways to help members experience a change that is consistent with the members' personal expectations and needs. These transformations require a strong "service culture."

9

Creating a Member Service Culture That Drives Member Experiences That Build Retention

Chapter Objectives

The previous two chapters looked at membership retention and how this factor is affected by a club's ability to create memorable experiences for its members. In turn, it was pointed out that a club's success in creating memorable member experiences relies heavily on having a service culture. This chapter details the role of service in creating memorable experiences for the club's members and what steps are needed to establish and sustain a service culture.

The Service Profit Chain

According to Leonard Schlesinger of Harvard University in his article, "How Does Service Drive the Service Company," the "service profit chain" lies at the heart of growing a business's profitability. Like a "chain," the process has several interrelated links. Profitability is driven by customer loyalty, which is influenced by customer delight. Customer delight is affected by outstanding external service to the customer, which, in turn, is driven by delighted employees who are the recipients of great internal service (refer to Figure 9.1). Simply stated, in club terms, profitability is driven by loyal members, who have a sense of delight that is derived by their having engaged in memorable

The "service profit chain" lies at the heart of growing a business's profitability.

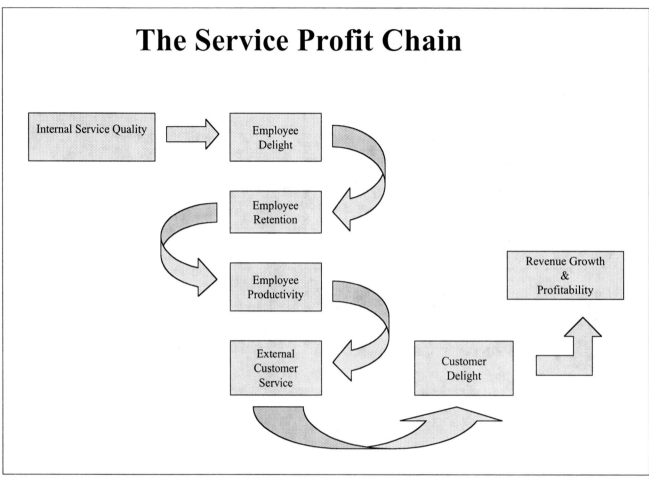

Figure 9.1. The service profit chain

Establishing a service culture therefore becomes one of the most essential elements in any health/fitness club's operating model.

experiences at the club. These member experiences are delivered by a staff with a strong internal and external service culture. It is the aforementioned "service profit chain" that lies at the center of membership retention and the ability of a club to create memorable member experiences.

Defining a Service Culture

The key to the club staff providing great service that is focused on delivering memorable member experiences starts with the establishment of a service culture. A service culture is a system of customs, habits, and conventions, the values, words, and works attendant to this culture help create and sustain a long-term environment in which the staff are passionate about and are empowered to deliver whatever is required to provide the club's members with a personally relevant and memorable experience. Establishing a service culture therefore becomes one of the most essential elements in any health/fitness club's operating model.

Creating a Service Culture in the Health/Fitness Club Business

Establishing an appropriate service culture in the club industry can involve a number of steps, including:

❑ *Create a Set of Core Business Values Around Service.* The core foundation of all cultures is a set of values. Whether it is a societal culture, such as the ones that exist in England, China, or Germany, or a business culture, such as witnessed at Ben & Jerry's, Starbuck's, Nordstrom's, or BMW, the heart of every culture is based on a set of values that lie behind every decision that is made. If a club wants to establish a service culture, its values must be consistent with the service expectations of its membership.

In every culture, the values and traditions that are attendant to that culture are sustained by leaders who embody those values and traditions.

For example, at ClubCorp, a Dallas, Texas-based private club company, the company's founder, Robert Dedman, established a service culture for the organization that featured several core values that were focused on service. The first value was, "the member and guest are king." With this one precept, Dedman established a framework for how he expected each employee to interact with the members of ClubCorp. Another fundamental ClubCorp value that Dedman constantly referred to was, "warm welcomes, magic moments, and fond farewells." When Dedman spoke of this underlying company sense of purpose, he was referring to the role that each employee plays in making sure all members receive a personalized welcome when they arrive, a personalized farewell when they leave, and a memorable and magic experience when they are in the club. Another core value established by Dedman was to call each member by their name at least four times when they were in the club. This practice was intended to reinforce the culture of personalizing each member's club experience. Over the years, the company values and attitudes instilled by Dedman have served ClubCorp very well.

In a similar approach, Red Lerelle, of Red's in Lafayette, Louisiana, has established some very basic business values for his company that speak to service. At Red's, every employee understands that they are to smile and say hello and goodbye to every member. At Red's, everyone knows that it is their job to do whatever it takes to take care of the members. These values, established by Red when he founded his club more than four decades ago, continue to set the framework for the club's service culture.

❑ *Create a Tradition of Service Values by Starting at the Top.* In every culture, the values and traditions that are attendant to that culture are sustained by leaders who embody those values and traditions. These leaders act in a manner that supports the core values of the culture. In the club business, one of the steps that can help create a tradition of great service is to reinforce the values in word and deed at all times. At Red's, for example, Red can be found training new employees on the importance of saying hello and goodbye to members of his club, most often by being seen throughout the club saying hello or goodbye. By the same token, at ClubCorp, when Robert Dedman visited a club, he could often be found talking with members and asking what he could do to help them. In both Red's and Dedman's world, the service values started with them. In other words, they did whatever it took to demonstrate the service values that they wanted to inculcate within their organization's culture.

❑ *Establish Courses of Action that Reinforce the Values and Service Culture.* In any culture, it takes more than one individual to spread the service culture. According to anthropologists, a culture is sustained by artifacts, tradition, myths, legends, and heroes. In other words, once an entity has the values of a culture established, it must have the people and stories to keep it alive and vibrant with the individuals who are part of that endeavor. As previously described, not only does it take leaders who will share relevant stories attendant to the service culture and believe in a manner consistent with the core values of the culture, it can require much more.

In the club business, for example, leaders must identify key staff members who embrace the service culture of the club and will "walk it and talk it." These employees become the club's storytellers and heroes. Accordingly, clubs should undertake an effort to collect employee recollections of the company's service culture so that they can be shared with the other employees. At ClubCorp, the company encourages employees and clubs to make note of stories that exemplify the service culture, and then to share those stories with their fellow employees by means of the company's web site and through daily staff lineups at each respective ClubCorp club. Sharing their own stories of a service experience during such a lineup can result in a "magic moment" for those staff who are conveying their remembrances. In the process, these individuals become one of the service culture's storytellers.

Among the other steps that can help reinforce the service culture within a club are the following:

- *Create a service recognition program.* Employees are far more likely to embrace a service culture when they are recognized for actions that align with the club's service culture. At ClubCorp, for example, this recognition program was called STAR Recognition. Other clubs have different names for their recognition programs. The key, however, is to recognize employees who live the service culture, irregardless of the term utilized to acknowledge the effort.

- *Develop an education program.* Clubs need to initiate an ongoing education program for all of their employees. At the heart of that training program should be a module dedicated to both the club's service culture and how employees can become the apostles for that

> Employees are far more likely to embrace a service culture when they are recognized for actions that align with the club's service culture.

service culture. At ClubCorp, the first educational effort an employee is exposed to is a video that explains the service culture at ClubCorp. Furthermore, it's essential that the club's educational program on its service culture is an ongoing one, not just a one-time delivery.

- *Loosen the knot.* One of the most common complaints from customers is that when they need something done, that employees have to ask their supervisors for instructions or permission to act. In reality, however, if a club wants to have a genuine service culture, it should empower its employees to act according to the culture. It should trust its employees to make the right decisions. At Nordstrom's, for example, employees are given the freedom to deal with customers, based solely on the company's service values. Fortunately, many clubs give its employees the freedom to make the right decision, based on an environment of trust. The key point that should be noted is that the process should be grounded in the clubs' service culture and how the clubs educate and support that culture.

- *All decisions need to be founded in the club's service values.* Many businesses establish service values, but then act outside them. For example, ClubCorp has a core philosophy that is based on the precept that the "member is king." If a situation subsequently occurs where the employee has to make a choice with regard to a particular action, that person's choice must be consistent with the value that the "member is king." If the employee's decision runs counter to that value, then the first link in ClubCorp's service culture chain has been broken.

- *Document the core values and practices of the club's service culture.* It is critical that the values and practices of the club's service culture be documented and shared with each of its employees. ClubCorp, for example, gives each of its employees the "basics card," which is a small, wallet-sized card on which are noted the values and philosophies that are at the heart of the company's service culture. The card that each employee of Red's receives lists eight specific values that are at the heart of Red's service culture. The card utilized at Red's serves as a statement of the service-culture standards at Red's. Not only does it help all Red's employees know the service culture expectations at Red's, it also furnishes them with a constant reminder of those expectations. The eight values listed on the Red's card include:

  ✓ The members are number one.

  ✓ Make eye contact, smile, and say "hello" and "goodbye."

  ✓ Show up on time and ready to work.

  ✓ If a member has a problem, solve it. Keep them happy.

  ✓ If you've got time to lean, you got time to clean.

  ✓ I don't know the answer; I'll find out, so check back with me.

✓ Have a positive attitude; be enthusiastic about your job.

✓ Stay in shape.

❑ *Provide a Means for Members to Communicate with Management About Their Experiences at the Club.* A service culture requires a high degree of openness by management. As such, management must be open to listening to the members and fostering an environment of trust between the members and the staff. Members must feel like they can share both their praise and their concerns openly and know that management and employees will respond to the members' efforts to communicate with them in a manner that helps ensure a better member experience. Among the approaches that clubs can utilize to elicit and enhance feedback from their members are the following:

- *Open door/open floor.* This approach to listening involves management leaving time for members to drop in and talk. It also mandates management should spend a portion of each day out in the club talking with members. The combination of getting out and talking with members and also leaving time on the schedule for members to walk in and meet with club staff allows the club to foster an environment of trust.

- *Member committees.* At ClubCorp, the ClubCorp clubs have committees made up of members. These committees serve dual roles. Not only do they provide valuable feedback on the experiences of the members, they also allow the members to become involved in identifying experience solutions. The number of committees varies from club to club. Some clubs only have a few committees, while others have more than a dozen, such as a social committee, racquet sport committee, membership committee, group-exercise committee, etc.

- *Focus groups.* Focus groups are an effective way for clubs to learn more about what their members feel. Focus groups allow a club to bring together groups of members in a non-intimidating environment and identify what they feel and believe about their experiences in the club.

- *Surveys.* Surveys are a practical method for assessing how members feel about the club experience. In this regard, surveys should be conducted at least once annually. Within the industry, numerous clubs, such as the Maryland Athletic Club in Timonium, Maryland, annually conduct surveys to find out how their members feel about key factors involving their experiences at the facility, particularly those that might affect their decision about maintaining or foregoing their club membership.

Members must feel like they can share both their praise and their concerns openly and know that management and employees will respond to the members' efforts to communicate with them in a manner that helps ensure a better member experience.

- *Comment box system.* Every club should offer members some version of the comment-box system that their members can use to share their concerns and praises. This effort could range from having boxes with comment cards left available throughout the club, to web-based feedback systems. Clubs, such as the MAC in East Lansing, Michigan, the ACAC in Charlottesville, Virginia, Club One in California, and the Western Athletic Clubs in California, all offer some type of a feedback system for their members to share their thoughts, concerns, and praises.

❑ *Eliminate the Sacrifices that a Member Has to Make.* The process of creating and sustaining a service culture requires that a club look at its operations and identify the sacrifices that members must make in order to use the club. In that regard, a member can sacrifice in a number of ways, including a loss of convenience, self-esteem, results, friendships, etc. When a club identifies sacrifices that its members must make, it should remove them. For example, many clubs require members to hand over their keys and ID just to get a towel. All factors considered, these clubs are asking members to make some degree of sacrifice just to use a towel. On the other hand, if members can obtain a towel without all of that inconvenience, it could easily be argued that they would feel much better. In reality, too many club operators construct barriers, thinking they will save money, but instead, they create member sacrifices that eventually help drive members away.

> The process of creating and sustaining a service culture requires that a club look at its operations and identify the sacrifices that members must make in order to use the club.

❑ *Create a Service Recovery Approach That Can Patch the Gaps.* Even in the best service culture, mistakes occur. According to the data shared by Dr. Leonard Schlesinger in his article, "The Service-driven Service Company," customers who have a bad experience can be turned around with the proper service-recovery process. The data on customer service indicates that up to 95% of customers will make a repeat purchase if their experience problem is addressed promptly and correctly. This type of information makes it imperative that a club's service culture includes a service-recovery process. In developing a service-recovery process, clubs should make sure to address each of the following steps:

- *Listen.* The first element of a service-recovery process is to listen to the member. This endeavor begins with having a system, featuring elements such as those discussed previously, that allows a club's members to voice their issues. It is imperative that the members be allowed to express their concerns either anonymously or not. Employees should be willing to listen attentively when members bring up an issue of concern to them. If the issue is brought up through a survey or other medium, then management needs to contact the member and hear what that person has to say.

- *Empathize.* Whenever a member shares an issue with the club's employees, they need to empathize and show that they understand the member's perspective on the issue. This attitude needs to be communicated clearly to the member.

- *Apologize.* It is imperative that the member with a relevant issue over their experience in the club receives an apology from the individual employee with whom they shared their concern. The apology from the employee should be imparted on behalf of the club, indicating that the club staff regrets the situation. The apology should be made promptly. If the concern is expressed to an employee in person, then the apology should occur at that time. If the issue comes to light at a later time (e.g., by a letter or other communication medium), then the apology needs to be delivered verbally and in person, if possible, as soon as the issue has come to the attention of management.

- *Respond.* Once the club has become aware of the issue and has apologized, it should take action to address the matter. As indicted on the aforementioned values card utilized at Red's, "solve it and keep them happy." If the issue has been brought to the attention of a line employee, the employee should be empowered to solve the issue. If the issue is beyond that person's scope of responsibility, then it should be immediately brought to the attention of an employee or supervisor who can solve the issue. If the issue cannot be resolved immediately, the club should make sure that someone gets back to them as soon as possible. The employees at Red's are instructed to respond to such a situation by stating, "I don't know the answer; I'll find out, so check back with me." If an issue is raised anonymously, management still needs to act promptly to address the situation. The key in service recovery is to empower the employee team to respond to issues promptly with solutions and when the employee does not have a solution to a particular problem, the club should make sure that the employee knows where to go for the solution. Finally, whenever and however the club is responding, the club should inform the member that it is taking action to address the situation.

- *Communicate the Response.* When an issue occurs that needs to be addressed, management should begin the process of solving the matter by letting the member know what action the club is taking, something that should be done at the time it learns of the issue. When the issue is raised anonymously, a note can be placed on a communication board in the club or on the club's website, informing the membership in general of an issue that has come to management's attention and of the action the club plans to take concerning the situation. If the issue is raised in person, members should immediately be informed of the action the club is taking. Members need to have prompt feedback that the club understands their issues and how it plans to deal with them.

> Whenever a member shares an issue with the club's employees, they need to empathize and show that they understand the member's perspective on the issue.

- *Follow-up.* The final critical aspect of the service-recovery process is for a club to make sure that once it has taken action on a member issue, that it clearly and promptly communicates to the member what the outcome of the action is. If the issue was raised anonymously, then the club should post the resulting action on a comment board at the club or on the club's web site.

It should be noted that the service-recovery process applies just as much to employee-related issues, as it does to member issues. Clubs that can properly and effectively address an employee-related issue are far more likely to have employees who are able to act in an appropriate manner when member-related problems occur.

Implementing Service Culture Values and Standards

Creating and sustaining a service culture is not an easy process. Examples of possible service values and standards that club operators might consider as they create their own service values and culture include the following:

❑ *Greeting Members*:

- Always smile and make eye contact.
- Call the member by name.
- Personalize the greeting by saying more than just "hello."
- Always greet members by standing and extending a hand.

❑ *Professionalism and Education*:

- Make sure the staff has the appropriate certifications and education and post that information for members to view.
- Always have the staff share information of value with members when the opportunity arises.
- Always have a solution or know how to find the solution.

❑ *Social Engagement and Member Interaction*:

- Never have staff walk by a member without saying hello and introducing themselves.
- Make it a practice to introduce members to other members.
- Ask members in a genuine fashion if they need assistance.
- Foster a relationship with the members and learn something unique about them.
- Focus on listening and empathizing with the members before responding.

Creating and sustaining a service culture is not an easy process

❑ *Programming of the Club*:

- Offer a variety of programs for a variety of needs.
- Be flexible in the club's program offerings.
- Find ways to determine the program interests of the members.

❑ *Justice and Safety for Members and Employees*:

- Don't play favorites; treat every member and employee as an equal.
- Become aware of the personal interests of both the members and employees and have the staff act appropriately.
- Talk about "we" and avoid using "me."
- Create an environment that is not intimidating for the members or employees.

Creating and sustaining a service culture is an absolutely essential aspect of a successful health/fitness club.

❑ *Self Esteem of Members and Employees*:

- Focus on knowing everyone's goals and make an effort to provide what it takes for them to be achieved.
- Never let a member or employee feel like their needs are a burden; instead let them know they are important.
- Provide an environment that speaks to greater perception of body and mind awareness and comfort.

❑ *The Facility*:

- Keep it clean and make it everyone's job to keep it clean.
- Keep all equipment in working order unless an alternative is provided.
- Make the facility convenient to use.
- Make the facility seem like a second home or office.

Creating and sustaining a service culture is an absolutely essential aspect of a successful health/fitness club. As such, this factor should be the first and foremost issue that club operators address if they want to create memorable member experiences and enhance their club's level of membership retention.

10

Programming for Health/Fitness Clubs

Chapter Objectives

According to consumer research on why people either join or leave a health/fitness club, programming plays an important role in both decisions. Since prospective members, current members, and former members all tend to view programming as a critical part of the health/fitness club membership equation, it is essential that club operators understand the dynamics involved in programming the activities that their club offers. Initially, this chapter explores the role that programming plays in membership. It then provides an overview of the variety of program opportunities that exist for clubs. Finally, the chapter concludes by presenting the key steps involved in successful programming.

A club that is interested in driving its level of membership sales and membership retention needs to become adept at programming.

Programming: Understanding the Basics

Programming involves engaging members in the club experience and creating opportunities for members to become actively involved in the club. Research indicates that individuals join clubs for a variety of reasons, including social engagement (women), group activities (women), challenge and competition (men), and achieving fitness goals (both genders). By the same token, research has also been able to identify some of the primary reasons members give up their club membership, including not being able to make social connections with other members, not feeling engaged by the club, losing the motivation, not having a training partner, and not using the club frequently enough. When those factors that affect the decisions concerning both joining and leaving are examined more closely, it becomes evident that programming lies at the heart of many of them. As a result, a club that is interested in driving its level of membership sales and membership retention needs to become adept at programming.

All factors considered, clubs should look at programming as the "play" or "theatre" that they put on to create the memorable experiences that members want to have. Hypothetically, creating such experiences is like putting on a play, with the facility being the stage for the play, the equipment serving as the play's props, and the staff as the actors in the play. In this scenario, programming becomes a series of one-act plays that the club's staff puts on to entertain and engage the members. Programming has the ability to create connections between members, help motivate individuals to achieve their personal goals, help members establish training partnerships, offer competitive challenges for members, and entertain the members. Programming is the club's most viable option for meeting and exceeding the expectations that most members have about being a club member. Furthermore, effective programming is also one of the best strategies a club has for differentiating itself from its competitors.

Program Offerings of the Health/Fitness Club Industry

Research shows that the health/fitness club industry makes a wide variety of program options available to its members. According to the IHRSA *2004 Profiles of Success*, for example, clubs offer over 60 different types of major programs to their members. A sampling of the top programs offered by clubs is included in Figure 10.1.

One interesting observation that can be made from the data presented in Figure 10.1 is that clubs tend to offer programs that are more individual- than group-oriented in their focus (e.g., personal training, counseling, and massage). An additional observation would be that, as a rule, clubs have still not picked

> All factors considered, clubs should look at programming as the "play" or "theatre" that they put on to create the memorable experiences that members want to have.

Program activity		Percentage of clubs that offer it	
Tennis leagues	5%	Basketball leagues	6%
Spa services	12%	Wellness classes	13%
Lower back classes	15%	Pilates	16%
Boot camps	19%	Tai Chi	21%
Volleyball	22%	Wallyball	26%
Physical therapy	28%	Children's programming	30%
Juniors programming	34%	Competitive sports	35%
Summer camps	36%	Martial arts	36%
Aquatic exercise	41%	Senior programming	42%
Kickboxing	42%	Group cycling	43%
Massage	59%	Weight management	63%
Nutrition counseling	66%	Yoga	67%
Step aerobics	87%	Fitness evaluations	89%
Personal training	91%		

Figure 10.1. Sampling of health/fitness club programming *(IHRSA's 2004 Profiles of Success)*

up on the importance of offering programs that are targeted at special-interest populations. Instead, most clubs tend to focus on programs that are geared to the general population. However, as the demographics of the country continue to change, especially as the role of baby boomers, echo boomers, and cultural fusion becomes even more prominent, a need will exist for clubs to intensify their efforts to develop and market programming that is targeted at specific groups of individuals.

Programming Options in the Health/Fitness Club Industry

A review of the various program categories and the types of programs that are currently offered by clubs indicates that clubs have an extensive array of programming opportunities. Among the various options that clubs have with regard to programming are the following:

❑ Aquatic Area. A number of club operators see the pool as a loss leader that can help sell the club. Beyond that limited perception, however, they tend to view pools as an operational challenge. Fortunately, many operators have chosen to make their pool(s) an asset, instead of a liability. In the process, they have developed dynamic programs around their aquatic facilities. In that regard, some of the most successful clubs at aquatic programming include the Baylor Tom Laundry Center in Dallas, the Michigan Athletic Club in East Lansing, Michigan, the Maryland Athletic Club in Timonium, Maryland, and Franco's in Louisiana. Among the more successful and interesting programs that are offered in aquatics are the following:

- *Masters swimming*. Masters swimming involves competitive swimming and training for older adults. Masters swimming is usually restricted to those individuals who are over the age of 25. A strong masters swimming program not only provides adults with a competitive outlet for their interest in swimming, but also a chance to meet others of a similar age. One of the best masters programs in the country is offered at the Baylor Tom Laundry Center in Dallas, Texas. One of the masters programs offered at this center, the Lone Star Masters, which was developed by Jim Montgomery, has over 200 participants.

- *Swim lessons*. Swim lessons are extremely popular, especially in a family-oriented market. The YMCA is probably the most successful in the industry in this programming area. The YMCA's program features multiple levels of skill acquisition, which enables children to acquire the necessary skills and then be recognized when they move up to the next higher level of skill. The American Red Cross also offers a structured format that clubs can utilize in a fashion similar to the YMCA's approach.

- *Aqua-exercise*. Providing opportunities to engage in physical activities that place a minimum of load force on the body's musculoskeletal system, aqua-exercise classes have grown in popularity over the years.

As the demographics of the country continue to change, especially as the role of baby boomers, echo boomers, and cultural fusion becomes even more prominent, a need will exist for clubs to intensify their efforts to develop and market programming that is targeted at specific groups of individuals.

In fact, multiple types of aquatic exercise options are currently being offered at clubs throughout the country, including water-step classes, water-based stretch classes, water-based Tai Chi classes, water-based yoga classes, water-based kickbox fitness classes, and even water-based Pilates classes. Lending credence to the value of aqua-exercise, the National Arthritis Foundation offers a certification for one type of water-based exercise class.

- *Flick-n-float parties.* "Flick-n-float" is a common term used by many clubs for a party-themed, aquatic event. Flick-n-float refers to the practice of offering film viewing at poolside, while also including such activities as swimming, floating on the pool, and having food delivered poolside. Arguably, this particular program offering can be thought of as a "party at the pool." These events are particularly popular with families that have young children.

- *Scuba and snorkeling classes.* Numerous clubs exist in the marketplace that have leveraged the public's interest in adventure-oriented programming and use their pool to deliver classes in snorkeling and scuba diving. The more creative clubs often tie in an adventure outing at the end of the scheduled classes so that their members can utilize their newfound skills to experience an out-of-the-club event.

- *Swim team.* Many clubs with pools leverage their efforts to target the family market by offering competitive junior swimming. Some clubs, for example, have as many as 200 to 400 kids who are actively involved in the club's swim teams. One of the keys to success with conducting a swim-team program is to be able to offer competition against other clubs. It is interesting to note that many health/fitness club teams will often find themselves in competitive leagues with teams sponsored by country clubs.

> Group-exercise programming represents the most significant opportunity for achieving programming excellence in the health/fitness club industry.

❏ *Group-Exercise Programs.* Group-exercise programming represents the most significant opportunity for achieving programming excellence in the health/fitness club industry. At one time, group exercise was somewhat limited in the opportunities it provided as a programming option when it was simply referred to as "aerobics." Since moving toward a group-exercise and group-fitness orientation, however, this area of programming has assumed a significant role for many clubs. For example, some clubs report that nearly 50% of their daily visits are driven by participation in their group-exercise programs. Clubs that have established a reputation as offering great group-exercise programming include Crunch, Equinox, Sports Club/LA, Bodies in Motion, and Healthworks. Among the most successful program offerings in group exercise are the following:

- *Group cycling.* Originally known as Spinning, group-cycling programming has evolved to include other licensed programs, such as

Precision Cycling and RPM, along with a host of other club-oriented names. While the group-cycling juggernaut has slowed down somewhat in recent years, it is still one of the most popular program options in the industry.

- *Yoga.* Since the 1990s, yoga has been one of the two fastest-growing forms of group exercise. In fact, in some clubs, yoga constitutes nearly 50% of their group-exercise programs. Yoga's popularity grew as a by-product of the focus that baby boomers had on mind-body exercise. Initially, yoga just involved Hatha yoga. Currently, however, there are over 20 varieties of yoga offered in clubs, including Hatha, Astranga, Ishevanya, Bikram, and Power Yoga. The yoga of today and the future will continue to evolve as an integrated form of the original Eastern art and the desires of western culture.

- *Pilates.* Pilates has been the fastest growing group-exercise program in the industry since the early part of the 21st century. Pilates, first developed in the 1920s by Joseph Pilates, has undergone several western modifications in the last few years. In the process, it has been integrated into the group-exercise arena. Formerly offered only on special equipment, Pilates is now offered in multiple formats for group exercise, including mat Pilates, prop Pilates, tower classes, and allegro Pilates.

- *Resistance-driven classes.* Over the last 10 years, the concept of resistance training in a group format has exhibited significant growth. Initially, resistance-training programming involved classes such as body sculpting, using resistance tubes and free-hand exercises, and then progressed into classes that utilized hand weights and weighted bars. One of the most popular classes of the latter type is taught with the body bar. In recent years, the industry has started to offer more structured or choreographed resistance-training classes, such as Body Pump, which is marketed by Les Mills, International.

- *Core and functional-fitness classes.* Programming involving core stability and functional-fitness conditioning is another highly popular form of group exercise. The introduction of the exercise ball created an entire series of exercise-ball classes that focused on developing the individual's core. In addition to exercise-ball classes, another highly popular and effective format for conditioning the core and enhancing an individual's level of functional fitness were classes that were created using foam rollers, an approach based on practices in the physical therapy arena. Other examples of core and functional-type classes include medicine-ball classes, bousa-ball classes, and core-board (Reebok program) classes.

- *Theme classes.* A recent trend in programming, which has been popularized by club groups such as Crunch and Sports Club/LA and modified by other club operators, are classes that are designed around

Pilates has been the fastest growing group-exercise program in the industry since the early part of the 21st century.

a specific theme. The basic underlying concept of a theme class is to remove members from the ordinary and take them on escapist adventures. Theme classes often make use of props and costumes to create a greater sense of theme-related reality. Examples of commonly conducted theme classes include:

✓ *Fireman's class*. This class offers exercise movements based on the activities that a fireman typically carries out. Some clubs even use props, such as hoses, stairs, etc. The first club group to popularize this type of class was Crunch.

✓ *S.W.A.T. class*. This class offers exercise movements that are based on the activities and physical requirements of police SWAT units.

✓ *Boot camp class*. This class is structured around the activities that the military uses to train its recruits in basic training. At Red's in Lafayette, Louisiana, for example, the boot camp classes are held in an outdoor training area that includes obstacles employed in many basic training programs.

✓ *Cardio striptease class*. This class, which is offered by Crunch in New York, is an extreme example of a theme class that appeals to a targeted audience that is looking for a real escape. The class would feature movements that might typically occur in a striptease establishment, for example, minor disrobing.

✓ *New York ballet workout*. This type of class was popularized at several New York clubs by a former ballet dancer. These classes incorporate the movements and conditioning exercises used by ballet dancers.

✓ *LA cheerleaders class*. This class was popularized by the Sports Club/LA based on the dance movements and routines of the Los Angeles Lakers cheerleaders.

Over the past several years, fusion classes have moved to the forefront of the industry's interest in group exercise.

• *Fusion classes*. Over the past several years, fusion classes have moved to the forefront of the industry's interest in group exercise. Fusion refers to the blending of dissimilar cultures and dissimilar class structures. This movement toward offering fusion classes is, in part, driven by the changing demographics in America and the desire to offer classes that provide a blend of styles and themes. Examples of fusion classes that are currently popular in the health/fitness industry include:

✓ *Yoga/spin classes*. These are classes that offer a blend of group cycling with yoga movements. Participants are given a chance to mix mind/body with intense cardiovascular movement.

✓ *Pilates/spin classes*. These are classes that offer the mix of high-intensity cardiovascular conditioning with the stretching and strengthening of Pilates.

✓ *Bousa/step classes*. A new twist on the step class is offered by incorporating the core conditioning benefits of a Bousa ball with the cardiovascular benefits of a step class.

✓ *Aqua tai chi*. This class, first offered in the New York market, blends the mind/body benefits of the ancient Chinese martial art with the enhanced resistance provided by exercising in the water.

✓ *Kickbox yoga*. This class, offered in some of the more progressive club markets, blends two martial arts, resulting in an activity that combines soft movement with more intense cardiovascular movement.

✓ *Cardio funk classes*. First offered at Crunch and presently an offering at many clubs, this class blends the movements of basic "aerobics" with the music and movements of funk.

✓ *Salsa step*. This class offers a blend of the Latin American dance steps of salsa with the more basic movements of "aerobics." These classes often include the use of band music (either live or recorded) to extenuate the theme of the class.

• *Equipment classes*. Equipment classes, which have been popular since the mid 1990s, are based on offering classes that are structured around the use of standard fitness equipment in a group setting. Among the equipment classes that clubs offer to its members are:

✓ *Trekking*. A registered program of Star Trac, trekking involves walking/running on a treadmill in a group format, choreographed to music.

✓ *Rowing*. These classes, featuring a group-exercise class format, involve the use of rowing ergometers.

✓ *Stairclimbing*. The company that manufactures StairMasters developed a registered program called, "stomp," which involves having individuals exercise on a stairclimbing machine in a group format.

✓ *Gravity*. Gravity classes involve the use of custom equipment resembling Pilates equipment.

❑ *Fitness Programs*. Fitness programming refers to a generic blend of program activities that target members who tend to only use the club for cardiovascular or resistance training. As a rule, these members use the club

Fitness programming refers to a generic blend of program activities that target members who tend to only use the club for cardiovascular or resistance training

on a more personal basis while pursuing their fitness goals. By offering fitness programming, clubs can provide avenues that allow those members to make connections with other club members who have similar interests and be better positioned to achieve their personal fitness goals. The primary goals of fitness programming are to create personal connections, stimulate competition, enhance motivation, and support the pursuit of each member's fitness goals. Among the examples of fitness programs that are currently offered in the health/fitness club industry are the following:

- *Personal training.* Personal training has become the most popular fitness program in the industry, as well as the leading source of incremental revenue for clubs. Personal training can be offered either on an individual basis or in a group format, an option that has increased in popularity over the past few years. Personal training allows a member to work individually or in a small group with a fitness professional who provides instruction and motivation. In some instances, personal training programs are developed around a particular theme, such as "women on weights."

> Personal training has become the most popular fitness program in the industry, as well as the leading source of incremental revenue for clubs.

- *Sports-performance training.* One popular fitness offering is to offer sports-specific conditioning programs in either a group or individual format. This type of programming targets members who have an interest in enhancing their level of performance in a specific sport. The most popular of these sports-performance programs include golf fitness, football conditioning, speed and quickness training, jump training, tennis fitness, and ski conditioning.

- *Special population fitness.* Over the past few years, with the aging of the baby boomers, clubs have begun to be aware of the value of offering fitness programs that target the needs of individuals who have certain health conditions. Examples of such programs include cardiac rehabilitation, arthritis exercise, physical therapy, senior exercise, and exercise for the obese.

- *Fitness games.* One of the most effective methods that clubs can use to increase member participation in their fitness programs is to provide games and challenges that allow the members to exercise independently, yet be part of a social and competitive event. Fitness games are often based on board games or more large-scale sports events. Examples of some of the more popular fitness games include:

  ✓ *Race across America.* This type of fitness event allows members to earn miles for the time they exercise. These miles then go towards their efforts to cover a certain distance, such as crossing America. Some clubs pair members up in teams in an effort to introduce members to other members.

  ✓ *Clue.* This particular fitness game involves having members move across a Clue board, based on the time they accumulate exercising.

This game is the same as the board game, except that it requires that a participant perform a predetermined amount of exercise to move, rather than based on numbers derived from the roll of a dice.

✓ *Monopoly.* This fitness game is based on the board game of Monopoly, with members getting the opportunity to move and buy and sell properties, based on their fitness activities.

✓ *Football challenges.* A popular theme for fitness games is to recreate a specific football classic, such as Texas vs. Texas A&M or Michigan vs. Ohio State. The game involves having members choose a particular team, and then having each team earn yards for the activities of the members on their teams. The game is held over a specific time period, and the team that crosses the goal line most often wins.

❑ *Health Promotion Programs.* Health promotion programs, often called "wellness" programs, are specialty programs that focus on activities and interventions intended to benefit the health and well-being of the individuals who participate in a given program. Health promotion programs can range from personal programs, such as nutritional counseling, to group programs such as stress management. The following examples illustrate several of the most common health-promotion programs that are offered by health/fitness clubs:

• *Health screenings.* Health screening programs can range from blood-pressure screening to mammograms. Most clubs coordinate with other healthcare institutions to offer these programs for their members and the community. The most popular health screenings include cholesterol screenings, blood-pressure screenings, cancer screenings, coronary risk-factor screenings, bone-health screenings, and diabetes screenings.

• *Health fairs.* Health fairs feature a more comprehensive form of health screening that is extremely popular among corporations and local communities. There are endless programs that clubs can include in their health fairs, including multiple offerings such as blood-pressure screenings, postural screenings, cholesterol screenings, massage, nutrition education, cooking demonstrations, body-fat appraisals, and exercise demonstrations. As a rule, health fairs are best offered once or twice a year.

• *Health education seminars and classes.* Members are often attracted to seminars and classes that focus on specific health-related themes. Such seminars usually involve a one-hour offering, in comparison to classes that might constitute a series of several sessions. The most popular health-education seminars and classes include:

Health promotion programs, often called "wellness" programs, are specialty programs that focus on activities and interventions intended to benefit the health and well-being of the individuals who participate in a given program.

As a rule, seminars and classes that focus on smoking cessation are very attractive to a club's corporate members, because most corporations are aware of the fact that smoking is one of the most costly health behaviors in which employees can engage.

✓ *Back care classes.* Back care classes, such as the YMCA's Healthy Back Program, are extremely popular with members and offer an opportunity for members to get professional instruction in dealing with their back problems.

✓ *Weight-loss classes.* Weight-loss classes and seminars are among the most popular programs offered by health/fitness clubs. Some clubs offer franchised programs, such as "Healthy Inspirations" or "Weight Watchers," while others design their own weight-loss programs that mix exercise, nutrition education, and monitoring.

✓ *Women's and men's health seminars.* Another popular health-education program offering involves seminars and classes that are targeted at gender-specific health concerns, such as prostate cancer, breast cancer, osteoporosis, heart disease, and diabetes.

✓ *Smoking cessation classes.* As a rule, seminars and classes that focus on smoking cessation are very attractive to a club's corporate members, because most corporations are aware of the fact that smoking is one of the most costly health behaviors in which employees can engage.

✓ *Alternative medical practices seminars.* Clubs have found that seminars in such medically-related endeavors as chiropractic care, acupuncture, herbal medicine, and physical therapy can be appealing to many members.

❑ *Recreational Programs.* Recreational programs refer to program activities that are structured around the various recreational facilities of a club. Recreational programs can be offered in a variety of competitive arenas, such as basketball, volleyball, racquetball, squash, handball, softball, soccer, badminton, tennis, and (for those clubs fortunate enough to have a course) golf. Most recreational programs are offered in one or more of the following formats:

• *Intra-club leagues.* An intra-club league is based on organizing teams from among the club's members and then having the teams compete among each other over a specified period of time. In sports such as racquetball and tennis, the competition can be held between individuals or teams.

• *Inter-club leagues.* An inter-club league is based on establishing teams from the club's members and then organizing competition against teams from other clubs. Such competition can be held between individuals or teams.

• *Tournaments.* Tournaments are normally one-day events that are conducted at the club level, but can also be conducted for a larger audience. Most tournaments are offered in a single-elimination, double-elimination, or round-robin format. A tournament can involve competition between individuals or teams.

- *Mixers*. Mixers are popular in tennis, but offer a great program structure for other recreational activities as well. In a mixer, members or teams of members are scheduled to play other members/teams in a less-competitive format. One of the keys to a successful mixer is to include a social component in the event, such as providing a meal, serving drinks, or including a dance.

- *Ladders*. Ladder competition is a popular format in both tennis and racquetball. In a ladder, the members' names are placed on a ladder, and the members schedule games with those above them on the ladder. The primary goal of this type of recreational programming is for a member to move up the ladder by defeating the members who are above them on the ladder.

❏ *Adventure Programs*. Many clubs have found that programming can move outside the four walls of their club's facilities and, in the process, address the outdoor interests of their members. With the emerging growth in the number of echo boomers and the increased focus of many Americans to connect with the outdoors, the value of adventure programming has increased in recent years. In England, Cannons—a large club operator—offers an incredible array of adventure-driven programs for which members can register. While individual adventure programs may not attract comparatively large audiences, when taken as a whole, adventure programs represent an exceptional opportunity to provide members with greater membership value. The most common types of adventure programs offered by health/fitness clubs include:

- *Bike tours*. Some clubs offer these events as one-day adventures, while others might schedule bike tours with a theme. For example, clubs in California, such as the Western Athletic clubs, offer wine-tasting bike tours.

- *Ski outings*. Ski outings are extremely popular among members. Clubs can schedule these events for small-member groups and offer them multiple times during the year.

- *Scuba outings*. Many clubs, particularly clubs in the South, have found that scuba and snorkeling outings are extremely popular with members.

- *Whitewater rafting*. Whitewater rafting is one of the more popular adventure programs offered by clubs. In most parts of the country, there are outside groups that will work with clubs in scheduling whitewater outings.

- *Rock climbing*. The popularity of rock climbing has driven many clubs to schedule special one-day or weekend rock-climbing outings.

- *Golf tournaments*. While golf might not be considered an adventure outing, many clubs have found that offering an annual club golf outing brings high member and guest participation.

While individual adventure programs may not attract comparatively large audiences, when taken as a whole, adventure programs represent an exceptional opportunity to provide members with greater membership value.

One of the best ways a club can support the interests and needs of members to create connections with other members is to develop social programs that place an emphasis on getting individuals together, rather than focusing almost entirely on exercise and health programming.

❑ *Social Programs*. Some club operators feel that because they are in the health/fitness club business, that their programming efforts should be focused entirely on fitness. What these operators don't seem to understand is that many members of a club are interested in making connections with other members. One of the best ways a club can support the interests and needs of members to create connections with other members is to develop social programs that place an emphasis on getting individuals together, rather than focusing almost entirely on exercise and health programming. Among the most successful social programs that clubs can offer include events that feature the hobbies, cultural interests, and sports interests of their members. In this regard, some of the most popular social programs include:

• *Beer, wine, and food tasting events*. Beer, food, and wine tastings are among the most popular social events that clubs can schedule for its members. Clubs can offer these evening beer, wine, or food tasting events as a means of bringing members and their guests into the club. In fact, a number of clubs combine these tasting experiences with other club activities as a means of prospecting for new members.

• *Theatre nights*. Many clubs have found value in coordinating special social events that involve taking a group of members to a particular cultural activity, such as a theatre event, symphony, play, or opera.

• *Sporting-event outings*. One of the most popular social events that a club can schedule is taking group outings to local sporting events. Furthermore, clubs can coordinate organized activities where members meet at the club, travel to a sporting event, and then return to the club afterwards for dinner or a reception. These outings involve attending a variety of sports-related activities, such as professional sports, college sports, or special sporting events.

• *Charity events*. Clubs can organize special events at their clubs to support a local charity. These events can be receptions, auctions, or dinners, using the club's facility areas, such as group exercise rooms or sport courts. For example, the Met in Houston, Texas takes a tennis court and converts it to a large ballroom for its annual charity event. Clubs can also consider hosting special runs for charity that begin and end at the club.

• *Clubs within a club*. "Clubs within a club" refers to the creation of special interest groups within the club. The basic concept underlying "clubs within a club" is to create small-niche interest groups that appeal to the interests of the club's members. In most cases, clubs within a club are built by identifying members with a passion for a particular hobby or activity and then working with those individuals to establish a club based on that activity. The best clubs within a club are those in which the members lead the clubs, but for which the club provides a degree of administrative and financial support. Among the types of "clubs within a club" that might be organized are the following: dancing club, photography club, gardening club, mountaineering club, running club, biking club, yoga club, card club, skiing club, swimming club, wine club, theatre club, bowling club, tennis club, golf club, etc.

The Keys to Great Club Programming

A number of critical steps are involved in the efforts by health/fitness clubs to develop and execute an effective program strategy that enhances membership retention and sales. Among the essential steps that can help provide club operators with a simple process for achieving successful programming are the following:

❏ *Have a Purpose and Vision.* The club's first step in developing its programming approach should be to establish a purpose and vision for its programming. This purpose and vision need to align with the club's overall mission. The purpose and vision should be based on its answers to the following questions:

- Is the club's programming designed to drive member involvement and participation?

- Is the club's programming designed to enhance the sale of memberships?

- Is the club's programming an integral part of the club's brand differentiation process?

- Is the primary purpose of the club's programming seen more as providing incremental revenue?

- Is the club's programming part of its experience theme?

At best, every club needs to establish a purpose and vision for its programming that can be stated in one paragraph and serve as the framework for its programming efforts. At ClubCorp clubs, for example, the purpose of programming is to drive member involvement in the club and create memorable experiences that can help enrich the lives of the members and build relationships.

❏ *Understand the Market Served.* Once the club has established the purpose and vision for its programming efforts, its next step should be to make sure that it understands enough about its members to provide the programming strategies that will allow it to successfully address the club's purpose and vision. The discovery process for a club to understand its members should begin with the club opening the lines of communication with its members and finding out their interests, needs, and wants. Conducting focus groups and surveys on a regular basis can help provide clubs with the basic information it will need in this regard. At a minimum, every club should ask

> The club's first step in developing its programming approach should be to establish a purpose and vision for its programming.

a series of questions of all new members that enables it to determine what their program and activity interests are. Another excellent step in this regard is to keep track of what activities members participate in when they are in the club. As this information is collected, the club should create a file on the interests and participation level of each member, as well as files on the programs. This information can facilitate efforts by clubs to provide member-centered programming.

❑ *Get the Members Involved.* One of the best-kept secrets about programming is that the more a club's members take ownership in the programming, the better it will be for the club. When its members take a sense of ownership in the club's programming, those individuals will be more likely to help the club design its programming efforts to meet their needs and assist the club in getting other members to participate in the club's activities. Among the steps that clubs that are relatively successful in getting their members involved in their programming are the following:

- Establish member committees that act as liaisons with the membership and serve as ideation centers for programming.

- Identify member loyalists and get them involved in the programming at a volunteer level.

- Provide recognition and rewards for the members who become involved.

One of the best-kept secrets about programming is that the more a club's members take ownership in the programming, the better it will be for the club.

❑ *Get the Employees Involved.* The club's ability to get its employees involved in its programming efforts is an essential factor in whether it will be able to deliver great programs. Employees who participate in the planning and execution of the club's programming are more likely to assume an enhanced sense of ownership and responsibility for the success of the club's programming. The club should initiate programming efforts by having the staff assigned to the task brainstorm about program ideas. Subsequently, the club should appoint employee teams to flush out the various programs in more detail. Finally, the club should assign particular programs or program initiatives to specific employees and hold them accountable for their efforts. Most importantly, clubs should never make programming a one-person show.

❑ *Create an Annual Program Business Plan for the Club.* Once the club understands and executes the aforementioned steps, it then needs to develop an annual program plan for the club. An annual program plan allows the club to establish goals, timelines, schedules, and accountability for its program offerings. The annual program plan serves as the club's roadmap for programming success. The essential components of such an annual program plan include:

- *S.M.A.R.T. objectives.* The club should begin the process of developing an annual plan for its programming efforts by identifying specific objectives that should be achieved yearly that are simple, measurable, attainable, realistic, and trackable. These objectives should be consistent with the club's overall purpose and values. Examples of S.M.A.R.T. objectives include:

  ✓Achieve an average of 3,000 participants each week in group exercise

  ✓Increase member retention from 65% to 70% by the end of the year

  ✓Generate an additional $30,000 each month over the prior year in program revenue

- *Establish a blended mix of programs.* The club should make sure the success of its programming efforts is not dependent on just one type of programming, such as group exercise. Its programming efforts should incorporate a variety of program options, including fitness programs, group-exercise programs, health-promotion programs, social programming, etc. Furthermore, the club's annual program plan should feature a mix of ongoing programs (i.e., programs that are offered on a daily or weekly basis, such as personal training, group exercise classes, etc.) and special-event programs (i.e., programs that are held once a month or at certain designated times, such as fitness games, adventure outings, etc.).

- *Create a program booklet and calendar.* Most highly successful clubs develop both an annual program calendar and a quarterly program calendar. Program calendars serve to provide a club's members with a timetable of its programs so they can arrange their personal and business calendars to participate in the programs that are of interest to them. Producing a program booklet that can be given to its members is another beneficial step that clubs can take. These booklets provide a description of the programs on the program calendar, thereby making it easier for the members to select the programs in which they are interested. These program calendars and booklets should be made available to the members through the club's web site, its newsletters, and the various distribution channels that the club uses to interact with its membership.

- *Establish core marketing and promotional strategies for each program.* As part of its annual program plan, the club should identify how it plans to market its programs to its members. The top three-to-five strategies should be detailed in the plan and then implemented to the degree possible. For example, some clubs employ posters and flyers to promote their programs, while others utilize their club's

Most highly successful clubs develop both an annual program calendar and a quarterly program calendar.

newsletters and websites. A number of clubs use displays and interactive media to promote their programs. Because most clubs will not be able to use every available marketing tool, they should make a concerted effort to identify the strategies that it plans to use and then do the best it can to execute them.

- *Assign each program to an employee with a timeline.* As part of its annual program plan, the club should assign an employee accountability for the delivery of the program. Many larger clubs have program directors who have overall responsibility for the club's entire programming effort. Unfortunately, however, many smaller clubs cannot afford a program director. In these instances, the club should appoint someone who is held accountable for each program.

- *Build a basic financial plan for programs as part of the program plan.* The final aspect of a club's program plan should include itemized revenue and expense goals for the overall program and for each of the programs offered. While the financial portion of the program plan does not need to be detailed, it should provide a framework for which employees can be held accountable.

❏ *Market, Promote and Sell Constantly.* Some clubs develop a plan for programming, get their members and employees involved, and have all the materials that they need to offer the various programs, and yet their members still don't participate. The question arises concerning how such a scenario could occur. In this regard, one of the biggest pitfalls for club programming is the failure of many clubs to let their members know what their programs are and when they are offered. Too often, clubs feel that if they simply put a poster up, that their members will sign-up for the activity. In reality, nothing could be further from the truth. Because members are constantly exposed to a variety of marketing materials, clubs need to be creative and disciplined in their approach to marketing and selling their programs. Among the steps that clubs can take to successfully market and sell its programs are the following:

- *Touch all the senses with its marketing efforts.* Most members of a club will respond to the club's marketing efforts if it blends the media it uses to promote its programs and these efforts touch the various senses of the individual members. For example, the club can stir a person's visual senses by employing flyers and posters. It can affect an individual's sense of hearing by using audio marketing through the club's audiovisual mediums. It can also market a particular program by addressing a person's sense of smell, through the use of such contrivances as lighted incense or scented candles. Still other clubs might appeal to the member's sense of touch by using an interactive display to promote their programs.

Because members are constantly exposed to a variety of marketing materials, clubs need to be creative and disciplined in their approach to marketing and selling their programs.

- *Think about targeting marketing efforts toward specific member audiences.* Instead of using generic posters, videos, or displays, clubs should develop direct-mail pieces, invitations, or e-mail blasts to enhance member awareness. By using its records of member interests and activity patterns, the club can create special invitations and e-mail blasts that are targeted to provide information on specific programs to specific member groups.

- *Create sales goals for each program.* The club should ensure that each program has a measurable target and then should share that information with its employees. Creating measurable targets for each program will make it easier to hold employees accountable for each program's success.

- *Teach employees the importance of leveraging their relationships to sell the club's programs.* For whatever reason, most employees are uncomfortable with "selling" and shy away from it. As a result, many clubs find that even the best-planned sales goals and marketing efforts often fall short. In reality, clubs need to educate their employees to understand the fact that the relationships that they have with the club's members is the best avenue for program sales. Accordingly, clubs should establish incentive and reward programs that support the sales efforts of their employees. Such programs can have a meaningful impact on a club's efforts to market and sell its programs.

Clubs need to educate their employees to understand the fact that the relationships that they have with the club's members is the best avenue for program sales.

❑ *Feedback is the Breakfast of Champions.* Even after the club has undertaken each of the aforementioned programming steps and the club's members have responded by participating in numbers never anticipated, the club has one more critical step to complete—obtain feedback from its members about its programming efforts. The most effective programmers make a concerted effort to get feedback from the members and employees at the conclusion of every program. By soliciting feedback from all parties involved, the club will help lay a framework for continuous growth in its programming success. Feedback provides information concerning what everyone really thinks and offers an objective look at the successes, opportunities, and possible limiting factors that exist within a club's programs.

THE HEALTH/FITNESS CLUB BUSINESS

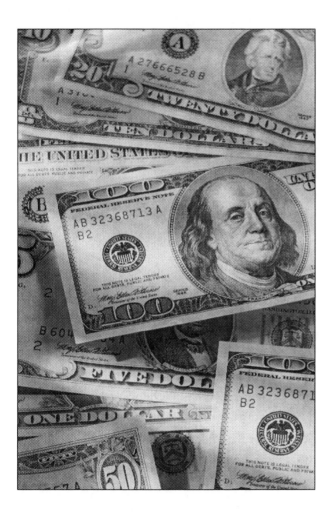

Part Four

11

Establishing a Health/Fitness Club Business

Chapter Objectives

The process of establishing a health/fitness club business can be relatively complicated. This chapter reviews the basic legal and business requirements for establishing a health/fitness club business entity and then examines how to develop the proper plans and systems that can help to insure that the business is successful. Initially, the chapter looks at the legal options for creating a health/fitness club. Next, the chapter discusses the types of club business models that are commonly employed. Finally, the chapter details the key steps that are necessary to help turn a business venture into a great business organization.

The Legal Business Structure: Understanding the Options

The first step in establishing any business is to determine which legal business structure makes the most sense for that particular business. The business structure selected will play a significant role in the degree of legal liability, taxability, distribution of profit, and ability to solicit investment capital that the new business will face. Not a decision to be taken lightly, it should always be pursued with the professional advice of both legal council and a certified public accountant. As a rule, individuals have five basic options concerning which legal business structure should be employed for a particular business: a sole proprietorship, partnership, corporation, cub-S corporation, and limited liability corporation.

> As a rule, individuals have five basic options concerning which legal business structure should be employed for a particular business: a sole proprietorship, partnership, corporation, sub-S corporation, and limited liability corporation.

❏ *Sole Proprietorship (SP)*. A sole proprietorship is the simplest form of business structure that can be established. A sole proprietorship has no formal legal requirements and involves a single owner, the individual who is forming the business. As a sole proprietorship, the individual can reference the business under their own name or indicate that they are doing business as (d.b.a.) under a specified name. If the decision is made to establish a sole proprietorship and operate under a d.b.a., then the owner will be required to file for a certificate "for doing business as" with the state government. The advantages and disadvantages of a sole proprietorship include the following:

- *Advantages*:

    ✓ The business is owned an operated by one person who has complete control of the business.

    ✓ The net profit of the business is taxed only once, and all expenses involved in operating the business can be deducted from the revenues by the owner.

    ✓ The owner can file to operate under another name other than that of the owner.

- *Disadvantages*:

    ✓ No insulation exists from liability, and all liability and debt are the responsibility of the owner.

    ✓ The assets of the owner are left vulnerable to the business, and therefore, the personal assets of the owner can have a lien placed on them.

    ✓ The business will terminate upon the death or incapacity of the owner.

The sole proprietorship structure might be an appropriate option if an individual was establishing a personal training business and chose not to have any employees beside themselves. For a business such as a health/fitness club, however, it is not the recommended option.

❑ *Partnerships.* Partnerships are another basic form of business structure. Partnerships can exist in several structural arrangements—general partnerships, limited partnerships, and limited liability partnerships:

- *General partnership (GP).* General partnerships can be written, oral, or implied and are intended to generate a profit. A general partnership can consist of two or more persons carrying on business as co-owners. In a general partnership, each partner is an agent of the partnership and can legally bind the other partner to any agreement entered into by the other partner on behalf of the business. In a general partnership, each partner has joint and severable liability, meaning that one individual or all of the individuals can be held accountable for the debt and legal liability of the business. In a general partnership, either partner has the ability to dissolve the partnership at any time. One common type of general partnership is a joint venture in which the partnership is intended to carry out a single business transaction.

> A general partnership can consist of two or more persons carrying on business as co-owners. In a general partnership, each partner is an agent of the partnership and can legally bind the other partner to any agreement entered into by the other partner on behalf of the business.

- *Limited partnership (LP).* Limited partnerships require a formal agreement between the involved parties and a certificate of limited partnership. A limited partnership has a general partner who usually manages the business and typically has the largest financial stake in the business. This type of business structure also has limited partners who have a financial stake in the business, but who are not involved in managing it. In a limited partnership, the partners can be individuals or corporations. Limited partnerships are similar to general partnerships in that the partners have joint and severable liability, meaning one or all partners can be held liable for the actions of the business. A limited partnership exists as long as the general partner is involved or until all partners agree to terminate the arrangement. Limited partnerships are commonly employed by such organizations as law firms, physician groups, and accounting firms. In the health/fitness club industry, limited partnerships can be created that can have ownership of the physical assets of club and then be operated as a management company under another type of business structure.

- *Limited liability partnership (LLP).* In a limited liability partnership, the general and limited partners are protected from liability beyond a collective limit of $100,000. To register as a limited liability partnership, the partners have to demonstrate that they have insurance to cover the $100,000 limit and must file a formal application with the state. In certain instances, the partners in a limited liability partnership are not always liable for the debts and obligations of the business. The registration for a limited liability partnership expires after one year.

When looking at each form of partnership, it should be understood that with the exception of the limited liability partnership, that each partner assumes liability for all obligations of themselves and the other partners. Furthermore, in this particular business structure, only the general partner has control of the business. The upside to such a partnership is the opportunity for a limited partner to participate in the success of a business without having to be involved in management. As was previously discussed, limited partnerships are an appropriate option for those individuals or businesses who are interested in owning a health/fitness club and do not want the responsibility of managing the business.

❏ *Corporations (C-Corp).* Corporations, also known as C-Corps, are legal entities created to conduct business and authorized to act with the rights and liabilities of a person. Such business entities can exist as general, professional, and non-profit corporations. Of the three options, general corporations are the most commonly found type in the health/fitness club industry. In a general corporation, the business is organized for profit and distribution of earnings to the officers and owners (stockholders). When a

> In a limited liability partnership, the general and limited partners are protected from liability beyond a collective limit of $100,000.

For many single-unit health/fitness clubs, the sub-S is an attractive legal alternative for structuring the business.

corporation is formed, it must file articles of incorporation, which include a listing of the owners, directors, and officers, with the state under which it is incorporated. A corporation is required to have both bylaws and annual meetings of its directors and officers, with the directors and officers representing the owners. A corporation may also issue stock, both common and preferred. Such an issuance enables numerous individuals and organizations to have an ownership stake in the business. A corporation may exist for perpetuity.

A corporation insulates its owners from personal liability and loss, which is much different than the situation that sole proprietors and partnerships encounter. In essence, a corporation allows the owners to walk away from the business with minimal liability for the company's liabilities and debt. The downside of the corporation is that earnings are taxed at both the corporate level and again at the individual level, based on the individual's stake in the business. In addition, a corporation requires a majority decision of its directors and officers for major business decisions, which is considerably different from other legal business structures. In the future, as registration and licensure of health/fitness professionals occurs, a time might come when personal trainers might incorporate as professional corporations, similar to physicians, lawyers, and architects.

❑ *Sub-S Corporations (Sub-S).* A sub-S corporation is a hybrid corporation that has certain features that do not exist with the typical corporation. For example, a sub-S corporation is restricted to a maximum of 35 stockholders and can only issue one kind of stock. Another unique aspect of a sub-S corporation is that it insulates the owners from personal liability associated with the business. At the same time, it avoids the double taxation of a typical corporation by allowing all earnings of the business to be distributed to the owners without any corporate taxation. As a result, all earnings are passed on to the owners, who are then taxed on their vested earnings. For many single-unit health/fitness clubs, the sub-S is an attractive legal alternative for structuring the business.

❑ *Limited Liability Corporation (LLC).* The limited liability corporation is a relatively new corporate structure that is seen as providing its investors and owners with a combination of benefits from the other legal entities previously described. For example, an LLC provides comparable, if not better, insulation from liability than a corporation, while at the same time offering the favorable tax advantages of a partnership. An LLC must create articles of organization with the state in which it forms and assign managers. Instead of stockholders, an LLC has members. An LLC can consist of a single member or multiple members. LLCs can have individuals, partnerships, or even corporations as members. Furthermore, one caveat of the LLC is that it can last no longer than 30 years and in

Category	Sole Proprietor	Partnership	Corporation	Sub-S Corporation	LLC
Personal risk	Unlimited	Share of total investment	Amount of personal investment	Amount of investmen & loans	Amount of investment up to a cap
Taxation	One time on business earnings	One time on share of earnings	Company earnings and then again on personal earnings	One time on all personal share of business earnings	One time on personal share of business earnings
Control of business	Very high	Moderate to limited	Depends on stock position	Moderate to limited	Moderate
Capital for growth	Owner's money	Loans from partners	Stock sale, bonds	Sell stock or loans	Sell stock or loans
Staffing	Poor	Poor to fair	Good	Fair	Fair to good

Figure 11.1. A comparison of the advantages and disadvantages of selected types of business structures

states such as Texas, it must provide the appropriate funding to cover a specified dollar level of liability coverage.

As is evident, health/fitness club owners have numerous options concerning their choice of which business structure to employ—each of which has its benefits and risks. As such, potential business owners need to weigh the council of lawyers, accountants, and other professionals to determine what structure will work best for their business. Figure 11.1 presents a comparison of some of the primary advantages and disadvantages attendant to each of the various types of business structures.

Business Operating Models

Once a decision has been made from a legal and tax perspective on the type of business structure under which the club will function, the next step is to identify which operating model the club prefers. In the health/fitness club industry, there are three basic models from which to choose: an independent club operator, a part of a multiple-club operation (regional or national), or a franchise (single or regional). A review of each of the three types of models can help reveal the benefits and risks associated with each option:

❑ *Independent Club.* An independent club model involves a business that operates independently of any other club or business association. As such, the development and operation of the club is solely dependent upon the club's ability to build the systems needed to operate itself. Over 50% of the health/fitness clubs operating in the U.S. are independently owned and operated, including industry leaders such as Red's in Lafayette, Louisiana, Franco's in Louisiana, the Maryland Athletic Club in Timonium, Maryland,

Potential business owners need to weigh the council of lawyers, accountants, and other professionals to determine what structure will work best for their business.

the Gainesville Health and Fitness Center in Gainesville, Florida, the Rochester Athletic Club in Rochester, Minnesota, and the East Bank Club in Chicago, Illinois.

Among the benefits of establishing the business as an independent club are the following:

- The club can be designed and operated as part of the local community, thereby creating a product unique to the demographics of the market in which it is located.

- The ownership group of the business has control of the club's destiny as a business and can create the systems and structures it deems necessary.

- The club can establish a brand for itself in the local community that is built on the values and goals of the ownership group.

- The club will not be burdened with some of the overhead costs normally associated with being part of a franchise or multiple-club operation.

Concurrent with the aforementioned benefits, the owner and operator of an independent club also faces several challenges that the other operating models do not have, including:

- Independent operators will not have access to the capital, operating, and marketing resources that the other operating club models can offer.

- Independent operators may find themselves at a disadvantage with the other club models when it comes to purchasing power, marketing clout, and talent recruitment.

While the health/fitness club industry was founded by independent operators whose talent and passion helped forge the $14 billion industry that presently exists, the current landscape portrays an environment that is less friendly to those individuals who operate independently.

> **While the health/fitness club industry was founded by independent operators whose talent and passion helped forge the $14 billion industry that presently exists, the current landscape portrays an environment that is less friendly to those individuals who operate independently.**

❑ *Multiple-Club Operation.* The multiple club business model exists today because it affords owners and operators several distinct advantages when it comes to accessing capital, recruiting talent, and controlling a particular market. Multiple clubs currently occupy about one-third of the entire club market. A multiple-club operation can be national, such as 24 Hour Fitness, Lifetime Fitness, or Wellbridge; regional, such as Town Sports International (Northeast corridor), Western Athletic Clubs (California), or Sport and Health (Washington, Maryland, and Virginia); or local, such as Wisconsin Athletic Clubs (Milwaukee), Fitness Formula (Chicago), Healthworks (Boston), or DMB Sports (Phoenix).

Being part of a multiple-club operation offers several business advantages when compared to being an independent club operator, including:

- Access to capital for growth

- Business systems and programs that can assist in operating a club more profitably

- Talent sources and intellectual capital that can enhance the opportunities in a given market and help grow local talent

- Cost efficiencies driven by volume purchases

- Branding and marketing as provided by the parent company

Concurrent with the aforementioned advantages, being part of a multiple-club operation also has several potential downsides about which a business operator should be aware, including:

- The business operator will normally have less control of their destiny and less freedom to operate their business as they desire, because they will need to fit their efforts into the systems, policies, and procedures of the parent company.

- The business operator may find that the club is less unique to its market than it would prefer or expect since it must function according to the branding and operational model established by the parent company.

- The business will most likely have to assume the name of the parent company and thereby forfeit any direct identity with its local market (e.g., 24 Hour Fitness, LA Fitness, Bally's, etc.). There are multiple-club operations, however, such as Wellbridge and Tennis Corporation of America, that allow their clubs to have individual identities.

❑ *Franchised Club Operation.* Owning and operating a franchised club provides some of the advantages of both an independent operation and a multiple-club operation. The franchising model is based on the principle that local business owners will have greater success connecting their club to the local community and making it successful if they have an ownership stake in the business. At the same time, these individuals will benefit from being associated with a recognized brand that provides operational and marketing assistance. The most established and possibly most recognized health/fitness club franchises are Gold's Gym, World Gym, and Powerhouse Gyms. Since 2000, specialty franchises, such as Curves, have established themselves as leading franchise operations and have helped to reshape the industry by establishing greater value to the franchise model. Multiple-club operations, such as Bally's, also provide franchise opportunities, especially on an international basis, for individuals and companies wanting to get involved in the health/fitness club industry.

Owning and operating a franchised club provides some of the advantages of both an independent operation and a multiple-club operation.

Most franchisers charge the franchisee an up-front franchise fee that can range from as low as $5,000 to as high as $25,000 and an annual fee that can run between $3,000 and $6,000 annually.

A franchise can be purchased for one club or an entire region. Most franchisers, such as Gold's, require potential investors to meet certain financial expectations before they can assume a franchise. These expectations include the requirement that the franchisee must demonstrate the level of financial backing that would be needed to build and operate the franchise. Most franchisers charge the franchisee an up-front franchise fee that can range from as low as $5,000 to as high as $25,000 and an annual fee that can run between $3,000 and $6,000 annually. In addition, there are other costs associated with having a franchise, including the cost of purchasing the operational and retail products needed for the club through the franchiser's business system.

The advantages to a health/fitness club operator who chooses to become a franchised operation include:

- Obtaining the rights to a nationally recognized brand that will immediately position the new business in the marketplace

- Access to the business systems created by the franchiser, such as design plans, equipment discounts, operations manuals, marketing templates, etc.

- Access to national marketing programs and the ability to share costs on marketing and advertising programs

- Access to educational programs and conventions operated by the franchiser

- Ability, as a local owner, to control the destiny of their business as long as they meet the criteria established by the franchiser

	Independent Club	Multiple Club	Franchisee
Branding	Local brand that has to be built by owner.	Aligned with a national brand, but still some branding required.	Instant brand recognition and marketing support of the brand
Operating Support	Entrepreneur. Owner has to develop all the systems.	Based less on entrepreneur and more on systems administration	Entrepreneur focus, but systems provided
Marketing support	None, except what is developed locally	Varies according to the parent company. Can range from high to very low.	Excellent support with templates and tie-in to national campaigns
Sense of Community	Very High	Low to moderate	Moderate to high
Cost Advantages	Few to none	Moderate to high	Moderate
Educational Support	None	Moderate to high	Low to moderate

Figure 11.2. A comparison of selected club operating models

Concurrent with the aforementioned advantages are some disadvantages, including:

- Upfront capital for the franchise fee, something the club would not have if it operated independently or was part of a multiple-club operation

- The annual cost of maintaining the franchise

- An association with a specific brand, especially if that brand proves to be the wrong one for the club's particular community. A club should be aware of the fact that the consumer will associate it with a specific brand, even if it operates differently than most of the others who use that franchise brand.

- Limitations in the club's flexibility to operate the business as it desires, because of the requirements of the franchise agreement

As the aforementioned discussions point out, the options for a club business model are as varied as are the legal options for setting up the business. Figure 11.2 provides a simple comparison of the three basic models for opening a club.

Deciding Whether to Buy or Build a Club

Once individuals have successfully navigated the decision-making path of what legal structure to assume and what type of club model under which they want to operate, the next major business hurdle they face is to decide whether they want to build a club or purchase an existing club. All factors considered, this decision is as important as any they will make and more than any other will impact their initial capital requirements and their ability to achieve profitability. It is essential that the individuals who are making these critical decisions (whether to build or buy) fully understand the various factors that affect each choice. Such an understanding can help them decide which option is the best course of action for them.

❑ *Building a Club.* If the decision is made to build a club, two standard courses of action can be taken. One is to purchase land, and then proceed to build a free-standing club structure. This approach to building requires not only that the land be purchased, but also that the club operators have the capital to build a free-standing building. This course of action is normally the most capital intensive, because it requires the funds both to purchase the property (ranging from $2 to $10 a square foot), and also to build a free-standing structure (ranging from $75 to $300 a square foot). By the time the process is completed, anywhere from $2 million to $20 million could be spent on the club. (It should be noted that some operators have spent over $30 million for clubs that exceed 100,000 square feet in size.) Besides the large outlay of cash, when a club is built

Once individuals have successfully navigated the decision-making path of what legal structure to assume and what type of club model under which they want to operate, the next major business hurdle they face is to decide whether they want to build a club or purchase an existing club.

	Free-standing building	Building in leased space	Purchase free-standing club	Purchase club in leased space
Upfront capital required	Very high—land costs and structure costs	Moderate to high, depending on landlord allowance	Moderate; depends on club's earnings performance	Low to moderate
Range of cost all in	$100 to $300 s.f.	$40 to $200 s.f.	4x to 8x EBITDA	1x to 5x EBITDA
Time to profitability	1-to-3 years, with average closer to three years	1-to-3 years, with average closer to two years	Immediately to one year	Immediately to one year
Risks	High capital costs; time to profitability; cost of taxes	Capital costs; limitations set by landlord; time to profitability	Capital costs moderately high; unknown liabilities not uncovered during due diligence	Condition of the space; unexpected liabilities or costs; restrictions set by landlord

Figure 11.3. Comparison of buying vs. building a club

from scratch, the membership also has to be built from scratch. As a result, the cash flow from the club's operations at its opening will normally not support the facility's operating expenses. It is common in the industry for free-standing clubs to not reach profitability until the end of their second or third year of operation and not begin to provide any return on their assets until at least their third year. Of course, exceptions to this rule exist.

Another option concerning building a club that operators have is to lease space in a strip mall, office park, or office building. In this instance, the club will still have to build out the facility, but the costs will be less. In this scenario, the landlord usually provides the shell structure, along with an allowance for tenant build out (usually ranging from $15 to $50 a square foot). This contribution by the landlord reduces the amount of upfront capital that is needed by the club's owner. Similar to a free-standing club, the time needed to generate enough membership to reach profitability will often take approximately two to three years. In this scenario, the owner's initial level of debt will not be as great. However, some additional built-in overhead—e.g., rent—will exist if this option is chosen.

❑ *Buying a Club.* An attractive alternative to building a club is to purchase an existing club. When individuals purchase a club, they have two options—one is to purchase the entire business and the other is to purchase only the assets of an existing club's business. Most attorneys will advise individuals to purchase only the business assets, an option that will allow them to avoid assuming the liabilities of the existing business. The primary advantage of purchasing an existing club begins with the cost of purchase. As a general rule of thumb, most clubs will sell for four times to six times their EBITDA (earnings before interest, taxes, depreciation, and

> It is common in the industry for free-standing clubs to not reach profitability until the end of their second or third year of operation and not begin to provide any return on their assets until at least their third year.

amortization). As a result, the majority of clubs normally sell for far less than they would cost to build. Another benefit of purchasing an existing club involves the fact that purchasers are also getting an existing membership and an existing cash flow. In other words, the time it will take a club to reach profitability and gain a return on assets or equity will typically be far shorter. On occasion, an existing club can reach profitability immediately and provide returns on the purchased assets as early as the first year. (It should be noted that the process of purchasing is far more complicated than the aforementioned discussion indicated and will be covered more thoroughly in chapter 14). Figure 11.3 provides an overview comparison of buying an existing club versus building a club.

The vision of any business revolves around three distinct narratives—the mission statement, the promise, and the theme.

Getting the Business Started

To this point, the chapter has addressed the primary challenges facing a prospective club owner, which revolve around the legal structural framework for the club, the type of club model employed, and whether to buy or build the club. The final critical step in starting a health/fitness club involves establishing the business framework that will enable the club to be successful. In that regard, several key steps can be undertaken by club owners that can help them establish an appropriate framework for their business, including:

❑ *Establish a Clear Vision of the Business.* The vision of any business revolves around three distinct narratives—the mission statement, the promise, and the theme. The mission statement is a succinct statement that clearly communicates to both a club's customer and its employees who and what the business is. At ClubCorp, their mission statement articulated the fact they would be the "world class leader in delivering the private club experience." This simple statement makes it clear what the intentions of the business are and whom they intend to serve. For any business, it is imperative that they provide a mission statement that allows their team and customers to understand the overall focus of the business.

The second essential narrative is the club's customer promise. The promise is the commitment that the club makes to each and every customer of its business. At ClubCorp, that promise was to "build relationships and enrich lives." The promise not only lets a club's customers know what to expect, more importantly, it enables the club's staff to be aware of what experience they are expected to deliver to the club's members.

The final piece of the vision puzzle is the theme. The theme is the driving force behind the experience the club intends to provide its members. Many businesses forget to establish a theme. As a result, their business tends to lose focus on the experience it is trying to create. An example of where a club is using a predetermined theme in an appropriate manner is at Crunch. Their theme speaks to "making no judgments." When individuals visit one of their clubs, they definitely can pick up on the fact that the Crunch employees are making an effort, with the help of their facilities and programs, to act out that theme.

❑ *Create a Culture and Strive to Maintain It.* Culture is often defined as the traditions and practices that make a country, business, or people unique. With regard to a business setting, its culture is what makes a business unique from any other. Culture for a business is like culture for a country; it speaks to what is unique and special about the business and in what each and every employee can take pride. Culture begins with the establishment of core values and traditions, which are then sustained through stories told by the "leaders and heroes" of the business. Over time, these stories become the myths of the business, and the heroes become the legends.

> Culture for a business is like culture for a country; it speaks to what is unique and special about the business and in what each and every employee can take pride.

The first step that a business must take in order to create a culture is to identify its core values. The core values serve as the foundation behind every decision a business makes. They are the roots of the business that nourish it and sustain it. At ClubCorp, their core values included a philosophy where the member/guest is king, a mandate for every employee to plan their work and work their plan, an unwavering commitment to integrity, and a firm belief in the necessity to exhibit character at all times. At Red's in Lafayette, Louisiana, their core values reflected such precepts as "greeting each member with a smile," "saying hello and goodbye," and "if you have time to lean, you have time to clean." Although simple, the aforementioned values are powerful influencers of positive business behavior.

The second step in creating a business culture is to establish specific philosophies and practices that, when replicated over time, will become traditions. At the Ritz Carlton, for example, they speak of "ladies and gentlemen serving ladies and gentlemen." Similarly, at ClubCorp, the discourse of "creating a refuge for the member, a home away from home" is commonly expressed. The philosophies of both companies serve as a framework for the actual practices in which their employees engage. Over time, as employees repeat these mantras and engage in these practices, they become traditions. Even more importantly, over time, employees will tell stories about how certain employees carried out these practices in a special way. When this occurs, myths and storytellers have been created, which are critical to sustaining the culture the business has developed.

❑ *Establish Long-Term and Short-Term Business Objectives.* Before the club ever opens its club doors to serve its future members, it needs to establish both long-term objectives (e.g., 10-to-20 years out) and short-term objectives (e.g., one-year, three-year, and five-year). Together, these objectives can help establish a road map for the club's business journey and help inform the club's investors and employees where it is planning to go and how it plans to get there.

The long-term business goals are often referred to as BHAG's (big hairy audacious goals). These goals represent what the club ultimately wants to achieve. While these goals should be clear and succinct, at the same time, they should not be as specific as those the club establishes for the short-term. An example of a BHAG for a health/fitness club might be "to be recognized as the premier health/fitness club in the market, as reflected by capturing 15% of the market." If this goal were part of a club's plan, then it should be relatively clear to everyone what the club planned to accomplish in the future. Just as importantly, it could also serve as a marker for the club's progress over the years.

The club's short-term business goals need to be S.M.A.R.T. (simple, measurable, attainable, realistic, and trackable). All factors considered, short-term goals serve as the benchmarks for the beginning of a club's business journey. Examples of short-term business goals might include:

- Achieve 2,000 members at the end of year one
- Achieve revenues of three million dollars at the end of the first year and seven million dollars by the end of the fifth year
- Achieve an annualized return on assets of 12% for each of the first five years
- Open up a second club by the end of the third year of business

By establishing its goals, the club is attempting to provide a meaningful framework for its success.

❑ *Establish Replicable Operating Standards and Systems.* When a business is young, the club owner can often oversee every step that is taken. As time passes, however, the business' success will not depend on the ability of a single person. Rather the club's staff must be able to replicate the practices that drive the club's success. In that regard, the club must have clearly defined standards and systems.

Standards set the expectations for how a specific practice should be carried out. Standards need to be simple and clear. In essence, standards convey a description of the outcome that the club expects from an operational practice. Standards do not tell employees the "how," but rather the "what" and "when" a particular practice/action needs to be achieved. An example of a standard might be, "Every member will receive an orientation to the fitness floor that includes an exercise prescription." As such, this standard communicates the expectation, but not the path to be taken.

Systems are the processes and resources that the club provides to its employees that enable them to achieve the standards. More importantly, systems create consistency in the club's service delivery across space and time. Systems can include such factors as employee education programs,

By establishing its goals, the club is attempting to provide a meaningful framework for its success.

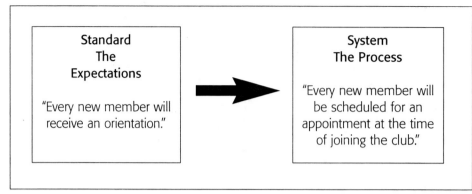

Figure 11.4. The relationship between a standard and a system

procedural documents for the handling of membership sales, procedural documents for accounting practices, etc. If the club does not establish business systems, even simple ones, it may find that its employees will tend to take the steps that are best for them and not necessarily the best for the business. Figure 11.4 helps illustrate the connection between standards and systems.

❏ *Establish an Accountable Organizational Model.* Every business, especially a health/fitness club business, needs to have an organizational structure that brings decision-making relatively close to the member or customer. This scenario involves creating a flat organization where as few layers as possible exist between the customer or member and the employee who is making the decision concerning what should be done. This process of creating an accountable organizational structure requires the following key steps:

- Create a clear structure showing the relationships of each position to the members and to the other employees. Make sure to have as few layers between the customer and the owner as possible.

- Create a job description for each position that is based on accountability and not on tasks.

- Establish a model for open communication up and down the organizational structure. Eliminate communication holes and traps by doing away with positions of power.

By addressing these issues up front, the club can create an organizational structure where every employee takes a sense of ownership in the success of the business. Samples of organizational charts and job models are included in the appendices.

❏ *Hire the Best and Then Provide a Continuous Learning Environment.* The truest indicator of how successful a particular club business will become lies in the talent of the people it employs. As a consequence, club owners and

> Every business, especially a health/fitness club business, needs to have an organizational structure that brings decision-making relatively close to the member or customer.

operators need to hire the best people. According to Jim Collins, author of *Good to Great*, the best employees are those individuals who embrace the company's values and culture and have disciplined focus, disciplined thought, and disciplined action. As such, it is imperative that business leaders take the time to select and hire the best individuals. Furthermore, to keep the best, the club needs to provide an environment that promotes continuous learning and growth. In addition, the club needs to establish a culture that encourages employees to learn new skills and provide the support, both financially and time-wise, for employees to take advantage of learning opportunities. In addition, clubs should budget for educational efforts and programs, bring in outside speakers, establish regular in-house education, expose employees to other job roles, and promote those individuals who demonstrate that they are leaders and achievers.

The best employees are those individuals who embrace the company's values and culture and have disciplined focus, disciplined thought, and disciplined action.

❏ *Remember That Service Delivery Stays Close to the Member.* Many businesses create hurdles and barriers that force their customers to sacrifice something as part of their experience. When individuals create a business, they should establish a framework that eliminates member sacrifice. More importantly, the framework should enable its frontline employees (i.e., those employees who directly interact on a daily basis with the members) to do the delivery and, if necessary, the recovery of the services. For example, if a member comes to a fitness instructor and has a concern about an issue, the member should not be made to wait while the instructor chases down a supervisor. Instead, the club should have a policy of empowering instructors to act on their own.

❏ *Create a Standard Financial Model and Budgets.* A final key to achieving success in a business is to create a financial model that everyone can understand and work with. The financial model should be based on establishing budgets that the respective club staff can work from and by which they can monitor the club's financial performance. As a matter of practice, club owners/operators should make the budget available to the appropriate staff members so that they know what has to be achieved and how they have performed over the course of the budgetary period, financial-wise. The club's financial model should also include simple reporting tools that enable the club to monitor the key financial indicators on a daily, weekly, monthly, quarterly, and annual basis.

Qualities of Great Clubs

A great club is one that, year in and year out, generates success for everyone involved in the facility—members, financial stakeholders, employees, and the community. In this regard, some of the most significant indicators are:

- Continuous growth in membership each year

- Continuous growth in revenues and earnings each year

- High levels of membership retention (well above the industry average)

- High levels of employee satisfaction

- Low employee turnover (less than the industry average)

- Tenured senior staff

- High levels of member satisfaction and member loyalty

- High levels of respect in the community

- Have been in business for at least 10 years, exhibiting the ability to sustain itself for an extended period

- Documented return on investment for the equity holders of at least 10% annually

Without question, additional indicators of success can be identified. Regardless of the ultimate mix of factors that is ultimately associated with a particular facility prospering, one observation is clear: great clubs always seem to have a full compliment of members and employees with tenure. More importantly, great clubs seem to perform well, year after year, even during periods when other facilities are struggling. As such, great clubs in the health/fitness industry tend to exhibit certain characteristics, including:

❑ *Location, Location, and Location.* Similar to the real estate business, location is one of the best predictors of success in the health/fitness club business. More often than not, great clubs are located in areas that are close to the right demographics and convenient to access. It is also important to note that while some of the current great clubs did not always have a great location, they did know that in the future their location would be an outstanding one. In reality, location involves more than just having the right demographics or even just the right street address. Rather, location involves building the club in a place where its visibility to the public is enhanced. Without the proper location, the process of achieving greatness can take considerably longer.

❑ *The Owners Constantly Reinvest in the Facility.* Great clubs invest their earnings into their facilities. By engaging in such activities as purchasing new equipment, repairing worn areas, adding the newest services, and making sure that the facility is never outdated, great clubs show their members and their staff that they are committed to providing a positive experience for everyone involved. According to statistics reported by IHRSA, most clubs devote approximately three percent of their revenue in capital upgrades. Great operations spend nearly double that. As a result, these clubs continue to grow and prosper.

> Without question, additional indicators of success can be identified. Regardless of the ultimate mix of factors that is ultimately associated with a particular facility prospering, one observation is clear: great clubs always seem to have a full compliment of members and employees with tenure.

❏ *Clean Facilities*. Really great clubs are incredibly clean. Just as importantly, all of the employees, including the manager, feel a sense of personal accountability for keeping every aspect of the club clean. From the top on down, all levels of staff should focus on cleanliness.

❏ *Vision, Values, and Strong Culture*. Great clubs have a clearly defined vision that identifies and articulates the target toward which they are channeling their resources and energies. Vision is what defines the future of the organization. It is the standard of excellence by which the efforts of everyone within the organization can be judged. It is the benchmark that keeps every staff member on track. An appropriate vision meets several criteria, including being achievable, tangible, and meet the expectations of the club's staff and members.

Great clubs see their employees as their greatest asset. In that regard, great clubs view their staff as the heart of the organization.

Great clubs also have a values-orientation. They exhibit a moral core that is based on ethically grounded principles. Their values inspire confidence and help rally staff to achieve a common purpose. Great clubs know the difference between doing their best and doing what is right. From top to bottom, employees in great clubs exhibit high levels of integrity, honesty, trustworthiness, loyalty, and pride in their mission and their accomplishments.

In addition, great clubs have a unique culture that is often easily distinguished from the other clubs in the market. A club's culture is similar to the culture of a country. It involves an integrated pattern of beliefs, behavior, customs, knowledge, and traditions. When a facility's leadership makes an effort to maintain a strong culture, everyone associated with the club benefits.

❏ *Investment in People*. Great clubs see their employees as their greatest asset. In that regard, great clubs view their staff as the heart of the organization. As such, they make a concerted effort to provide a work environment that enables their employees to achieve at their maximum level of productivity and potential. One step that great clubs employ to help attain that objective is to develop and support a program of ongoing education for their employees. Such a program can include such activities as bringing in outside speakers to address the staff, encouraging employees to attend professional meetings, requiring staff to be certified by an accredited organization, recognizing and rewarding employees for their efforts at lifelong learning, providing financial support for learning-related endeavors, etc. The key point that should be noted is that great clubs are aware of the fact that an investment in their staff is an investment in the facility's future.

Great clubs are able to communicate effectively with both their members and their employees.

❏ *Teamwork.* Every great club is a unified team. A team is another name for a group of two or more individuals who are interacting in pursuit of a common goal. In that regard, great clubs have an enhanced level of esprit de corps. They feature a workplace environment that, all factors considered, is more "worker friendly." This atmosphere helps reinforce parochial attitudes in the staff. Employees are more willing to do whatever it takes to do the job that needs to be done. Furthermore, they are more likely to accept responsibility for their efforts (personal accountability) and take pride in the final outcome. In team-oriented situations, an aura of collected responsibility is ingrained. If the team succeeds, everyone succeeds. On the other hand, if the team fails, everyone fails.

❏ *Tenured Staff.* Great clubs typically have employees who have been with them for an extended period of time. Having a tenured staff can benefit a club in a number of ways. First and foremost, tenured staff tend to know the nuances of their jobs and fulfill their roles within the club very well. Retaining staff means time and resources don't need to be devoted to attracting and training new employees. Tenured staff are more likely to be team-oriented and less likely to act in a self-interested manner. Perhaps most importantly, tenured staff tend to inspire loyalty from the club's members. The members know them, like them, and trust them. Such loyalty enhances the experience a member achieves at the facility, as well as improves the club's membership retention levels.

❏ *Two-Way Flow of Communication.* Great clubs are able to communicate effectively with both their members and their employees. They appreciate and understand the need for a two-way flow of communication. In that regard, they develop systems that allow members to easily communicate with management about their experiences at the club, good or bad. They also make it a practice to always respond to member's feedback within at least a 48-hour time period, if not before. As such, these clubs are constantly seeking feedback from their members through the use of such tools as focus groups, surveys, and one-on-one discussions. Great clubs clearly communicate their policies, rules, and related practices to their members, as well as their employees. Furthermore, they understand that the ability to communicate effectively involves more than just verbal skills. They are able to utilize their entire array of communication skills (including listening, feedback, memory, and non-verbal), depending on the situation, to reinforce their message

❏ *Everyone Knows the Numbers.* Great clubs share their important "numbers" with their staff. They understand that a key factor in achieving the desired results is to have employees who take ownership of the numbers. Sharing this information sends a very positive message to staff members. It enhances their feelings of importance and self worth. It helps inspire loyalty and commitment to the club's mission/vision. In that regard, such proprietorship can serve as an exceptional catalyst for inspired performance. Great clubs ensure that the department heads and other employees know the key numbers. As a result, these department heads know what their performance targets are and how they have performed against them. Their employees are aware of how membership sales are going. One step that some clubs take to share their numbers with the staff is to have a scoreboard in the employee break room that reflects all of the club's key performance indicators.

❑ *Member Apostles.* Member apostles are individuals who are very loyal to the club and believe so strongly in the value of the club that they enjoy referring friends and associates for membership. Creating these member apostles is a by-product of a culture that focuses on treating each member the same by treating them differently. Great clubs embrace the belief that once a member joins a facility, it is the responsibility of every employee of the club to do everything in their power to create a positive experience for that person. When this attitude is put into practice, members are more likely to take a sense of ownership in the club and fervent advocates (i.e., become the sales people) for the club. Great clubs obtain many of their new members from member referrals.

Great clubs embrace the belief that once a member joins a facility, it is the responsibility of every employee of the club to do everything in their power to create a positive experience for that person.

12

The Health/Fitness Club Financial Model

Chapter Objectives

Initially, this chapter reviews the basic financial tools that are used to measure financial performance in the health/fitness club industry. It then presents an overview of benchmark financial data from the industry.

The Basic Financial Tools Used by the Health/Fitness Club Industry

As the health/fitness club industry has matured, the tools for measuring financial performance have also become more sophisticated. The three most important financial tools and the information each provides are as follows:

❑ *The Balance Sheet* (refer to Figure 12.1). The balance sheet provides a quick snapshot of the financial health of the club on a day-to-day, week-to-week, and period-to-period basis. The balance sheet tells the business exactly how healthy its finances are at any point in time. The balance sheet lets the club know what its assets are, what its liabilities are, and what its equity in the business is.

- *Assets*. The assets of a business are the cash value of its business holdings—property, equipment, land, etc. In turn, its holdings are defined as either short-term (current) assets or long-term (non-current) assets. The club's short-term assets are those assets or holdings of the business that can be turned into cash over the next 12-month period of time. Examples of short-term assets include:

    ✓ Cash in the bank and cash equivalents

    ✓ Short-term physical assets that could be sold over the next year, such as small equipment

As the health/fitness club industry has matured, the tools for measuring financial performance have also become more sophisticated.

160

Balance Sheet for Club XYZ

Category	Current Year	Category	Current Year
Current Assets		**Current Liabilities**	
Cash & Equivalents	$250,000	Accounts Payable	$100,000
Short Term Investments	$150,000	Notes Payable	$50,000
Accounts Receivables	$100,000	Current Portion Long Term Debt	$100,000
Current Imstallments of Contracts	$50,000	Accrued Expenses	$50,000
Notes Receivables	$0	Deferred Revenue	$50,000
Total Receivables	$150,000	Deferred Rent	$0
Inventories	$140,000	Deferred Taxes	$25,000
Prepaid Expenses	$20,000		
Deferred Income	$20,000		
Total Current Assets	**$730,000**	**Total Current Liabilities**	**$375,000**
Non- Current Assets		**Non-Current Liabilities**	
Land	$1,000,000	Notes and Similar Liabilities	$3,500,000
Building	$5,000,000	Obligations Under Capital Lease	$100,000
Leasehold Improvements	$0	Deferred Rent (long term)	$0
FF&E	$750,000	Other Long Term Liabilities	$200,000
Less Accumulated Depreciation	$250,000		
Security Deposits	$0	**Total Non-Current Liabilities**	**$3,800,000**
Intangibles	$100,000		
		Owner's Equity	**$3,155,000**
Total Non-Current Assets	**$6,600,000**		
Total Assets	**$7,330,000**	**Total Liabilities and Owners Equity**	**$7,330,000**

Figure 12.1. The balance sheet

✓ Accounts receivables that are due and not collected (i.e., the money members owe the club, but have not paid yet, such as dues and personal training fees)

✓ Prepaid expenses (i.e., expenses the club has paid ahead of time to save money, such as utilities or phone expenses)

✓ Inventory items (e.g., merchandise with a shelf life of less than one year)

✓ Deferred taxes

In most successful health/fitness club businesses, the club's current assets should represent between 15% and 30% of its total assets.

In most successful health/fitness club businesses, the club's current assets should represent between 15% and 30% of its total assets. Just as importantly, the majority of its current assets should be either cash or cash equivalents. If the club's current assets are more heavily weighted towards inventory, it may end up having to write that off the inventory as an expense and potentially have to pay taxes on that inventory. By the same token, if the club has a large accounts receivable, then it is in a position of losing a portion of that to bad-debt expense and having to write that portion off.

The club's long-term assets are those holdings and financial instruments of the business that are not expected to be collected over the next 12 months. Examples of long-term assets include:

✓ Property (land and buildings)

✓ Leasehold improvements (e.g., the capital the club has placed into a leased space to make it operational, such as new carpeting, new showers, etc.)

✓ Equipment (e.g., treadmills, resistance training equipment, etc.)

✓ Security deposits and lease deposits

✓ Loan fees

✓ Depreciation (deducted)

A rule of thumb with regard to current liabilities is that they should never exceed the value of the club's current assets (current ratio) and, ideally, should be equal to 50% of the value of the club's current assets.

The non-current assets of a financially healthy health/fitness club should range between 70% and 85% of its total asset value. Just as importantly, the club's long-term assets should lean toward property, equipment, and deposits because these are assets that are more easily sold. If the club has substantial dollars tied up in leasehold improvements, it is less likely to recoup them.

- *Liabilities.* The club's business liabilities are the financial obligations it has—in essence, the money it owes to others as part of operating its business. Liabilities are defined as either short-term (current) liabilities or long-term (non-current) liabilities. In the best of cases, the club would prefer that its total liabilities not exceed more than 75% of the value of its total assets, with less being better.

The current liabilities of the club are those obligations that will be due and payable within the next 12 months. Examples of current liabilities include:

✓ Accounts payable (these are invoices that the club has not paid for, but for which the club has already used the service)

✓ Notes payable (e.g., any loans that come due during the current year)

✓ Income taxes that are due

✓ Deferred revenue (this is revenue from contracts or agreements that have been collected, but not earned. For example, if the club sells three-year membership contracts, it must reflect two years of that revenue as a liability)

✓ Deferred rent (any rent the landlord agrees can be paid at a later date)

✓ Deferred taxes

A rule of thumb with regard to current liabilities is that they should never exceed the value of the club's current assets (current ratio) and, ideally, should be equal to 50% of the value of the club's current assets.

The long-term liabilities (debt) are those obligations and expenses, while not due during the next 12 months, are due some time thereafter. In the health/fitness club industry, it is recommended that the club's long-term debt not exceed a value of 40% to 50% of its total assets. On the other hand, there are some club companies that are underwritten by venture capital that look favorably on carrying a high debt load, since it is one way to generate business growth. The downside of this approach is the liability of such debt and the strain it can place on a club's operating cash flow. Examples of long-term debt include:

✓ Future interest and principal payments on loans from financial institutions

✓ Deferred revenue from long-term contracts (an example might be a five-year corporate membership contract)

✓ Deferred rent (oftentimes, a landlord will agree to provide a tenant with a window of no rent with the stipulation that the rent must be paid at a later date when the club is more profitable)

✓ Deferred taxes

- *Owner's equity.* Owner's equity represents the owner's actual investment in the club, which can include any initial dollars invested, as well as dollars earned over the life of the business. Owner's equity can vary, depending on whether the club was established as a corporation, a limited liability corporation, a partnership, or a sole proprietorship. Owner's equity is determined by subtracting the total liabilities of the business from the total assets of the business. In the case of a financially sound club, the owner's equity will usually be in the neighborhood of 20% to 30% of the total asset value. In the case of more mature clubs, however, it may be closer to 50% of the total assets. Situations also exist, especially in highly leveraged clubs (i.e., clubs carrying a high level of long-term debt), where the owner's equity might be as low as 10%. Examples of owner's equity are as follows:

  ✓ *Corporations.* In corporations, the owner's equity can exist in a number of forms, including capital stock (common or preferred), paid in capital (actual cash put into the business), and retained earnings not distributed to the stockholders (money the business makes and then puts back into the business).

  ✓ *Partnerships, limited liability corporations (LLC), and sole proprietorships.* In these business structures, the owner's equity can exist as contributions in cash or kind (sole proprietor or partnership) and cash generated by the withdrawal of assets (partnerships).

Investors and lending institutions will look at a club's balance sheet as one way of evaluating its current financial health and its ability to be profitable over

> There are some club companies that are underwritten by venture capital that look favorably on carrying a high debt load, since it is one way to generate business growth.

the long run. In doing so, there are a few critical financial ratios or key indicators, based on the information furnished on a club's balance sheet, that can be used to provide a quick glimpse of a club's overall financial health. The most frequently used balance sheet-based indicators are current ratio, acid-test ratio, debt-equity ratio, return on equity, and return on fixed assets.

✓ *Current ratio.* The current ratio is an indicator of a club's financial liquidity (cash in hand) within the next 12-month period. The current ratio is determined by dividing the value of the club's current assets by the value of its current liabilities. For example, if a club had a total of $1,000,000 in current assets and $500,000 in current liabilities, then its current ratio would be two. A current ratio above two is considered excellent; a ratio between one and two is considered good; a ratio between .6 and one is fair; and a ratio that is less than .6 is considered poor.

✓ *Acid-test ratio.* The acid-test ratio is a measure of a club's "quick" liquidity or its ability to generate cash immediately. The acid-test ratio is determined by taking the club's current assets and subtracting out that portion attributable to inventory and prepaid expenses, and then dividing by its current liabilities. A financially sound club operation should have an acid-test ratio of one or higher. For example, if the club has $1,000,000 in current assets, of which $300,000 is in inventory and $200,000 is in prepaid expenses, and has $500,000 in current liabilities, then its acid-test ratio would be one.

✓ *Debt-to-equity ratio.* The debt-to-equity ratio is a good measure of a club's leverage (in other words, the value of the owner's equity in comparison to the total liabilities that the club carries). The debt-to-equity ratio is measured by taking the total liabilities of the business and dividing them by the total owner's equity. For example, if a club has $4,000,000 in total liabilities and the owner's equity was $1,000,000, then the debt-to-equity ratio would be four. The average debt-to-equity ratio in the club industry is approximately 1.1, although it ranges from .1 to 3.3. The higher the ratio, the greater the debt is in comparison to the owner's equity, and the more likely the club is highly leveraged.

✓ *Return on equity.* Return on equity is a measure that is used by investors to assess the value of their investment. Return on equity is determined by taking the net income (earnings before taxes) and dividing it by the cash or equity invested. In an investor's mind, this ratio tells them how well their investment is working for them in generating cash flow. On average, most venture-capital groups look for returns in excess of 40%, while other investors are likely to be satisfied with returns of 20% to 30%. For owners who reinvest in their own club, such as when undertaking an expansion

The average debt-to-equity ratio in the club industry is approximately 1.1, although it ranges from .1 to 3.3.

of an existing facility, they may be satisfied with a return of 15% to 20%. For example, if a club owner were to invest $250,000 for a fitness-center expansion and, as a result, generated an additional $50,000 in cash flow as a by-product of having more members and spending more money, their return on equity would be $50,000/$250,000 or 20%.

✓ *Return on fixed assets.* Return on fixed assets is another a measure used to assess the value of an investment. Return on fixed assets represents the profitability of a business measured against the amount the business holds in its fixed (non-current) assets. To some investors, this measure is considered a more valuable indicator of how well their money is working for them than is the return-on-equity ratio. For example, if a club had $2,000,000 in fixed assets and, as a result, produced an additional $200,000 in cash flow for the club, then the return on fixed assets would be $200,000/$2,000,000 or 10%. While many club investors look for returns on fixed assets of 20% to 25%, ranges of 10% to 15% are considered acceptable. The basic reason investors and owners see this measure as a more realistic assessment of their return is because they have their money tied up in the assets of the business. In turn, the cash they generate is a result of how well that equity is doing for them.

As can be seen, understanding the nuances of a club's balance sheet is essential to understanding of the value and financial health of that business.

The standard practice in the health/fitness club industry is to produce both monthly and year-end profit-and-loss statements.

❑ *The Profit-and-Loss Statement or Statement of Income* (see Figure 12.2). The profit-and-loss statement is a financial tool that is used to reflect a club's operating performance over a given period of time. The standard practice in the health/fitness club industry is to produce both monthly and year-end profit-and-loss statements. There are several club chains that divide the year into 13 operating periods of four weeks each and compile a profit-and-loss statement for each of the four-week periods, as well as an annual statement. Finally, there are a few clubs that actually provide a weekly profit-and-loss statement that reflects their operating performance on a weekly basis. Some businesses refer to the profit-and-loss statement as a statement of income or a statement of operations.

The profit-and-loss statement is designed to show the club operator how well the club is performing financially over the designated time period by providing information on actual performance, planned performance, and the variance-to-plan performance. With each profit-and-loss statement, the club operator can get an accurate update on how the club is performing, both actually and against budget, for the given period, as well as year-to-date. This type of information allows the operator to make decisions regarding such factors as membership sales, revenue strategies,

Club XYZ Profit & Loss Statement
Version 1.0

Department/Category

Revenue & Expense Departments	Month			Year - to Date		
	Actual	Plan	Variance	Actual	Plan	Variance
Membership Revenue	$1,000,000	$990,000	$10,000	$2,000,000	$1,950,000	$50,000
Membership Expense	$100,000	$125,000	($25,000)	$250,000	$250,000	$0
Membership net	$900,000	$865,000	$35,000	$1,750,000	$1,700,000	$50,000
Fitness Revenues	$125,000	$130,000	($5,000)	$500,000	$489,000	$11,000
Fitness Expenses	$125,000	$100,000	$25,000	$450,000	$400,000	$50,000
Fitness Net	$0	$30,000	($30,000)	$50,000	$89,000	($39,000)
Spa Revenue	$21,000	$20,000	$1,000	$100,000	$110,000	($10,000)
Spa Expenses	$15,000	$16,000	($1,000)	$75,000	$80,000	($5,000)
Spa Net	$6,000	$4,000	$2,000	$25,000	$30,000	($5,000)
Tennis Revenue	$50,000	$40,000	$10,000	$400,000	$385,000	$15,000
Tennis Expenses	$45,000	$40,000	$5,000	$180,000	$178,000	$2,000
Tennis Net	$5,000	$0	$5,000	$220,000	$207,000	$13,000
Net Operating Profit	$911,000	$899,000	$12,000	$2,045,000	$2,026,000	$19,000
Undistributed Expenses						
G&A Expenses	$100,000	$95,000	$5,000	$400,000	$390,000	$10,000
Housekeeping Expenses	$100,000	$100,000	$0	$375,000	$382,000	($7,000)
Marketing Expenses	$125,000	$125,000	$0	$275,000	$250,000	$25,000
Capital Repair	$10,000	$5,000	$5,000	$75,000	$80,000	($5,000)
Utilities	$50,000	$60,000	($10,000)	$150,000	$160,000	($10,000)
Insurance	$5,000	$5,000	$0	$20,000	$20,000	$0
Property Taxes	$10,000	$10,000	$0	$50,000	$50,000	$0
EBITDAR	$511,000	$499,000	$12,000	$700,000	$694,000	$6,000
Rent	$75,000	$75,000	$0	$150,000	$150,000	$0
EBITDA	$436,000	$424,000	$12,000	$550,000	$544,000	$6,000
Principal & Interest	$30,000	$30,000	$0	$80,000	$80,000	$0
Depreciation	$25,000	$25,000	$0	$45,000	$50,000	($5,000)
Capital Addition	$0	$5,000	($5,000)	$15,000	$20,000	($5,000)
Net Income	$381,000	$374,000	$7,000	$440,000	$434,000	$6,000

Figure 12.2. The profit-and-loss statement or statement of income.

and expense control in a timely and effective manner. It is important to remember that the profit-and-loss statement is based on an accrual system. In other words, it measures financial performance based not only on both the cash generated and spent, but also on allocations for cash yet to be received or yet to be spent during a given period of time.

As such, the profit-and-loss statement provides a reflection of both planned performance and actual performance. One of the most useful tools in the health/fitness club industry, for understanding the profit-and-loss statement is the book—*Uniform System of Accounts for the Health,*

Racquet, and Sportsclub Industry—which was developed under the leadership of IHRSA. This document establishes specific categories within the profit-and-loss statement for budgeting and monitoring financial performance in the industry. The key profit-and-loss categories (revenues, department expenses, undistributed expenses, fixed expenses, EBITDA, and EBIT) that the industry employs to monitor and evaluate a club's financial performance include the following:

- *Revenue categories.* The revenue portion of the profit-and-loss statement is intended to provide the club operator with a means of budgeting and tracking the revenue-producing aspects of the business. The primary revenue areas or revenue departments on a profit-and-loss statement include:

    ✓*Membership.* The membership revenues are those revenues that are generated through the membership dues paid by members on a monthly basis and the initiation fees that members pay upon joining a club. A club must record all revenues from these two areas on the profit-and-loss statement under the category assisgned to the membership revenue department. In the instances where a club uses membership contracts, the club can only reflect on its profit-and-loss statement the amount of revenue from the contract that has been earned during the period of time reflected on the profit-and-loss statement. For instance, if a club receives $1,200 from a member upon joining for one-year's dues, then on the monthly profit-and-loss statement, only $100 of those dues can be reflected on the statement. In the health/fitness club industry, according to IHRSA's *2004 Profiles of Success*, approximately 66% to 84% of all club revenues come from the membership department. The industry is trying to reduce its dependence on membership revenue by promoting other revenue sources. In that regard, some clubs report that they generate closer to 50% of their overall revenue from their membership department.

    ✓*Fitness.* The fitness department generates the second largest amount of revenue in the club industry. Revenues earned from personal training, group-exercise classes, Pilates classes, and locker rental are examples of income that could all be attributed to this particular department. In many clubs, the fitness department generates upwards of 15% of the total revenues. In fact, some clubs claim to generate as much as four million dollars annually in personal-training revenue.

    ✓*Spa.* The spa department contributes revenues by providing such services as massages, facials, pedicures, manicures, and related activities that are delivered in a spa environment. In the last few years, the spa department has developed into a significant revenue source for many health/fitness clubs. In fact, spas can generate as much as $10,000 per treatment room per month.

According to IHRSA's *2004 Profiles of Success*, approximately 66% to 84% of all club revenues come from the membership department.

Most food-and-beverage departments are fortunate if they achieve a 10% to 20% margin.

✓ *Tennis*. The tennis department generates revenues through court fees, instructional lessons, and programming. In multipurpose clubs, tennis might be the second largest contributor of revenues. Industry data shows a tennis department can easily generate between $25,000 and $50,000 in revenue per outdoor court and $50,000 to $100,000 per indoor court on an annual basis.

✓ *Pro shop*. Financially, the pro shop is the source of the net revenues that are generated by merchandise sales. In most clubs, this contribution is relatively small when compared to total club revenues. In some clubs, the pro shop may generate as much as $500,000 to one million annually, though, on average, most generate less than $100,000 in annual revenues.

✓ *Food and beverage*. The food-and-beverage department generates revenues through the sale of food-and-beverages and by conducting special functions, such as parties. In most health/fitness clubs, the food-and-beverage operation is not a comparatively large contributor to the club's revenues, because their operations usually don't consist of much more than a snack bar or smoothie bar. There are clubs, such as the East Bank Club in Chicago, that generate millions of dollars in food-and-beverage revenue through multiple outlets, including private parties. That said, most food-and-beverage departments are fortunate if they achieve a 10% to 20% margin.

✓ *Youth services*. The youth department is a relatively recent undertaking for most of the clubs in the industry, but one that shows promise as a meaningful source of revenue. The youth department generates revenues by holding parties, providing youth programming, and offering childcare services.

✓ *Other revenue*. A number of clubs generate revenue from services that do not fall into the standard accounting categories on the profit-and-loss statement. In these instances, these revenues are often reflected under the category of "other revenues." The most significant sources of other revenue in the health/fitness club industry are revenues from space rental, physical therapy, and other medically related services. There are club chains such as Western Athletic Clubs that lease space to physical therapy businesses. The revenues from these leases are normally reflected as other revenue on the club's profit-and-loss statement.

• *Departmental Expenses*. Departmental expenses are that part of the profit-and-loss statement where the expenses incurred by each of the operating revenue departments in the delivery of their respective services and the generation of their respective revenues are listed. According to *IHRSA's 2004 Profiles of Success*, a club's departmental expenses typically run approximately 21% of revenues and may range from four percent to 30% of revenues. In other words, the departments of membership, fitness, spa, tennis, pro shop, food and beverage, and youth all have expenses that are directly associated with the services they provide and the revenues they generate. On the profit-and-loss statement, the expenses generated by each department are placed in an account that best reflects its activity or function. Examples of the accounts that are reflected in each department include:

✓ *Payroll.* The payroll expense represents the cost of employee wages and commissions. Payroll includes such items as salaries, hourly wages, commissions for employees, incentive pay for employees, etc. For example, the commission that the club pays a personal trainer would be considered wages, just as would the wages paid to a group-exercise instructor by the club, or the commission given to one of the club's sales representatives. Payroll (benefits and payroll taxes included) alone can represent approximately 40% of a club's total operating expenses and as much as 75% to 80% of any given department's operating expense.

✓ *Benefits.* This expense category represents the cost of providing basic benefits to the club's employees. These costs will vary, depending upon the benefits a club offers to its employees. The standard benefit package normally includes health benefits (hospitalization, dental, vision) and federally and state mandated payments, such as FICA, FUTA and SUTA (the payments made for social security, medicare, etc.). Additional employee benefits that many clubs offer include such items as club contributions to a company-sponsored savings plan (401 K), life insurance, long-term disability insurance, etc. Normally, the cost of employee benefits can range from as little as 15% of a club's total payroll expense to as high as 30% of its total payroll expense.

✓ *Education and training.* This expense category involves the expenses associated with the ongoing education of the club's employees. This category can include the cost of sending employees to conventions and conferences, funding continuing education credits, providing in-house training, and providing scholarships for pursuing coursework at local colleges. As a whole, the industry does not apply any standard allocation to this area. It would be in the club's best interest, however, for club operators to consider allocating funds equal to one-to-three percent of payroll for this expense category.

✓ *Supplies.* This category of expense varies from club to club. As a whole, this category includes expenses associated with cleaning supplies, general maintenance supplies, paper supplies, locker room

The cost of employee benefits can range from as little as 15% of a club's total payroll expense to as high as 30% of its total payroll expense.

amenities, etc. The industry average for this category is approximately two percent of the total revenues generated by a club.

✓ *Advertising/promotions/marketing.* This expense category represents the costs associated with marketing, promoting, and selling a department's products and services. For a particular department, such as fitness, this expense would include such items as the cost of flyers, posters, pamphlets, post cards, and other marketing pieces used to promote the department's services. Expenses emanating from efforts to promote activities in the membership department would involve internal departmental promotions, rather than external club promotions. Normally, the cost of external marketing is allocated to an undistributed expense category for marketing.

✓ *Printing.* This expense category is used to allocate expenses associated with printing efforts by the club, including club brochures, letterhead, envelopes, newsletters, and other hard-copy documents.

✓ *Dues and subscriptions.* This category is used by clubs to expense items such as club subscriptions for newspapers, magazine subscriptions for the club, subscriptions to special-interest publications, etc. The largest part of this expense category would arise from the costs involved with providing professional membership dues for employees (e.g., ACSM, NSCA, etc.), association dues for the club (e.g., IHRSA, ISPA, IDEA, etc.), and dues for local and community associations and groups (e.g., Chamber of Commerce, Rotary, etc.).

✓ *Contract labor.* This expense category is used to allocate the costs associated with retaining the services of outside professionals. For example, contract labor could include such items as attorney fees, accounting firm fees, outside speaker fees, special instructors, etc. In fact, many club operators pay their personal trainers and group-exercise instructors out of a contract-labor account, based on their mistaken belief that these providers are not employees, but rather independent contractors. As a result, they attempt to save on the cost of providing benefits to these individuals. Unfortunately, most club operators are misinformed about what constitutes an independent contractor. As such, they are running a risk in expensing these costs to this particular account. (Note: The issue of independent contractors is addressed in chapter 15 of this book).

✓ *Maintenance and repair.* This category of expense is associated with the general costs of maintaining the club's facilities and providing minor repairs to the facility. For example, if the club hires an exterminator to service the club, this expense would fall under

> Many club operators pay their personal trainers and group-exercise instructors out of a contract-labor account, based on their mistaken belief that these providers are not employees, but rather independent contractors.

this category. Another example of an expense assigned to this category would be if the club had to purchase some parts to repair a treadmill.

✓ *Cost of goods sold.* This category only applies to departments that sell retail items. The cost of goods sold represents the cost of an inventory item that is removed as it is sold from the inventory. For example, if the club purchases 500 shirts for $10 each, it would have a total of $5,000 in inventory. Later, if it sold all 500 shirts for $10,000, then its inventory cost for the shirts would be $5,000 (50% of the total revenue received from the sales). In most clubs, the cost of sales usually runs between 60% and 80% for their retail operations (e.g., the pro shop), though the inventory cost at many clubs runs much higher. As a rule, the cost of sales can be relatively high when a club holds too much inventory of an item and is later forced to write it off or it experiences shrinkage of inventory.

While the aforementioned expense categories are the primary departmental expense categories that exist on the profit-and-loss statement of most health/fitness clubs, they are not the only ones that occur. Clubs that want to monitor their costs in detail should create even more definitive expense categories. Establishing such categories can help them maintain an even firmer grasp on their expenses.

- *Undistributed expenses.* These are expenses that are associated with the overall operations of the club, rather than for running any specific department. In most club operations, these are expenses that emanate from the successful operation of the club that have no direct association with a specific department. In these situations, clubs allocate such expenses to the undistributed-expenses category. According to the most recent data published by IHRSA in its *2004 Profiles of Success*, the industry average for undistributed expenses is 46% of revenues, with a range of 30% to 60%. The most significant categories for undistributed expenses typically include the following:

  ✓ *Sales and marketing.* This expense is generated by efforts to market the club, such as advertisements in the media, websites, direct-mail pieces, and related sales materials. On average, most health/fitness clubs spend approximately four-to-five percent of their revenues on sales and marketing. In fact, major multiple-club operators, such as Bally's, 24 Hour Fitness, Sports Club/LA and Town Sports International, frequently devote considerably more of their resources to this undertaking, often reaching as high as 10% to 15% of their revenues.

  ✓ *Utilities.* Utility expenses include the costs of such items as electric, gas, water, and telephones. Most clubs lump these items as an

On average, most health/fitness clubs spend approximately four-to-five percent of their revenues on sales and marketing.

undistributed expense, while some club operators might distribute them as departmental expenses. The industry average for clubs is to spend between four and six percent of operating revenues on utilities. For clubs in the Northeast and West, especially California, utility expenses can often run as high as 10% of their revenues.

✓ *Member services.* This cost is an undistributed expense that is associated with the delivery of special member services and member relations. Expenses that fall into this category might include the cost involved in conducting focus groups, surveys, member-reward programs, and member-appreciation functions.

✓ *G and A (general administration and accounting).* This undistributed expense is generated by the costs involved in running the accounting department and in providing general management (e.g., manager, assistant manager, office assistant, etc.). It should be noted that in many clubs, the management and accounting areas are actually set up as departments, with their own expenses, and are treated as a separate department. Besides payroll, costs such as postage, credit-card charges, bad-debt expense, and EFT (electronic funds transfer) charges are normally debited to this accounting category.

> On average, in the club industry, a facility spends approximately five-to-eight percent of its total revenues on capital replacement and repair.

✓ *Capital replacement and repair.* This undistributed expense involves the costs associated with funding the ongoing upkeep and repair of the club's facilities. In most instances, capital costs involve items that either cost more than $500 or have a depreciation period of at least three years. Examples of capital replacement costs include such expenses as the funds allocated for buying new exercise equipment, buying computers for the staff, replacing carpet, expanding an area within the club, or replacing or repairing a piece of equipment (e.g., an air conditioner). On average, in the club industry, a facility spends approximately five-to-eight percent of its total revenues on capital replacement and repair. As a rule, some clubs may find that they need to allocate up to 15% of their revenues every five-to-seven years to handle their larger capital needs. In reality, many successful club operators handle this situation by accruing expenses over a few years to make sure that the funds are available for these larger capital requirements.

• *Fixed expenses.* Fixed expenses are considered those expenses that are not directly impacted by a club's operation, but rather the expenses that are recurring and relatively consistent year in and year out. According to IHRSA's *2004 Profiles of Success,* fixed expenses in the industry typically range from five percent to 20% of revenue. The standard fixed-expense categories for the profit-and-loss statement include:

✓*Insurance.* This particular category includes the costs associated with providing property, general liability, key-man, and professional liability insurance. In the club industry, these costs average between two percent and three percent of the club's total operating revenues. In fact, a few club operators feel insurance is not a fixed expense, but rather an expense that can be controlled through risk-management practices. Accordingly, they categorize insurance as an undistributed expense.

✓*Rent.* Rent is probably the largest single expense for most clubs, other than payroll. The industry average for rents is between 10% and 20% of the club's total operating revenues. In order for a club to be profitable, it should make every effort to keep its total rent payments below 15% of its total revenue. In most instances, rent is derived from the lease a club operator enters into, many of which run at least five years and more often for 10 years. A number of landlords also include what are called CAM costs into the rent. CAM costs are the landlord's costs for common area maintenance. In fact, class A office spaces (i.e., office space located in highly desirable locations and newer buildings) in many large, urban markets can have CAM costs that run as high as $10 to $15 a square foot. As such, it is essential that club operators get clarification of the CAM costs for a particular space and not make an operating or lease decision purely on the quoted rent cost.

> **The industry average for rents is between 10% and 20% of the club's total operating revenues.**

✓*Real estate/property taxes.* These are the expenses that the club pays local government for its property. If the club owns its land and building, then its property taxes are based on the assessed value of the property and building. On the other hand, if the club leases a space, its property tax will be based on an assessment of the leasehold improvements on the facility.

✓*Management fees.* Management fees are expenses that usually only occur in clubs that operate under a multiple-club operation. In a multiple-club operation, the ownership group or the management parent normally charges a management fee for the expertise, services, and guidance that it provides to each particular club. In addition, some independent clubs exist where ownership creates a separate management company for the business that then charges a fee to the club for the services of the owner. The majority of multiple-club operators charge a base management fee, which typically ranges from three-to-six percent of a club's total operating revenue.

✓*Depreciation.* Depreciation is the actual cost that a business incurs as a result of the loss in value of its fixed assets. Most clubs utilize a standard depreciation table to determine the depreciation schedule for its fixed assets, with property and buildings being depreciated over 20 years and equipment over five-to-10 years.

As a rule, the club industry utilizes broad EBITDA benchmarks to indicate the operating effectiveness of a club.

✓ *Principal and interest.* Principal and interest represent the cost associated with paying down debt and include both the interest on the loan balance, as well as the amortized amount of principal.

• *EBITDA (earnings before interest, taxes, depreciation, and amortization).* EBITDA is determined by taking the total revenues of the club and deducting the departmental expenses, undistributed expenses, and fixed expenses. The only expenses not counted in this regard are the costs of depreciation, capital replacement, and capital repair. Reflective of a club's profitability and earnings, this number is used by investors and owners as a benchmark for valuing a company and benchmarking its operating efficiency. For example, if a club that generates four million dollars in revenue has two million in department expenses, $500,000 in undistributed expenses, and $500,000 in fixed expenses, its EBITDA would be $1,000,000 or 25% of revenues. As a rule, the club industry utilizes broad EBITDA benchmarks to indicate the operating effectiveness of a club (refer to Figure 12.3).

Efficiency	EBITDA Range
Fair	15% to 20%
Good	20% to 25%
Excellent	25% to 30%
Extraordinary	30% or above

Figure 12.3. EBITDA benchmarks in the health/fitness industry

Under most circumstances, a club that is leasing space will find it a challenge to ever exceed and EBITDA of 25%, due to the impact that its rent has on its overhead.

• *EBIT.* EBIT stands for earnings before interest and taxes and represents the net cash flow before interest and taxes that the club owner is able to earn. EBIT is derived by taking the calculated EBITDA and then deducting the expenses associated with capital replacement, depreciation, interest on loans, and amortization of a loan (the principal that is paid). On average, a club operator can expect this factor to range between five percent and 10% of the total revenues, with a range of six-to-eight percent the most likely scenario.

❑ *The Departmental Income Statement*

The departmental income statement represents a detailed profit-and-loss document for a specific department. While the profit-and-loss statement provides a look at the financial performance of a club for a specified period of time, a departmental income statement provides each operating department

Departmental Income Statement
Fitness Department

Category	Actual - to - Date	Plan - to - Date	Variance
Revenues			
Personal Training	$750,000	$710,000	$40,000
Classes	$50,000	$20,000	$30,000
Activity Programs	$100,000	$75,000	$25,000
Locker Rental	$100,000	$100,000	$0
Other	$10,000	$12,000	($2,000)
Total Revenues	**$1,010,000**	**$917,000**	**$93,000**
Expenses			
Wages	$250,000	$248,000	$2,000
Commissions	$375,000	$360,000	$15,000
Bonuses	$60,000	$56,000	$4,000
Total Wages	**$685,000**	**$664,000**	**$21,000**
Payroll Costs	$76,000	$71,000	$5,000
Hospitalization	$20,000	$16,000	$4,000
Workers Compensation	$20,000	$17,000	$3,000
Related Benefits	$10,000	$10,000	$0
Total Payroll and Benefits	**$811,000**	**$778,000**	**$33,000**
Advertising and Promotions	$50,000	$58,000	($8,000)
Printing	$15,000	$17,000	($2,000)
Postage	$7,000	$6,000	$1,000
Dues & Subscriptions	$5,000	$5,100	($100)
Supplies	$76,000	$75,000	$1,000
Maintenance	$23,000	$20,000	$3,000
Education	$5,000	$4,000	$1,000
Total Other Expenses	**$181,000**	**$185,100**	**($4,100)**
Total Department Expenses	**$992,000**	**$963,100**	**$28,900**
Department Net Contribution	**$18,000**	**($46,100)**	**$64,100**

Figure 12.4. Sample departmental income statement for the fitness department

within a club a detailed summary of the revenues, expenses, and net cost of operating that particular department. For the club operator, the departmental income statement can be a useful tool for helping evaluate the performance of a specific department and holding the respective department head (supervisor) accountable for the financial performance of that department. Many of the top club operators in the industry expect their department heads and supervisors not only to develop a departmental income budget, but also to then use the departmental income statement as a tool for monitoring the success of their department.

IHRSA's book, *Uniform System of Accounts for the Health, Racquet and Sportsclub Industry*, provides a detailed description of the various departmental income statements that are employed in the industry.

IHRSA's book, *Uniform System of Accounts for the Health, Racquet and Sportsclub Industry*, provides a detailed description of the various departmental income statements that are employed in the industry. A list of the most common departments within the club industry includes membership, aquatics, fitness, spa, pro shop, racquet sports, food and beverage, and children's programs. For each of these departments, a complete accounting of the revenues, expenses, and net cost of the department can be determined and then compiled in a departmental income statement. Figures 12.4 and 12.5 provide a sample departmental income statement for the fitness and spa departments respectively. Having such detailed accounting for each department can help a club operator hold each department head accountable for the financial success of that individual's respective department.

Spa Departmental Income Statement			
	Actual YTD	**Budgret YTD**	**Variance**
Revenues			
Body Treatments	$23,000	$22,100	$900
Facials	$50,000	$45,000	$5,000
Manicures	$14,500	$14,000	$500
Massage	$100,000	$98,000	$2,000
Pedicures	$17,200	$20,000	($2,800)
Merchandise sales	$24,000	$22,100	$1,900
Total Revenue	**$228,700**	**$221,200**	**$7,500**
Cost of sales	$17,500	$16,000	$1,500
Gross Profit	**$211,200**	**$205,200**	**$6,000**
Expenses			
Salaries and wages	$30,000	$30,000	$0
Commissions	$81,000	$79,000	$2,000
Benefits	$6,400	$6,100	$300
Payroll costs (SUTA, FUTA, etc.)	$9,000	$8,600	$400
Total payroll and costs	$126,400	$123,700	$2,700
Dues and subscriptions	$2,375	$2,350	$25
Licenses	$1,400	$1,400	$0
Laundry	$7,350	$6,575	$775
Uniforms and towels	$8,150	$8,100	$50
Supplies	$12,345	$13,100	($755)
Other expenses	$2,100	$1,500	$600
Total other expenses	$33,720	$33,025	$695
Total Expenses	**$160,120**	**$156,725**	**$3,395**
Department Net	**$51,080**	**$48,475**	**$2,605**

Figure 12.5. Sample departmental income statement for the spa department

Benchmarks for Financial Performance in the Industry

A summary of the key industry benchmarks for financial performance is provided in Figure 12.6. The data reflected in Figure 12.6 is based on material from the IHRSA report, *2004 Profiles of Success*, which features the results of a survey of the industry. (Note: Individuals who would like to obtain a more detailed compilation of the basic financial indicators for the health/fitness club industry should contact IHRSA.)

Benchmark Category	All Clubs		Multipurpose Clubs		Fitness Only Clubs	
	2002	2003	2002	2003	2002	2003
Revenue (000s)	$1,974	$2,099	2,151.8	2,245.9	1,377.8	1,618
Revenue per Member ($)	630	654	676	758	584	559
Revenue Indoor per S.F. ($)	45	47	38	41	56	69
Non-dues Revenue as % of Total Revenue	27%	28%	29%	30%	22%	23%
EBITDA as % of Revenue	18%	18%	11%	17%	9.5%	14%
EBIT as % of revenue	1%	6%	1%	6%	.7%	5.4%
Payroll as % of Revenue (includes benefits)	43%	44%	42%	43%	47%	45%

Figure 12.6. Key financial-performance benchmarks for the health/fitness club industry

13

Budgeting, Forecasting, and Driving Profitability in the Health/Fitness Club Industry

Chapter Objectives

The previous chapter reviewed how the industry keeps score of its financial performance, but not how it establishes its financial targets or drives the achievement of those financial targets. This chapter initially offers an overview of the budgeting and forecasting process, and then concludes with an examination of the most effective industry practices for driving profitability and achieving budget targets.

Budgeting in the Health/Fitness Club Industry

Creating a budget is the first step in driving a successful financial plan and achieving profitability.

The practice and process of budgeting exist in every business. Creating a budget is the first step in driving a successful financial plan and achieving profitability. Budgeting is simply the process of creating financial targets for the business, based on an understanding of the underlying forces that shape the operations of the business. In the club industry, budgets are done on an annual basis, usually beginning three-to-fourth months prior to the start of the next fiscal year. A club budget is a best estimate of its financial performance, based on a thorough knowledge of the market and the operational forces that impact it. At all times, a budget is a living, breathing document that serves as a roadmap for a club's financial targets.

Most clubs initially create a five-year budget prior to opening for business and then once they're open and operating, develop an annual operating budget. Two primary approaches to budgeting exist in the industry: zero-based budgeting and trend-line budgeting.

❏ *Zero-Based Budgeting.* Zero-based budgeting involves the process of building a budget from scratch, using such factors as information on pricing, market forces, expected usage levels, expected staffing levels, etc. When a club develops a zero-based budget, it uses its knowledge of the market

Two primary approaches to budgeting exist in the industry: zero-based budgeting and trend-line budgeting.

Revenues	Expenses
1. What will be the expected number of members or memberships at the beginning of the year and the end of the year?	1. What will be the club's total hours of operation?
2. What will be the net gain in membership each accounting period?	2. What will be the total number of FTE (full-time equivalents) that will be required for each area of club operations (fitness, spa, front desk, classes, etc.)?
3. What will be the average monthly and annual dues for each membership?	3. What will be the average hourly rate for each FTE by area?
4. What will be the average enrollment fee collected with each membership?	4. What percentage of revenues, based on industry averages, will be allocated to payroll?
5. What percentage of memberships will participate in personal training services?	5. What will be the cost of benefits as a percentage of total wages?
6. What will be the average fee collected for personal training services?	6. What will utilities be, based on square footage and an average cost per square foot?
7. What percentage of membership will participate in services such as massage, atheletic leagues, court reservations, group classes, special events, etc.?	7. What are the expected unit costs for various expenses, such as supplies, uniforms, printing, etc., as a percentage of revenue?
8. What will be the average price for each service at the club (e.g., massage, classes, leagues, court fees, event fees, etc.)?	8. What are the expected unit costs for insurance, property tax, capital repairs, etc., per square foot for the club?
9. How many guests will use the club and what will be the average guest fee?	9. What is the total club square footage?
10. What percentage of the revenues does the club want to derive from dues, personal training, etc.?	10. How many members will the club have?
11. What revenues does the club expect per member or per square foot of the facility?	11. What is the club's target for EBITDA and EBIT as a percentage of revenue?

Figure 13.1. Examples of basic assumptions and questions used in the zero-based budget process

Assumption	Volume	Unit Cost	Weekly Budget	Annual Budget
Level of membership	2,000	NA		
% of members each week taking personal training	5% (100)	$50	$5,000	$260,000
Average fee for personal training	$50	NA		
% of members taking paid exercise classes each week	5% (100)	$10	$1,000	$52,000
Average fee for classes	$10	NA		
% of members taking other fee-based services each week	10% (200)	$5	$1,000	$52,000
Average fee collected for other services	$5	NA		
Total Revenue			**$7,000**	**$364,000**
# FTE for department	10 (400 hours)	$10	$4,000	$208,000
Average hourly rate for FTE	$10	NA	NA	
% of commission on personal training	50%	50%	$2,500	$130,000
Benefits as % of payroll wages	15%	15%	$600	$31,200
Other expenses as % of department revenues	25%	25%	$1,000	$52,000
Total Expenses			**$8,100**	**$421,200**
Department Net				**-$57,200**

Figure 13.2. An example of a zero-based budget for a fitness department

and market conditions to build a template of what it expects to occur and what these circumstances will mean from a financial perspective. Zero-based budgeting is used most often when developing a new club or making a significant change in the operation of an existing club. When a club uses the zero-based approach to budgeting, it must take into consideration a host of assumptions, examples of which are shown in Figure 13.1.

The questions included in Figure 13.1 are the types of queries that club operators must ask and be able to answer if they want to pursue a zero-based budget process. Figure 13.2 presents an example of a zero-based budget for a fitness department.

As can be seen in Figure 13.2, a zero-based budget requires that the club operator make accurate assumptions with regard to several factors, including membership levels, pricing, volume of traffic for services, and selected other categories. Many club operators believe that using zero-based budgeting forces them to stay attuned to the factors that are impacting their market and business. As a consequence, they are more likely to achieve their budgetary predictions or estimates.

❑ *Trend-Line Budgeting.* Trend-line budgeting is the most commonly used budgeting practice for multiple-club operations and independent-club operations. The trend-line budget process is based on the principle of clubs building their next year's budget off the past financial trends of their business and then extrapolating forward, based on those trends. This method of budgeting is assumed to be more accurate and predictable, because it relies on a known history of financial-performance trends and then applies certain assumptions to those trends. A downside of this approach is its overreliance on past performance trends and its shortsighted view of current and future market forces. In any event, trend-line budgeting is an effective approach to budgeting, one that is much easier to apply when working with multiple-club entities. Figure 13.3 illustrates the revenue, expense, and EBITDA trends, in millions, for a club over a five-year period.

As can be seen in Figure 13.3, the club's revenues have grown consistently over the past five years at a rate of approximately $100,000 annually. At the same time, expenses have also grown consistently and at a faster pace than revenues. As a result, the EBITDA has remained flat. For the next calendar year, using the trend-line budgeting process and assuming that its revenues and expenses will increase in proportion with the results of prior years, the club could assume that its EBITDA will drop as a result of the trends in revenues and expenses. When using the trend-line budgeting process, club operators need to consider a number of assumptions and questions (for ease of understanding, the data in Figure 13.3 serves as a reference for the assumptions and questions). Figure 13.4 lists several of these assumptions and questions.

Many club operators believe that using zero-based budgeting forces them to stay attuned to the factors that are impacting their market and business. As a consequence, they are more likely to achieve their budgetary predictions or estimates.

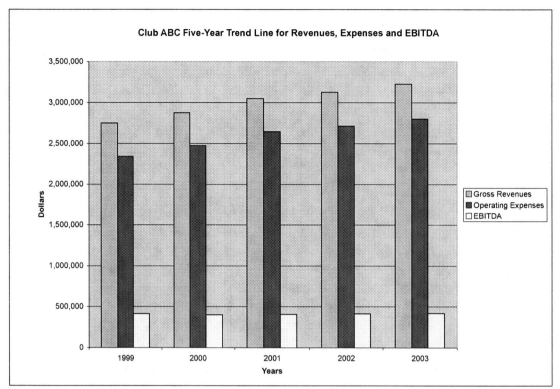

Figure 13.3. Revenue, expense, and EBITDA trends for a sample club.

The main difference between budgeting (an annual process) and forecasting (normally a quarterly process) is that with forecasting, the club is looking at its budget, then taking the most recent external and internal business events, and finally using those factors to create a more accurate estimate of its financial performance for the upcoming period (usually a quarter).

As Figure 13.4 illustrates, the trend-line budgeting process requires both an understanding of a club's prior year's financial-performance trends and the ability to foresee both the expected and unexpected with regard to external and internal business forces.

Forecasting in the Health/Fitness Club Industry

Forecasting is an extension of the budgeting process. It is normally undertaken to more accurately predict financial performance over a shorter period of time than an annual budget, such as on a quarterly or monthly basis. The process of forecasting is a mainstay of both the public market and those club operators desiring to enter the public market. In recent years, many, if not most, multiple-club operators have moved toward quarterly forecasting as a means to create more accurate financial predictions than they normally obtain from their annual budgets. The main difference between budgeting (an annual process) and forecasting (normally a quarterly process) is that with forecasting, the club is looking at its budget, then taking the most recent external and internal business events, and finally using those factors to create a more accurate estimate of its financial performance for the upcoming period (usually a quarter). By forecasting, the club can better predict its future financial performance and cash position. Forecasting is also an excellent tool for developing club leaders

Revenues	Expenses
1. What is the average percentage rise in revenues for each of the last five years?	1. What has been the average percentage increase in expenses each of the last five years?
2. What is the expected or assumed percentage increase for revenues in the upcoming year due to CPI?	2. What is the expected or assumed percentage increase in payroll and other expenses due to CPI?
3. What is the expected or assumed percentage increase in revenues due to either pricing or usage increases?	3. What is the expected or assumed percentage increase in payroll due to merit increases or the addition of new staff?
4. Is the club adding a new service that will bring new revenues?	4. What are the expected or assumed percentage increases in other expenses, such as utilities, benefits, hospitalization, etc., due to unexpected or rumored market conditions?
5. Is a new competitor moving into town that might pull members from the club?	5. Does the club have any outstanding liabilities that are expected to come due?
6. Is there an indication of a new business or residential development coming in that would cause a higher-than-expected bump in membership levels?	6. Does the club have any delayed capital repair that it must address in the coming year?

Figure 13.4. Examples of basic assumptions and questions used in the trend-line budgeting process

who are able to take greater accountability for the club's financial performance. Figure 13.5 illustrates a club budget, examples of recent business events, and their application to a quarterly forecast.

As Figure 13.5 indicates, the forecast for the next quarter has been adjusted from the original budget, because the operator has taken into account several recent external and internal business changes. As a result of the forecast, the operator is better prepared to manage the club's cash flow for the upcoming quarter and to make adjustments in the club's operations, if they're needed, to compensate.

Industry Practices for Driving Revenues

❑ *The Sources of Revenue.* Research conducted by IHRSA indicates that the largest source of revenue for clubs comes from membership dues. In its *2004 Profiles of Success*, IHRSA reports that between 66% and 80% of a club's total revenue is derived from membership dues. As a result,

> **IHRSA reports that between 66% and 80% of a club's total revenue is derived from membership dues.**

Category	Annual Budget	Next Quarter's Budget	Recent Events	Quarterly Forecast
Membership dues	$2,000,000	$500,000	In the last quarter, the club lost 50 members at annual dues of $50,000.	$487,500
Gross operating revenues	$3,000,000	$750,000	Price increase occurred in all services of 10%	$762,500
Payroll	$1,200,000	$350,000	Wage increases go into effect at 5%.	$367,500
Other expenses	$1,000,000	$250,000	As predicted	$250,000
Total expenses	$2,200,000	$600,000	See above	$617,500
EBITDA	$800,000	$150,000		$145,000
Loan payment	$300,000	$75,000	No payment for quarter	$0
EBIT	$500,000	$75,000		$145,000

Figure 13.5. An example of forecasting, using an existing annual budget

membership sales and retention play a critical role in driving a club's overall revenue. The other 20% to 34% of a club's revenue is normally provided from a number of sources, including:

- *Personal training.* Personal training is the second largest source of revenue in the industry, with the possible exception of tennis revenue in those clubs that offer tennis. According to anecdotal research, most clubs report that between five-and-ten percent of their membership participates in personal training on a weekly basis. In fact, with regard to personal training, a few clubs indicate that they are able to penetrate close to 20% of their membership. In other words, if the club has 1,000 members, it can expect to see 50-to-100 sessions involving personal training a week, and if the club has 5,000 members, it can expect to see 250-to-500 personal-training sessions a week. As a rule, personal training fees tend to range from $40 to $75 an hour, with the highest rates found in New York, Los Angeles, and San Francisco. With these types of numbers, it is not unreasonable for a club of 1,000 members to generate as much as $7,500 a week in personal-training revenues or $360,000 annually, while a club of 5,000 members can derive as much as $37,500 a week or $1,950,000 annually from

Personal training is the second largest source of revenue in the industry, with the possible exception of tennis revenue in those clubs that offer tennis.

personal training. In fact, some clubs, such as Equinox and Sports Club/LA, consistently do in excess of $2 million a year in personal training in their large clubs and have even reported income of over $4 million annually in this area.

- *Tennis services*. In clubs that have tennis courts and tennis services, tennis is often the largest source of revenue. In clubs with tennis, the largest single generator of revenue is providing tennis lessons (individual and group). Lesson revenue can account for as much as 80% of all tennis revenues. Other sources of revenue for tennis include court fees (indoor courts), youth programs, leagues, tournaments, and pro-shop sales. A club with outdoor courts can annually expect to generate between $25,000 and $50,000 in revenue per court, with the best clubs approaching $75,000 per court, while a club with indoor courts can expect to derive $35,000 to $100,000 per court. Club operators usually generate an average of $40,000 for an outdoor court and $75,000 for an indoor court. The reason indoor courts generate significantly more revenue is due to court fees. As previously indicated, lesson revenue is the top source of tennis revenue, with the average fee charged for a one-hour private lesson ranging from $40 to $60 an hour. Court fees range from a low of $10 per court hour to as high as $100 per court hour, depending upon the market in which the club is located. It should be noted that 10% to 40% of a club's members may be actively involved in tennis lessons on either an individual or group basis.

- *Spa services*. Spa services have grown into a prime source of revenue for the health/fitness club industry. In some clubs, this source of revenue might only involve the delivery of massage, while in other clubs, it might involve a number of activities, including massage, facials, body treatments, pedicures, manicures, and even hair service. According to research conducted by ISPA (the International Spa Association), massage is the leading revenue source in the spa-service category, followed (in order) by facials, pedicures, manicures, and body treatments. In most instances, massage will account for at least 50% of the spa-service treatments. Research conducted by the spa industry shows that a typical treatment room could generate as much as $10,000 a month, while a pedicure station usually generates approximately $3,000 a month. In the club industry, anecdotal research indicates that a club can expect to generate about $3,000 to $10,000 a month from a single treatment room. This same research also shows that between one percent and five percent of a club's members will be active users of its spa services. With regard to pricing, a one-hour massage can range from as low as $40 in some midwestern clubs to as high as $120 an hour in some of the high-end clubs in the more affluent markets.

Research conducted by the spa industry shows that a typical treatment room could generate as much as $10,000 a month, while a pedicure station usually generates approximately $3,000 a month.

As a rule, clubs have three core strategies that they can employ to increase their revenue output from the aforementioned revenue sources: increasing the pricing, increasing the usage rate of the services that they offer, and adding new products and services.

- *Youth programs and services.* In the last several years, the children's program and activity areas have become a significant source of revenue for many health/fitness clubs. Activities conducted in these area, such as birthday parties, sports camps, dance classes, martial arts, tumbling, after-school camps, holiday camps, swim lessons, and swim teams can provide significant revenues. In fact, youth programs in suburban clubs, such as the Pacific Athletic Club in Redwood City, California, Franco's in Mandeville, Louisiana, and East Hills in Grand Rapids, Michigan, all generate revenue that is as significant as those revenues that the facilities derive from providing services such as personal training or tennis.

- *Pilates.* One of the newest sources of revenue for the industry has evolved from offering Pilates to club members. By combining both private instruction and group instruction, many clubs have seen Pilates become their second largest source of revenue. For example, Health Works, a women's-only chain of clubs located in Boston, has a Pilates center that grosses close to a million dollars a year. One multiple-club company, Equinox, has Pilates studios that occupy 600-to-800 square feet per studio, each of which (according to sources at Equinox) generates between $20,000 and $50,000 a month in revenue.

- *Other revenue-generating programs.* In addition to the aforementioned four sources, clubs have developed a variety of services that can contribute to revenue growth. For example, clubs, such as ClubCorp's Rivers Club in Pittsburgh, Pennsylvania and the University Club in Houston, Texas generate over $200,000 annually in locker-rental income. The East Bank Club in Chicago derives over five million annually in food and beverage revenue. Many clubs (e.g., Western Athletic Clubs, etc.) have found that leasing space to a physical therapy operator can bring in as much as $100,000 annually from fixed leases and revenue sharing. Still other clubs have leveraged activities such as special events, leagues, adventure programs, and social events into significant sources of new revenue.

❑ *Increasing the Revenue Stream from Each Revenue Source.* As a rule, clubs have three core strategies that they can employ to increase their revenue output from the aforementioned revenue sources: increasing the pricing, increasing the usage rate of the services that they offer, and adding new products and services.

- *Price increases.* Many club operators assume that the best approach to driving revenues is to increase the price of a service. While price increases can generate significant bumps in revenue, especially if applied to membership dues or personal training, such increases can also have a negative impact if club operators do not take into consideration their club's market position and the value of the club's product offering. Many clubs make it a practice to increase their dues or personal training fees two-to-three percent every year, irrespective of market conditions, while others carefully consider the dynamics of the marketplace and their club's niche before passing on any price increases. In reality, if the club is delivering a great product and its members are satisfied, then an annual price increase equal to the consumer price index (CPI) or slightly higher can usually be accommodated.

- *Increasing volume.* Another effective approach for driving revenues is to increase member and guest participation in fee-based services. While the health/fitness club industry, as a whole, tends to shy away from this approach, all factors considered, it is the most effective strategy for generating relatively large increases in revenue. For example, multiple-club operators, such as Equinox, 24 Hour Fitness, and Bally's, focus most of their non-dues revenue efforts on internal selling. To effectively increase member usage of fee-based services, clubs should consider the following approaches:

    ✓ Sales management. The best clubs closely manage the sales of their primary revenue sources, such as personal training, massage, and other services, just as they do membership. The top revenue-producing clubs establish sales targets for their teams and each individual employee, and then closely monitor each entity's sales performance. Not only do these clubs establish challenging sales goals for both the sales teams and individuals, they then hold the teams and employees accountable for their performance against these goals.

    ✓ Sales training. Fitness staff (e.g., trainers, instructors, therapists, etc.) tend to be relationship people who shy away from sales. As a rule, many individuals view sales in a negative light. Accordingly, many top club operators make a concerted effort to provide continuous sales training for their employees that can help make them more comfortable about selling themselves and the services of their clubs.

    ✓ Selling upfront. The top revenue-producing clubs have learned that the best time to sell a service, such as personal training or massage, is when the member first joins the club. Many club groups, such as Equinox, 24 Hour Fitness, and Western Athletic Clubs, bundle special-service packages that the membership sales team makes new members aware of when they join the club. This process is often referred to as up-selling the club's services. Club operators should keep in mind that, all factors considered, new members represent the best audience for sales.

The top revenue-producing clubs have learned that the best time to sell a service, such as personal training or massage, is when the member first joins the club.

While driving revenue is critical to growing a club's profitability, controlling expenses also plays a vital role.

✓ Internal marketing. All too often, some clubs believe that by putting a poster on the wall, their members will automatically sign-up for the offering. In reality, to effectively make members aware of the services it offers, the club should utilize a variety of marketing tools, such as interactive displays, direct-mail invitations to members, web-based marketing, newsletter messages, and audio-visual messages, utilizing the club's internal audio-visual entertainment equipment.

✓ Relationships and making the call. Members who respect and trust the employees of the club are much more likely to purchase a service from those employees. The same can be said about members who know and respect other members. The top revenue-producing clubs make an effort to utilize their employees and members as sales people. Having employees make sales contacts or extend invitations to the members that they know can contribute significantly to revenue generation. Members who are provided an incentive will often serve as apostles for the services offered by the club and invite their friends to join them to participate in a fee-based service.

• Adding new products and services. The third strategy for effectively driving revenues is to introduce new products and services to the club's members. For example, if the club does not offer spa services, adding these services can generate new revenue streams. By the same token, if the club does not offer Pilates, including a Pilates center in the facility can help drive revenues for the club. In reality, the opportunities for adding new products and services are virtually endless. One proven strategy for identifying new sources of revenue is to create a club-based revenue team, consisting of employees from different areas of the club. This revenue team should then be empowered to meet on a regular basis and brainstorm new ideas for generating revenue. When the revenue team identifies a revenue idea that has consensus, then management can work with them to develop an execution strategy.

Industry Practices for Controlling Expenses

While driving revenue is critical to growing a club's profitability, controlling expenses also plays a vital role. The process of controlling expenses involves having systems and practices in place that can help prevent the club from needlessly wasting money. At the same time, the process can help the club invest its money more wisely in its people and assets.

❑ *The Leading Expense Categories.* According to IHRSA's *2004 Profiles of Success*, the top expense categories for clubs are wages and salaries, benefits, utilities, lease costs, and capital replacement and repair costs.

- *Wages and salaries.* According to the most recent industry studies, wages and salaries comprise approximately 45% (a figure that includes employee expenses) of every dollar in revenue that the club generates. If the related benefit costs are subtracted, then payroll is probably closer to 30% of gross revenues. This figure approximates to the total of all other departmental undistributed expenses combined. Wages and salaries include the salaries of supervisors, the hourly wages of the non-exempt employees, commissions paid to personal trainers and other instructors, wages paid to group-exercise instructors, and bonuses provided to any employee of the club. For most clubs, the wages paid to group-exercise instructors and the commissions paid to personal trainers and others constitute the largest single payroll expense.

- *Benefits.* Benefit costs can range from 15% to 25% of the actual wages and salaries. These costs include club contributions to social security taxes, hospitalization benefits, disability insurance, retirement type accounts, and education. The single largest contributor in recent years has been hospitalization costs, which have grown at rates over 12% annually the last several years.

- *Utilities.* Utility costs normally range between five percent and 10% of a club's operating revenue, depending upon its geographic location. The largest contributors to utility costs are heating, and air conditioning, and expenses attributed to the operation of the pools and whirlpools.

- *Leases.* For clubs that rent space, the cost of rent can be a club's second largest expense after wages. According to *IHRSA's Uniform System of Accounts* and its *2004 Profiles of Success*, lease rates can run as high as 20% of a club's revenue. Successful club operators look to keep their lease rate under 15% of revenues and preferably closer to 10% of their operating revenue. Many clubs get lulled into a state of complacency by assuming that they have a fixed based rent and they fail to consider the common area maintenance (CAM)—costs that landlords pass through, which represent the club's share of the building operating costs assumed by the landlord. In most markets, landlords like to offer triple-net leases, which means the club pays the landlord a base rent, CAM costs, utilities, and property taxes. In most markets, the lease rates for class "A" space run approximately $20-to-$40 a square foot per year, while the lease rates for class "B" space tend to be in the neighborhood of nine-to-$15 a square foot per year. CAM costs can run another six-to-$15 a square foot, depending upon the market in which a club is located. In smaller markets rent rates for space in strip malls run in the neighborhood of eight-to-$15 a square foot.

- *Capital replacement and repair.* According to industry surveys, clubs should allocate approximately five-to-six percent of their gross revenues on an annual basis to capital replacement and repair. Every fifth year, the percentage should be increased to as much as 15% of

Wages and salaries comprise approximately 40% (a figure that includes employee expenses) of every dollar in revenue that the club generates.

the club's gross revenues. These numbers represent a significant amount of a club's revenues and, if not budgeted for correctly, can have dire consequences for the club. Many club operators try to save money by not spending the capital replacement dollars. In the long run, however, such an approach almost always results in poorly kept facilities and lost revenues. According to *IHRSA's 2004 Profiles of Success*, clubs who invest more into their club have the highest membership retention rates. Capital replacement dollars are used to purchase new equipment, repair worn areas of the club, and fund expansion efforts when they are needed.

Controlling the Leading Expense Categories

Achieving profitability requires that the club operator put systems in place for controlling the large and small expenses that can often erode the revenue gains that a club makes. Among the most effective strategies that the industry employs to help monitor and control operating expenses, thereby facilitating growth in profitability, are the following:

❑ Managing Wages and Benefits Expense. Since wages and benefits contribute, on average, close to 45% of all operating expenses, it makes sense that by effectively managing its payroll, the club can also better manage its expenses. Examples of the most effective strategies for managing payroll include:

- *Scheduling for less than 40 hours.* Smart operators avoid scheduling their full-time employees for 40 hours and instead schedule them for 35-to-37 hours a week. This approach has two advantages. First, it provides leeway if an employee is asked to serve a few more hours, and second, it allows the clubs to avoid both overtime and overlapping schedules.

- *Not scheduling employees during low-usage periods.* Many clubs save wages by limiting their level of scheduling during low-usage times. While it is important to be fully staffed during peak-usage periods, during times when members are not using the facility, management can limit their scheduling of employees to only provide the necessary level of employee coverage. As needed, if additional staffing is required when special functions are held, these situations can be handled with salaried supervisors.

- *Monitoring and avoiding overtime.* Since overtime costs a club 50% more than regular time, wise club operators make it a practice to carefully monitor employee hours to avoid overtime. In this regard, software programs are available that will provide the club with reports that indicate when its employees are approaching overtime. In which case, the club can make whatever adjustments are necessary in its employee schedules to avoid overtime situations.

> Achieving profitability requires that the club operator put systems in place for controlling the large and small expenses that can often erode the revenue gains that a club makes.

- *Going to flat rates versus percentage commission.* Personal trainers and massage therapists are often paid a commission on the revenue they generate. The industry norm for commissions tends to vary from 40% to as high as 75%. Instead of paying a commission, many clubs pay a flat rate for personal training and/or massage. This approach enables the club to avoid providing wage increases every time the fees for services offered by the club are raised.

- *Group-exercise classes.* For many club operators, the cost of offering group-exercise classes can be very substantial. The average wage for a class instructor can vary from an average as low as $18 a class in some mid-western markets to $60 per class in the large urban markets, such as New York and San Francisco. When the fact that some clubs offer as many as 100 classes a week is considered, the enormity of the potential costs involved becomes apparent. The top club operators make it a habit to establish specific attendance requirements for a class to continue and when attendance falls below those specified levels, the class is eliminated. The primary goal of most clubs is to offer only the classes that appeal to members and thereby only pay the wages for those classes that bring value to each club's program offerings.

> **Instead of paying a commission, many clubs pay a flat rate for personal training and/or massage.**

- ❑ *Managing Operating Supply Costs.* In most clubs, the costs associated with operating supplies, printing, and other miscellaneous supplies can run as high as 10% of revenue and, if uncontrolled, much higher. The most effective approaches to managing these expenses include:

  - *Using a purchase-order system.* A purchase-order system requires that before employees can purchase an item for the club, they need to obtain a price quote and submit it to management for approval. If subsequently approved by management, the purchase order becomes the basis for an order. This approach allows management to monitor expenses against budget to insure that funds are not expended for unnecessary items.

  - *Par stock and inventory.* A par stock is a term that connotates a process that involves purchasing sufficient quantities of supplies and creating an inventory of those items for the club to pull from in times of need. In reality, many clubs unfortunately wait until they run out of an item before attempting to restock the item by purchasing it. With a par-stock process, the club purchases items based on usage experience and keeps an inventory sufficient to cover a particular period of time. Under the par-stock process, when the club's inventory drops to a certain level, it purchases the standard reorder quantity. This approach is similar to an open-to-buy system in retail. The par-stock method allows the club to buy in bulk, which saves money, but it also allows it to closely monitor the usage of products and control its shrinkage (e.g., inventory loss due to theft).

- *Preferred vendor arrangements.* Clubs can negotiate with vendors to obtain preferred status and thus gain discounts. If a club is willing to purchase its supplies from one or two vendors, it can often negotiate a discounted price schedule. In large multiple-club operations, this approach can involve a significant savings opportunity. In this regard, independent-club operators, should consider using industry-association programs, such as the programs offered by IHRSA.

❑ *Utility Costs.* As previously discussed, utility costs can amount to as much as 10% of a club's operating revenue. Most clubs can save on their utility costs by incorporating one or more of the following strategies:

- *Converting electric heating appliances to gas.* Gas is usually less expensive than electric, especially when it comes to heating pools, water heaters, whirlpools, and washers.

- *Using light-saver switches.* Many clubs use automatically controlled lighting systems that turn off lights in rooms when they are not in use. Far too many clubs waste money by keeping lights on in particular areas, even though those rooms are not in use. These clubs rely on their employees to turn off the lights as appropriate, an approach that is not always as effective as automated systems.

- *Installing water restrictors in the showers.* Water restrictors are devices that can be added to showers that reduce the total volume of water that is dispensed. Over time, these implements can save considerable costs in water bills.

- *Insulating the club.* Most utility companies will provide the club with incentives if it upgrades the level of insulation in the club. In many cases, utility companies will even cover most of the cost for such improvements. The upside for the club comes with the reduced cost of heating and cooling.

- *Negotiating with the utility company for a flat rate.* Club operators can often negotiate with the utility company to establish a flat utility rate that is reviewed on a semi-annual basis. Not only can this practice save money, more importantly, it can also enable the club to more accurately forecast its utility costs.

- *Install low-energy lighting.* Many utility purchasing groups offer incentives to businesses that install low-energy lighting systems. Such incentives allow a business to spend less in the conversion process, with savings subsequently being realized on their monthly utility bill.

❑ *Leases.* In most cases, leases are non-negotiable once they're in place. At least, this situation is what most operators assume. As a result, many club

If a club is willing to purchase its supplies from one or two vendors, it can often negotiate a discounted price schedule.

owners pay higher-than-needed rent and CAM costs. The first step for the club in managing its lease expense is to know its lease terms inside and out. By knowing the terms of its lease, the club can identify when unnecessary costs are passed through, such as high CAM costs and rent increases, when none exist in the lease. Even more important than knowing its lease, the club should be fully aware of a situation when the opportunity exists to renegotiate its lease. Landlords are open to renegotiating leases under several possible circumstances, including: when a new building owner becomes the landlord, when the landlord is looking to extend leases, and when lease rates for other spaces are going at a lower rate than what the club currently pays. All factors considered, if the club has established itself as a worthy and reliable tenant and has built a good relationship with the landlord, then the club is in a better position to renegotiate more favorable lease terms.

❑ *Capital Repair.* IHRSA's *2004 Profiles of Success* indicates that clubs should allocate between five-and-six percent of their revenues for capital replacement. As indicated previously, this outlay represents a significant allocation of cash for most club operators. Some operators feel that by limiting their allocation for capital reserve that they can bring more of their existing revenue to the bottom line. At first glance, this attitude might make sense, since it decreases the out-of-pocket cash that a club has to spend, thereby increasing the EBIT of the club. Unfortunately, this reasoning ends up costing clubs money, both in the short-term and even more so in the long-term. By allocating three-to-six percent of its revenues to capital repair and replacement and then using it, the club is investing in its physical assets, an approach which, in turn, helps to drive revenues and prevent costly operational maintenance costs. By investing the full capital replacement on an annual basis, the club also prevents having to spend much larger sums in future years, when a particular physical asset reaches a point where it requires major renovation and repair.

By allocating three-to-six percent of its revenues to capital repair and replacement and then using it, the club is investing in its physical assets, an approach which, in turn, helps to drive revenues and prevent costly operational maintenance costs.

Key Points to Consider

By incorporating annual budgeting and quarterly forecasting, a club operator can create realistic and achievable financial targets for its revenues, expenses, and earnings. These financial targets can then be used to foster individual and team accountability for the club's financial performance. Once in place, these targets can assist the club operator in determining which revenue-enhancement and cost-control strategies are needed to achieve particular financial targets.

14

The Art of the Deal: Buying, Leasing, Selling, and Raising Capital for a Health/Fitness Club

Chapter Objectives

As the industry continues to evolve and become more financially sophisticated, club owners and operators need to acquaint themselves with as many of the overriding issues surrounding the purchasing, financing, and sale of health/fitness clubs as possible. In that regard, this chapter will review the information and processes that a club operator should know concerning how to raise capital for the club, how to buy a club, how to sell a club, or simply how to properly evaluate a lease for the space that a club might occupy. Initially, the chapter discusses the key issues attendant to raising capital and then concludes by examining several of the most relevant factors involving buying, leasing, and selling clubs.

Raising Capital for a Health/Fitness Club

For independent-club operators just starting a club or an experienced multiple-club operation looking to expand its business, raising capital is an important factor in achieving success. As a rule, club owner/operators have three primary options for raising capital for their business: bank financing, private investor financing, and private equity-firm investment (venture capital). Besides the aforementioned sources of funding, larger multiple-club operators, with a proven track record of success, can also pursue an initial public offering (IPO), a process that raises capital through the issuance of public stock. Clubs that own their land and building also have a fifth option—selling the land and

For independent-club operators just starting a club or an experienced multiple-club operation looking to expand its business, raising capital is an important factor in achieving success.

building to raise capital and then leasing the property back from the investors to whom they sold the land and building.

❑ *Private Investor Capital.* Many independent-club operators pursue this approach to raising capital. This method involves having the owner of the proposed business venture (club) develop a business model that is subsequently presented to private investors for raising capital. In most instances, the owner needs to form a limited partnership, limited liability corporation, or corporation to serve as the legal entity for raising the capital. In attracting private-investor equity, the club operator must offer the investor stock, membership shares, or a similar ownership position. In essence, the club operator must allow the investors an ownership stake in the business if they intend to provide the capital.

> When club operators obtain private-equity investment, they should be aware of the fact that the investors assume an ownership position in the business that is proportional to their invested capital, both in equity and debt.

Private investors look for a minimum annual return on their invested capital (ROIC), also referred to as return on equity invested (ROE). In most cases, investors are looking for returns of 10% to 15% on their invested capital, though higher return expectations of 20% to 25% are not unusual. For example, if private investors provide one million dollars in capital in a club, they will normally expect an annual return of at least $100,000 to $150,000. This return is based on the free cash flow of the club after all expenses are accounted for. In raising capital through this approach, club operators may need to consider and attract several private investors, especially if they are looking to raise several million dollars. It should be noted that private investors could be individuals or partnerships.

❑ *Private-Equity Investment Firms (Venture Capital, Funds, etc.).* Clubs that pursue private-equity firms usually are trying to raise millions of dollars in capital. As a rule, it is not likely that an independent-club operation would pursue this option. Rather, this approach is a method that a multiple-club operation, seeking capital for acquisitions or rapid organic growth, would tend to favor. All factors considered, this option is far more suited to capital requirements exceeding $25 million than smaller capital requirements of only a few million dollars. When club operators obtain private-equity investment, they should be aware of the fact that the investors assume an ownership position in the business that is proportional to their invested capital, both in equity and debt. As a result, the original owners can often lose controlling interest in their business and, as such, be relegated to more of a management role. Accordingly, clubs should give careful consideration concerning whether to pursue this capital strategy.

Most private-equity firms that invest in a club business do so by investing both cash and assuming additional debt. For example, a private-equity firm may invest $40 million dollars in a club—which consists of $20 million in cash and $20 million in assumption of debt. Private-equity firms tend to view their investment far differently than a private investor, because

When looking for a bank to finance its business, a club should attempt to find a bank that defaults on no more than .5% of its loans. In other words, it makes the right financing decision 99.5% of the time.

their primary goal is normally to either sell their invested stake or take the business public in a period of five-to-seven years. Most private-equity firms tend to look for two factors when considering whether to invest. Not only do they expect the club(s) to achieve double digit growth in EBITDA on an annual basis (normally a range of 15% to 25%), they also anticipate to cash out after five-to-seven years with a compounded annual return between 20% and 30%.

In reality, there are some private-equity firms that have return expectations of 30% to 40%. For example, a private-equity firm invests $40 million in capital (which consists of $20 million in cash and $20 million in debt) for a business that generates $10 million in EBITDA. Over the next five years, they invest another $20 million, through cash and debt, to bring their total capital invested to $60 million. In return, hypothetically, they would expect the EBITDA of the business to grow from $10 million at the time of purchase to $12 million after one year, $14.5 million after two years, $17.3 million after three years, $20.7 million after four years, and $25 million by the fifth year. After the fifth year, they would want to sell the business for approximately four-to-eight times the club's EBITDA, thereby generating a total of $100 to $200 million in cash. After deducting their $60 million of investment, they would receive $40 to $140 million in cash earnings to distribute to their investors, which would amount to a return in excess of 20%. If a private-equity group does not see the expected EBITDA growth or the possibility of exiting the business with an appropriate level of return on its investment, it will often take control of the business and try to push earnings growth, through cost reductions, while looking for a suitable investor to buy the company.

❑ *Bank Financing (Debt Capital)*. Bank financing is one of the most common approaches employed to raise most of the capital needed to develop and operate a small or large business. Because banks are regulated, they tend to be very careful in their lending practices. When looking for a bank to finance its business, a club should attempt to find a bank that defaults on no more than .5% of its loans. In other words, it makes the right financing decision 99.5% of the time. Clubs should understand several basic factors about banks and financing, including:

- For banks, its loans are its assets, which means that every loan application is normally reviewed very carefully.

- Banks look for individuals, partnerships, and businesses with good credit ratings.

- Banks expect to see a business plan that has reasonable assumptions, reasonable budget projections, a qualified leadership team (management expertise and experience), and detailed value of the collateral that will be put up to secure the loan (the collateral must hold value to the lender).

- Banks expect full disclosure from the company to which they are going to make a loan.

- Banks will normally apply covenants to a loan. Covenants help protect the bank's investment in the loan. These covenants can be restrictive and if the business breaks the covenants, the bank can demand immediate payment of the debt balance, or take over control of the assets of the business, and even sell the business if necessary.

- Banks prefer that the owner(s) of the business have equity in the company. For new businesses, banks like to see one dollar in equity for each dollar being lent. For mature businesses that have a track record of success and can be secured with real estate, banks will normally loan out four-to-five dollars for each dollar of equity (in other words, owners are required to provide 20% to 25% equity to secure the loan). For example, if the club wanted to take out a loan for $2,000,000, it would need to put up $400,000 to $500,000 in equity.

- Most banks like the debt-to-EBITDA ratio of the business to fall between three and four (i.e., a club's total debt should not exceed four times its EBITDA). For example, if a club has an EBITDA of $1,000,000, its total debt should not exceed $4,000,000 and should fall between three and four million dollars. If its debt exceeds four times its EBITDA, then the club would be considered as heavily leveraged, which places a financial strain on the business, not to mention exposes it to the danger of not complying with the bank covenants for the loan.

- Cash-flow loans are loans that banks provide that are not secured by real estate. In these instances, banks tend to limit the amount of the loan to a total that does not exceed 50% of the value of the business (a value that is determined by a multiple applied to the club's EBITDA).

- The bank expects the club to educate it on both the industry as a whole and on the club's business model.

- In the case of small independent operations, the bank will tend to require full financial disclosure of any stockholders or partners with 20% or greater ownership in the business. Furthermore, these owners will often be required to sign a personal guarantee for the loan amount being pursued.

For new businesses, banks like to see one dollar in equity for each dollar being lent.

It is a common practice for most start-up clubs to obtain equity through private investors and then raise the balance of the funds needed through debt. Larger multiple-club operations, on the other hand, usually utilize private-equity investment firms to raise the equity and even source the debt.

Buying and Selling a Health/Fitness Club Business

The health/fitness club industry is a dynamic enterprise in which clubs and club companies are bought and sold regularly. One approach that individuals use who are considering entering the business is to acquire an existing club. In that regard, a club that wants to grow its business, acquisition may be a suitable option, rather than building a new club. On the other hand, if investors (or an individual) want to cash out of the business or to become part of a larger business by being the acquiree rather than the acquisition, then selling the club may be appropriate. Among the key factors that should be considered when buying or selling a club business are the following:

❑ *Selling the Club.* If owners decide to sell their club, they need to understand some of the basic factors that apply to the sale process, including:

- Most clubs are valued by applying a multiple to the club's EBITDA. For clubs that are in a leased space, that multiple can range from three times EBITDA to as high as six times EBITDA. In the majority of instances, it will likely be four-to-five times the club's EBITDA. For example, a club that has an EBITDA of $500,000 would be valued at two-to-three million dollars. Clubs that are freestanding and own the land on which they are located will have a projected value that ranges from three times its EBITDA to eight times its EBITDA. In the majority of instances, its value will be five-to-seven times its EBITDA. In other words, a freestanding club with an EBITDA of $500,000 would be valued at $2.5 million to $3.5 million. In most cases, the EBITDA that is used to project a club's value is what is termed "trailing EBITDA" (i.e., the EBITDA for the most current 12-month time period and not for a specific financial year).

- Even after a club is valued using the multiple of EBITDA, the seller should be aware that most buyers will deduct the value of the liabilities from the calculated EBITDA value before determining a price, especially if they are buying the business and not its assets. For example, if a club has an EBITDA of one million and liabilities of $1,500,000, then the buyer will likely value the club at five times its EBITDA minus the liabilities, or a projection that is determined by first multiplying one million by five, and then subtracting $1,500,000 to derive a calculated value of $3,500,000.

- If someone sells a club, the preference of most individuals is to sell the business and therefore release themselves from the liabilities of the business. The buyer is more likely to want to buy the assets at the mutually agreed upon price, while the seller remains responsible for the club's liabilities.

- If the seller owns the land on which the club sits, the seller should consider holding onto the land and selling the business, and then leasing the land to the new owner. This approach enables the seller to generate more cash out of the sale. For example, if a business is valued at five million dollars (of which the asset value of the land is one

Clubs that are freestanding and own the land on which they are located will have a projected value that ranges from three times its EBITDA to eight times its EBITDA.

million), an individual might sell the business for $4.5 million, but then lease the land to the new owner for $100,000 a year.

- Sellers should make sure that they complete their own due diligence before selling and have an accurate recording of their assets, liabilities, and EBITDA for the past three years, etc.

- Sellers should have an attorney involved and possibly a broker.

❑ *Buying a Club.* If their goal is to buy a club, then the individuals who are considering purchasing the business should make sure that they understand certain basics of buying a club business, including:

- Buyers should perform their due diligence and audit the books and operations in their entirety. They should also make sure the accuracy and authenticity of the accounting is correct. Finally, they should make sure that they are fully aware of any liabilities that the business might have, in particular, any hidden account payables or legal suits against the existing club.

- Most clubs in leased spaces will sometimes sell for three-to-six times their EBITDA, with four-to-five times more likely. Clubs that are freestanding will usually sell for between three-and-eight times their EBITA, with a range of five-to-seven times most likely. More often than not, sellers try to start at the high end of the price range, while buyers typically start at the low end and then work up.

- If possible, buyers should purchase the business assets, based on the cash flow value, rather than the business itself. When individuals purchase the assets of a business, they are acquiring both the short-term and long-term assets of the club, as well as purchasing the owner's equity. What they don't buy and don't really want are the liabilities.

- When purchasing a club, the buyers should make sure that the debt they finance does not exceed four times the trailing EBITDA.

- If the individuals purchasing the debt decide to buy the entire business rather than just the assets of the business, they should then make sure to deduct the liabilities from the overall price they agreed upon using a multiple of EBITDA.

- The buyers should remember that if they purchase a club that sells annual membership contracts, that when they purchase the assets and cash flow of the business, they might not be receiving the expected level of dues if the previous owner collected the annual dues before the sale. If the buyers know that a club collects annual dues, then they need to consider lowering the price that they are willing to pay for the business or ask for consideration for those dues already collected in

Buyers should remember that if they purchase a club that sells annual membership contracts, that when they purchase the assets and cash flow of the business, they might not be receiving the expected level of dues if the previous owner collected the annual dues before the sale.

the asking price. All too often, buyers end up purchasing a club that does not produce dues for a considerable period of time because of such a scenario.

- The buyers should retain the right to retain or dismiss employees of the former club.

Leasing and Sale Leasebacks

For most first-time club owners and operators, as well as the majority of existing club operations, leasing space for their club is a common practice. Leasing is usually the option most operators choose, especially since obtaining the land to build a freestanding club is often difficult to find and too expensive to purchase. In most situations, leasing requires less upfront capital. In turn, the club has less of a need to assume debt. On the other hand, on occasion, situations exist where independent and multiple-club operators actually purchase land and build a freestanding club under one company and then lease it back to the actual operating-club entity. By the same token, there are also clubs that will take the land and building they own and sell it to an investor, with the agreement that investor will turn around and lease the building space back to the club operator. Such a practice is called a sale-leaseback and is often used to raise capital. Leasing can involve several factors, including:

- As a rule, leases have minimum time requirements. In most urban markets, the landlords of class A and class B buildings look for a minimum time period of 10 years, while in suburban settings, especially strip-mall centers, leases will usually be for five-year periods at a minimum. Prospective tenants should look for a five-year lease with an optional five-year extension period. If they are confident in their business model, then they should consider a 10-year lease.

- Most leases can be negotiated to include clauses that allow tenants to renegotiate their lease rates at a predetermined timeframe within the lease. It is a prudent business owner who makes sure to negotiate this stipulation as part of their lease. A common practice would be to have a window of time for renegotiation in the second or third year in a five-year lease and the fifth year in a 10-year lease. This negotiating practice could also be employed to establish time periods for extending leases.

- Some landlords will offer a straight lease, which means that the tenant only pays the lease rate and the approved common area maintenance costs (CAM), but does not pay utilities and property tax. This type of lease is less common in today's market because of the high upfront costs and the carrying costs that many real estate owners assume. The more common lease is a triple-net lease, which is a contracted arrangement where the tenant is responsible for the lease, CAM costs, utilities, and property taxes on the space. Accordingly, prospective

For most first-time club owners and operators, as well as the majority of existing club operations, leasing space for their club is a common practice.

tenants should make sure that they know what type of lease is being offered and what the costs will be for each type.

- Most leases have a base rate that varies by building type (class A, class B, class C, strip mall), by location, and, of course, by market demand. In most markets, strip-mall space will carry base lease rates of between eight dollars and $20 a square foot. In urban markets, the base lease rate can range from as low as $10 a square foot to $50 a square foot. The most common range is between $20 and $30 a square foot. All factors considered, club operators should try to keep their base rent under $20 a square foot or less than 15% of their club's expected revenues.

- Tenants should know what their CAM costs will be. While in most leased spaces, it will range from three-to-six dollars a square foot, there are buildings in some cities, such as Chicago and New York, where the CAM rates can reach as high as $15 or more a square foot.

- Most landlords provide tenants with a tenant-improvement allowance (TI) when the tenant moves into a space. As a rule, it is common for these allowances to run between $15 and $25 a square foot. In most instances, tenants will have the option of negotiating a higher TI allowance, especially if they are willing to pay a higher lease rate. For individuals who are having trouble raising capital to build the space, negotiating with the landlord to provide higher TI allowances, in exchange for higher rent, can prove helpful.

- If tenants are paying utilities either as part of their lease or separately, they should make sure that they request separate metering of the utilities for their space. Most landlords prefer to bill their tenants for the cost of their utilities. At the same time, a few landlords will add some overhead and profit to the actual utility costs that they pass through to their tenants.

- Tenants should make an effort to have their HVAC operated separately from the buildings they lease. In many cases, landlords have set times during which they turn their building's HVAC on and off. Turn-off times are normally based on the operating hours of a typical business. As such, all factors considered, tenants who occupy buildings in which they have independent access to the HVAC for their space and have HVAC, which is independently metered, are better off. In the event that the club's space is tied into the building's HVAC, the tenant should be aware that they would probably need to negotiate after-hours access to the HVAC, which might result in higher costs to them.

- Tenants should establish a good relationship with the landlord and the landlord's representatives. Furthermore, they should make it a practice to meet with their landlord's representatives on a monthly basis.

If tenants are paying utilities either as part of their lease or separately, they should make sure that they request separate metering of the utilities for their space.

- Tenants should know the details of their lease. Many leases require landlords to provide a certain degree of maintenance on tenant spaces. On occasion, some landlords will try to downplay this factor if they can, especially if their tenants have a relatively large space and pay a lower lease rate. Accordingly, tenants should always be fully aware of all of the conditions in their lease.

- In some instances, landlords may be willing to provide tenants with several months of free rent. Tenants should understand, however, that landlords recover these "lost" revenues in the actual rent that they subsequently charge them. As a rule, individuals who are starting a club would be wise to try and negotiate between six months and a year's free rent as part of their lease. The extent of the period of free rent is dependent upon the length of the lease and what they pay for rent, with those who have higher rents and longer leases receiving a longer period of time before their rent kicks in.

As a rule, individuals who are starting a club would be wise to try and negotiate between six months and a year's free rent as part of their lease.

A sale-leaseback is another method that individuals employ to acquire space for their business. In a sale-leaseback, the club owner/operator will sell their property and building to another investor who then leases the space back to the club owner/operator for the business. This strategy is often used by club operators who wish to raise capital for expansion or renovation purposes. One of the primary benefits of this strategy is that it allows club owners to pull their equity out of the assets and use it for growing their business.

For many club operators, the financial aspects of the business can be the most challenging. On the other hand, by taking the time to understand the basic issues involved in these factors, individuals who operate health/fitness clubs will be better prepared to address these matters in an appropriate manner.

STAFFING ISSUES IN THE HEALTH/FITNESS CLUB INDUSTRY

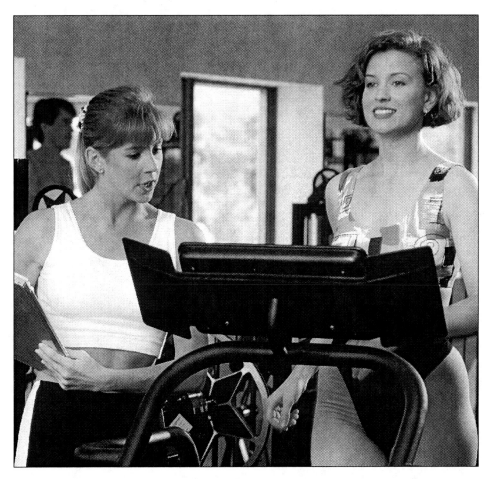

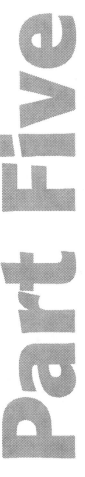

- Chapter 15: The People Factor: Employees in the Health/Fitness Club Industry
- Chapter 16: Building and Leading a Successful Health/Fitness Club Team

15

The People Factor: Employees in the Health/Fitness Club Industry

Chapter Objectives

The health/fitness club industry is a people-intensive industry. As indicated in the previous chapters on the industry's financial model, most clubs allocate upwards of 40% of their revenue towards wages and salaries. When a business allocates 40% or more of its resources to one area, that area takes on critical importance to the success of the business. In the health/fitness club industry, the employees create and sustain the experiences that the members have. In that regard, they directly influence a club's overall profitability. One of the most frequently heard comments in the health/fitness club industry is that its employees are the heart of the industry. These essential individuals deliver the services, create magic moments for the members, and foster the relationships that are so vital to a club's success. According to an article written by Leonard Schlessinger, *The Service Profit Chain*, employees are the key link for any business that desires to deliver great service to its customers.

This chapter initially begins by defining the differences between an employee and an independent contractor, as well as detailing the differences between an exempt and a non-exempt employee. Next, it provides an overview of the various positions in the industry and the role each position has in delivering the club's experience. Then, it outlines the compensation norms and educational expectations for each of these industry positions. Finally, it concludes by reviewing the various organizational structures that independent clubs and multiple-club groups utilize in operating their business.

> In the health/fitness club industry, the employees create and sustain the experiences that the members have. In that regard, they directly influence a club's overall profitability.

Similar to the separation between church and state, the lines between employees and independent contractors represent a challenge for the health/fitness club industry.

Employee Versus Independent Contractors

Similar to the separation between church and state, the lines between employees and independent contractors represent a challenge for the health/fitness club industry. All too often, clubs decide to have independent contractors provide a portion of their service delivery, not knowing that they are actually creating an employee environment. It is critical, however, that club operators clearly understand the difference between an employee and an independent contractor. Figure 15.1 details several of the basic differences between the two types of workers.

The fundamental differences between an employee and an independent contractor are quite significant. State and federal rules and regulations are very adamant about businesses adhering to the policies and procedures concerning the separation of employees and independent contractors. Clubs that attempt to pay people as independent contractors, but treat them as employees, open themselves to significant fines. If the club identifies someone as an independent contractor, but that person is characterized by any of the factors listed in the employee column in Figure 15.1, then that person is an employee and must be treated as such.

Exempt Versus Non-Exempt Employees

Another potential minefield for club operators involves whether an individual should be treated as an exempt or a non-exempt employee. An exempt

Employee	Independent Contractor
Schedule is established by the club.	Sets own schedule
Expected to follow employee policies and rules, including wearing a uniform	Only required to adhere to contractual obligations
Club can set rates for services the employee provides	Sets own rates for services that are provided
Must punch the clock or otherwise record all hours of work	Keeps own schedule and record of hours worked
Must be paid for overtime (all hours over 40 a week) and for club-recognized holidays	No overtime or holiday pay
Eligible for all club-sponsored benefits, such as holiday pay, vacation pay, insurance benefits, etc.	Not eligible for club-sponsored benefits
Covered by club-sponsored insurance such as disability, liability, etc.	Not covered by insurance and must provide evidence of liability insurance
Receives a W2 at year-end and club pays portion of social security taxes	Responsible for all taxes and receives a 1099 form showing earnings at year-end
Receives compensation via payroll	Receives earnings through a vendor check

Figure 15.1. Selected differences between employees and independent contractors

Exempt Employee	Non-Exempt Employee
Must supervise two or more employees.	Usually no supervisory responsibility or less than two.
Must allocate at least 50% of job responsibilities to supervision.	Supervision is less than 50% of the job responsibilities.
A commissioned employee can be exempt if a significant portion of their earnings is commission based.	More dependent upon a fixed hourly rate of pay for compensation.
Examples: Manager, sales manager, sales person, fitness director, tennis director.	Examples: Fitness instructor, program director, front desk staff, massage therapist, accountant

Figure 15.2. Selected differences between exempt and non-exempt employees

employee is a professional who receives a base salary (weekly, monthly, etc.), while a non-exempt employee is an individual who is paid an hourly wage for the provided service. In other words, an exempt employee is normally not eligible for overtime, while a non-exempt employee is almost always eligible for overtime pay. In 2004, federal legislation was passed by congress and subsequently signed by the President that applied tougher rules to the issue of overtime pay, extending overtime eligibility to certain exempt positions at lower pay levels, and extending additional overtime opportunities to hourly non-exempt employees. Historically, the club industry has tried to create exempt positions, in an effort to avoid having to pay overtime, a practice still carried out by some smaller independent clubs. In most large independent clubs and multiple-club operations, however, the line between exempt and non-exempt employees is very clear. Figure 15.2 provides a basic overview of the factors that delineate exempt from non-exempt employees.

The Position Players in Health/Fitness Clubs

The health/fitness club industry requires a diverse array of talent to deliver the experiences that members desire, expect, need, and deserve. As such, clubs must have employees who have an appropriate blend of social/relationship skills and technical expertise. Because the services that clubs provide cover such a broad spectrum of experiences, a vast pool of talent with expertise in a broad range of services is required. Figures 15.3 to 15.5 detail the key positions in the industry and offer a brief synopsis of the responsibilities of each of those positions.

As figures 15.3 to 15.5 illustrate, the health/fitness club industry involves a multiplicity of positions. While the various positions in these Figures are detailed in general terms and responsibilities, club operators can decide for themselves whether to develop positions that are consistent with the aforementioned

Historically, the club industry has tried to create exempt positions, in an effort to avoid having to pay overtime, a practice still carried out by some smaller independent clubs.

Position	Description
General manager	Oversees the entire operations of a club, with responsibility for all aspects of the club including membership, accounting, and all operational departments
Operations manager	Usually found in large club operations. Supervises the operating departments (front desk, house maintenance, pro shop, pools, etc.)
Sales manager	Usually found in larger clubs. Responsible for managing the sales staff and the sales efforts
Fitness director	Oversees the employees and activities of the fitness department, which includes personal training, fitness floor, and group exercise.
Tennis director	Oversees the employees and activities of the tennis department, often including programming, pro shop, and related tennis activities
Maintenance director	Found in most clubs. Oversees both maintenance and housekeeping employees and activities. In some clubs, also has responsibility for locker rooms and grounds.
Food and beverage director	In clubs with an F&B function, oversees all aspects of the food and beverage operation, including the employees and activities of the kitchen and dining areas

Figure 15.3. Selected examples of typical exempt positions in the health/fitness club industry

Position	Description
Activity/program director	Found in larger clubs. Responsible for coordinating all club activities and programs and the employees involved in those endeavors
Youth director	In clubs with extensive youth programming. Oversees the employees and activities involved in the youth department
Personal-training director	A mainstay of clubs with large personal-training programs. Oversees the personal trainers and personal-training program
Group-exercise director	Normally a part-time position, but in large clubs is often a full-time position. Oversees the group-exercise instructors and programs
Aquatics director	In clubs with a large aquatic program. Oversees the pool and aquatic employees and the aquatic programs and activities
Controller	In clubs with large accounting departments. Oversees the accounting department employees and the activities of the accounting department

Figure 15.4. Selected examples of club positions that could be either exempt or non-exempt employees in the health/fitness club industry, depending on the state and federal laws and regulations involving wage and hour requirements for employees in a particular geographic area

Position	Description
Aquatic/swim instructor	Provides swimming instruction for members and guests on individual and group basis
Personal trainer	Provides fitness instruction and coaching to members for a fee
Fitness instructor	Provides supervision of the fitness floor, general orientation of members to the fitness centers' equipment and programs, and some personal instruction
Group-exercise instructor	Teaches group-oriented exercise and fitness programs for members and guests
Front-desk staff	Works the front desk. Greets members, monitors usage, answers phones, disseminates club information, and schedules appointments for club services
Accountant/bookkeeper	Handles the basic accounting functions at clubs, including payroll, billing, accounts payable, and accounts receivable.
Maintenance/housecleaning	Provides cleaning, housekeeping, and general maintenance for the club. In many clubs, also handles the basic laundry functions as well.
Locker room	In clubs with large locker rooms, provides the general care and housekeeping of the locker rooms, but also greets members and delivers services, such as shoe shines, laundry, etc.
Child care/nursery	Provides supervision of the youth areas, including the nursery activities, but not licensed day care.
Tennis professional/instructor	Provides individual and group tennis instruction to members and guests. Also supervises leagues, mixers, camps, etc.
Activity instructors	Specialized professionals who provide individual or group instruction/coaching in their respective areas, including the martial arts, gymnastics, squash, racquetball, etc.
Massage therapists	Are professionals who are licensed by the state to provide massage therapy. Can also provide other spa services covered by their training and licensing.
Estheticians	Are professionals who are licensed to provide spa services such as manicures, pedicures, and facials.
Food-and-beverage service staff/waiters	Provide service to members and guests in the food-and-beverage area. May include waiters and bartenders.
Kitchen staff/cooks	Provide the cooking services
Pilates/yoga instructor	Specialized instructors with advanced certifications to instruct Pilates and yoga on either an individual or group basis
Lifeguard	Proves supervision of the pool and aquatic areas. Responsible for member/guest safety. May also have basic pool operational responsibilities.

Figure 15.5. Selected examples of non-exempt positions in the health/fitness club industry

descriptions or make adjustments in the various job specifications and define
the positions in slightly different ways.

Position	Description
Chief Executive Officer (CEO)	The CEO is the leader of the company and responsible for establishing the strategic direction of the company, serving as the public face of the company, involved with the company board, and often actively engaged in the new business development of the company. The CFO, CDO, CIO, and possibly one other position will report to the CEO.
Chief Operating Officer (COO)	The COO position and the position of President are often one in the same. The President/ COO takes responsibility for overseeing all aspects of the day-to-day operations of the business, with direct leadership over the levels of management supporting the clubs.
Chief Financial Officer (CFO)	The CFO is responsible for the financial aspects of the business, including cash management, budgeting, financing, financial reporting, etc. The CFO also works closely with the financial stockholders of the business.
Director of Marketing and Sales Vice President or higher position	The majority of multiple-club operations have an individual who oversees the marketing and sales efforts of the company. This individual will normally provide strategic direction to the company's marketing and sales efforts and guide the systems used in marketing and sales.
Director of Human Resources Vice-President or higher position	This individual will normally oversee all aspects of the company's human capital, including employee recruitment and selection, employee development and training, employee benefits, employee resources, etc.
Chief Information Officer (CIO) Senior Vice President or higher position	The CIO is responsible for the technology systems and support in the company. This position is involved in both the strategic direction of the company as it relates to technology, but also the oversight of all the employees who support the technology needs of the business.
Chief Development Officer (CDO) Senior Vice President or higher position	The CDO is responsible for all aspects of new business development. In many multiple-club operations, this position oversees new business, acquisitions, leasing, and construction.
Regional Operations Director or Vice-President of Operations	Multiple-club operations that have a large number of clubs typically assign a freestanding manager who has direct responsibility for the operations of a set group of clubs. Normally, the regional position will oversee between six and 12 clubs, with the mangers of the clubs reporting directly to that position.
Regional Membership Sales Director	The regional membership sales person usually reports directly to the vice-president of operations (the regional operations director) and indirectly to the director or vice president of Marketing and Sales. This position is responsible for sales management for a designated group of clubs, including supporting all corporate initiatives, as well as assisting in the recruiting and training of club sales staff.
Regional Controllers	The Regional Controller normally reports to either the CFO or the Vice-President of Operations. These individuals are responsible for supporting the club's accounting and bookkeeping staff, as well as assisting in financial reporting for the respective regions of clubs.

Figure 15.6. Selected examples of exempt offsite positions in multiple-club operations

Offsite Position Employees in Multiple Club Operations

With the continued growth of the health/fitness club industry, multiple-club operators represent close to 50% of the industry at the present time. The positions of accountability in these multiple-club operations are somewhat similar to those that exist in independent clubs at the club level. On the other hand, when the offsite support of these clubs is considered, the dynamics of employee accountability differ considerably. For example, most multiple-club operations usually allocate between three-and-eight percent of their total revenues to non-club or offsite overhead positions. Figure 15.6, while not inclusive, presents an overview of the offsite positions that most commonly exist in multiple-club operations.

> **Most multiple-club operations usually allocate between three-and-eight percent of their total revenues to non-club or offsite overhead positions.**

Compensation for Various Positions in the Health/Fitness Club Industry

The degree to which a club can attract and retain great employees is, in large part, dependent upon the package of compensation and benefits it provides. Figures 15.7 and 15.8 illustrate the average compensation levels for both exempt and non-exempt positions in health/fitness clubs.

Position	Base Salary			Total Compensation		
	Average	25th Percentile	75th Percentile	Average	25th Percentile	75th Percentile
GeneralManager	$60,307	$41,000	$75,000	$71,224	$50,000	$85,500
Sales Director	$33,150	$23,875	$42,000	$44,517	$31,375	$53,615
Membership Sales	$20,367	$12,740	$24,500	$34,807	$24,819	$38,900
Fitness Director	$36,136	$27,500	$42,000	$43,116	$32,000	$50,000
Group Exercise Director	$27,938	$20,000	$34,250	$30,984	$23,500	$36,000
Tennis Director	$33,032	$18,000	$40,000	$64,578	$44,625	$85,000
Program Manager	$33,651	$27,250	$41,125	$39,522	$29,250	$47,100
Controller	$46,631	$34,625	$56,457	$49,119	$35,000	$62,250
Front Desk Supervisor	$25,886	$20,000	$32,000	$27,608	$21,375	$32,520
Aquatics Director	$28,242	$20,500	$33,750	$30,924	$23,765	$35,840
Children's Director	$28,457	$21,500	$35,000	$31,881	$24,000	$36,700
Maintenance Director	$35,883	$27,625	$41,750	$37,938	$29,000	$44,750

Figure 15.7. Average salaried compensation and benefits across all club types—exempt employees (based on *IHRSA's 2003 Compensation and Benefits Survey*)

Position	Full Time			Part Time		
	Average	25th Percentile	75th Percentile	Average	25th Percentile	75th Percentile
Aquatic Instructor	$15.27	$9.38	$18.50	$14.60	$9.09	$17.56
Personal Trainer	$21.72	$13.00	$28.00	$20.63	$14.00	$26.04
Fitness Instructor	$11.47	$9.00	$12.00	$10.73	$8.00	$11.00
Tennis Pro	$25.47	$20.00	$30.00	$22.72	$16.75	$28.25
Group ExerciseInstructor	$23.58	$16.75	$30.00	$21.23	$15.00	$25.00
Pilates Instructor	$31.60	$25.00	$40.00	$26.94	$20.00	$32.75
Yoga Instructor	$32.52	$22.50	$40.00	$26.22	$18.00	$30.00
Front Desk	$8.85	$7.94	$10.00	$7.98	$7.00	$8.75
Bookkeeper	$13.81	$11.12	$16.25	$13.26	$9.00	$14.62
House Cleaning	$10.35	$8.00	$12.00	$9.03	$7.50	$10.00
Child Care	$8.28	$7.00	$9.00	$7.47	$6.70	$8.00

Figure 15.8. Average hourly compensation and benefits across all club types—non-exempt employees (based on *IHRSA's 2003 Compensation and Benefits Survey*)

With regard to exempt employees, most of these individuals are paid a base salary and incentive compensation. The incentive portion of the compensation tends to be position-specific, ranging from 48% of the overall compensation for tennis directors, 41% for sales representatives, 25% for sales directors, 16% for fitness directors, and 15% for managers to five-to-six percent for front-desk managers and controllers. The incentive portion normally consists of either a commission-based incentive (sales representatives, tennis directors, fitness directors) or a bonus, based on achieving predetermined performance targets (manager, front desk manager, controller). Ideally, all exempt employees should have a total compensation package that includes both a base salary and incentive compensation. Those exempt employees who are in sales-related positions, such as membership, tennis, or fitness, should have an incentive compensation that is tied to their sales performance.

Ideally, all exempt employees should have a total compensation package that includes both a base salary and incentive compensation.

Position	Basis of Commission		Amount of Commission	
	% Revenue	Set Fee	%	Fixed
Personal trainer	68%	32%	52.5%	$26
Tennis/racquet pro	63%	37%	66%	$26

Figure 15.9. Average commissions in the health/fitness club industry for personal trainers and tennis/racquet professionals

With regard to non-exempt employees, most of these employees are paid an hourly wage, with very few being eligible for incentive compensation. Three categories of non-exempt employees exist in the industry who are normally paid on a commission structure: personal trainers, massage therapists/estheticians, and racquet/tennis professionals. These positions are considered commissioned, because the services provided directly drive incremental revenue, which, in turn, is directly impacted by the sales performance of the individual employee. The *IHRSA 2003 Industry Compensation and Benefits Survey* reported the following average commissions for personal trainers and tennis/racquet professionals (refer to Figure 15.9):

Although IHRSA did not collect data on the compensation level for massage therapists or estheticians, the International Spa Association (ISPA) reports the following information concerning the compensation of these positions:

- On average, 37% of the massage therapists earn between $30,000 and $50,000 annually, while 32% earn between $20,000 and $30,000. These earnings are based on the therapists working full time. It should be noted that the average massage therapist earns a commission equal to 40% to 60% of the massage fee.

- On average, 40% of the estheticians earn $30,000 to $50,000, while the earnings of 33% range from $20,000 to $30,000. Estheticians are paid a commission that is similar to that earned by massage therapists.

As a rule, the compensation package that a club offers its employees is based upon a number of factors, including the club's geographic location, its market position, and, most importantly, the level of education and experience it expects its employees to have.

As a rule, the compensation package that a club offers its employees is based upon a number of factors, including the club's geographic location, its market position, and, most importantly, the level of education and experience it expects its employees to have.

Benefit	Fully Paid	Partially Paid	Not Provided
Medical – employee	25%	63%	12%
Medical – family	9%	39%	52%
Life insurance	34%	18%	48%
Dental insurance – employee	17%	44%	40%
Optical – employee	10%	31%	61%
Long-term disability	19%	14%	67%
Educational assistance	9%	44%	47%
Employee discounts	25%	55%	21%
Child care	14%	27%	59%
Retirement	12%	16%	72%

Figure 15.10. Average benefits for exempt employees

Benefit	Fully Paid	Partially Paid	Not Provided
Medical – employee	8%	49%	43%
Medical – family	1%	31%	68%
Life insurance	18%	15%	67%
Dental insurance – employee	4%	36%	59%
Optical – employee	2%	25%	74%
Long-term disability	10%	10%	81%
Educational assistance	5%	35%	60%
Employee discounts	19%	48%	33%
Child care	9%	23%	68%
Retirement	8%	11%	81%

Figure 15.11. Average benefits for non-exempt employees

As a rule, the health/fitness club industry is not as generous with benefits as are other industries, either at the management level or the hourly, non-exempt employee level.

Benefits Provided in the Health/Fitness Club Industry

As discussed previously, benefits are second only to wages in terms of their ability to attract top-performing employees. The primary benefits offered by most club operators include: medical, life insurance, dental, vision, short-term disability, long-term disability, employee discounts for services, paid vacations, and retirement. Some clubs also include additional benefits in the benefits package for their employees, such as continuing education support and even child-care assistance. Figures 15.10 and 15.11 detail several of the major benefits that are offered to both exempt and non-exempt employees in the health/fitness club industry.

As a rule, the health/fitness club industry is not as generous with benefits as are other industries, either at the management level or the hourly, non-exempt employee level. As Figure 15.10 illustrates, the management level, life insurance, medical benefits, and employee discounts are the most commonly offered fully paid benefits in the club industry, while employee discounts and

Position	High School	Associate's	Bachelor's	Master's	PhD
Manager	6%	8%	64%	21%	1%
Sales manager	14%	12%	65%	8%	0%
Fitness director	8%	9%	61%	22%	1%
Group exercise director	22%	13%	57%	7%	1%
Tennis director	6%	6%	83%	4%	2%
Controller	14%	10%	54%	18%	4%

Figure 15.12. Average level of education in the health/fitness club industry – exempt positions

dental benefits are next in line. For non-exempt, hourly employees, Figure 15-11 shows that the most significant fully paid benefits that the industry provides to this particular group of employees are employee discounts and life insurance.

Education and Skill Competency Required of Health/Fitness Club Professionals

The health/fitness club industry is a somewhat unique business when it comes to the required educational and experience competencies of its employees. Some of the positions in the industry that were described earlier in this chapter require a relatively high level of academic qualifications (manager, accountant, fitness director), while others place more focus on the more non-traditional forms of education, such as certification (personal trainer, group exercise instructor, massage therapist). Still other positions involve a greater emphasis on work experience. The degree to which health/fitness club operators establish high academic/certification or experience standards will determine, to a large extent, their position in both the marketplace and the mindset of the customers that they are attempting to serve. Figures 15.12 and 15.13 provide an overview of the average level of education possessed by specific positions in the industry.

The degree to which health/fitness club operators establish high academic/certification or experience standards will determine, to a large extent, their position in both the marketplace and the mindset of the customers that they are attempting to serve.

It is evident that, for most exempt positions, the health/fitness club industry places a relatively high degree of importance on having at least a four-year college degree. As Figure 15.12 illustrates, at least 65% to 85% of the exempt professionals have either a four-year degree or higher. The highest level of education in the industry is possessed by those employees who serve as fitness directors, with over 20% having at least a master's degree. On the other hand, with regard to the non-exempt professional positions that provide members with instruction in fitness, recreation, or sports-related activities, the existence of a college degree in these employees falls dramatically. Somewhat amazingly, in this particular category of employees, tennis pros are most likely to have a four-year degree, while less than 40% of fitness instructors and less than 30% of personal trainers have attained a comparable level of education.

Position	Bachelor's	Certifications			
		ACSM	ACE	AFAA	Other
Personal trainer	24%	14%	39%	14%	9.5%
Fitness instructor	37%	8%	23%	17%	15%
Tennis pro	39%	0%	0%	0%	USPTA, PTR
Group exercise instructor	9%	8%	40%	35%	8%
Yoga instructor	8%	6%	19%	28%	40%

Figure 15.13. Average level of education in the health/fitness club industry – professional non-exempt positions

❑ *Certification and Education for Fitness Instructors, Group-Exercise Instructors, and Personal Trainers.* Personal trainers, fitness instructors, and group-exercise instructors are the positions within the health/fitness club industry that provide members and guests with instruction, counsel, and advice in fitness- and health-related issues. As such, these non-exempt professionals typically are required to have a basic understanding of exercise physiology, human movement, healthy lifestyle, behavioral change, and nutrition. While the knowledge base that these professionals need is relatively high, the actual practices of the industry often fall way short of requiring these professionals to truly demonstrate that they possess the education and training attendant to such knowledge. As shown in Figure 15.13, less than 40% of personal trainers, fitness instructors, and group-exercise instructors have any four-year college degree, let alone a four-year college degree in an area of study related to either fitness or exercise science.

To compensate for the industry's less-than-emphatic emphasis on these professionals having a college education, the industry has moved towards a certification-based model of competency. In the certification model of competency, fitness professionals are required to demonstrate their overall level of competency by successfully passing the certification requirements for one or more of the various fitness-professional domains (e.g., group-exercise instructor, personal trainer, lifestyle, and weight-management counselor, etc.). As of 2004, over 100 certifications for personal trainers and close to as many certifications for various types of group-exercise instructors existed. In most instances, these certification programs require prospective fitness professionals to sit for either a written exam only or both a written exam and practical exam. As a rule, most of these programs accord certification on those candidates who achieve a score greater than 70% on the required examinations. Once certification is achieved, most programs require that the professionals maintain their level of certification by annually earning a predetermined number of continuing education credits.

A number of state legislatures have begun to push for either licensure or registration of personal trainers.

In 2003, the International Health, Racquet, and Sportsclub Association (IHRSA) set a benchmark, a much-needed standard for the certification of health/fitness professionals by proclaiming that, effective January 1, 2006, it would only recognize certifications that had third-party accreditation (e.g. the National Organization for Competency Assurance [NOCA] and its accreditation arm, the National Commission for Certifying Agencies [NCCA]). A direct link must be demonstrated between the certification offered and the competency requirements of a particular fitness position. IHRSA's actions were a necessary first step in bringing greater credibility to these fitness professional positions. Concurrent with IHRSA's position, a number of state legislatures have begun to push for either licensure or registration of personal trainers. Eventually (hopefully) the combined efforts of IHRSA, the certifying organizations, and state governments should bring about a greater level of demonstrable competency in each of the basic fitness professional positions in the industry.

Certifying Group	Sampling of Certifications	Description
American College of Sports Medicine (ACSM)	Fitness Instructor Exercise Specialist Personal Trainer Clinical Exercise Physiologist	ACSM certifications have been in existence for over 30 years. Its certifications are developed by physiologists, health-care specialists, and physicians who are active members of the college. It offers both preventative tract and clinical tract certifications. As a rule, the certifications tend not to be for entry-level fitness professionals.
American Council on Exercise (ACE)	Group Fitness Instructor Personal Trainer Lifestyle and Weight Management Consultant Clinical Exercise Specialist	ACE certifications have been in existence for over 15 years. ACE certifies more professionals than any other agency in the fitness industry. ACE is an industry leader in promoting exercise. Its certifications are targeted for entry-level fitness professionals.
Aerobic and Fitness Association America (AFAA)	Primary Group Exercise Personal Fitness Trainer Fitness Practitioner	AFAA certifications have been in existence of for over 25 years. AFAA at one time certified more group-exercise professionals than any other organization. Its offerings represent a front-line certification for entry-level fitness professionals.
National Academy of Sports Medicine (NASM)	Group Trainer Personal Trainer Performance Enhancement Specialist Sports Fitness Specialist	NASM has been in existence for over 10 years. Its certification program has a physical therapy/athletic trainer focus that places more emphasis on the instruction of modalities for flexibility and muscular strength and endurance. Its certifications are geared for both entry-level professionals and higher levels.
National Strength and Conditioning Association	Certified Strength and Conditioning Specialists (CSCS) Certified Personal Trainer	NSCA's first certification was awarded over 20 years ago. NSCA's initial certification efforts focused on resistance training and conditioning for athletes. By the early 1990s, it created the personal trainer certification, which focused the skills of prescriptive resistance training for average people.
Cooper Clinic	Physical Fitness Specialist Specialty Certifications for Biomechanics of Resistance Training, Optimal Performance Training, and Pre/post Natal Fitness Instructor	The Cooper Clinic and Aerobic Activity Center, founded by Dr. Kenneth Cooper in the 1970s, has been offering a variety of professional certifications since its inception. The certifications range from fitness instructor specialty certifications in such areas as back care, resistance training, weight management, etc.

Figure 15.14. Examples of certifying agencies in the health/fitness club industry

As previously discussed, the health/fitness industry currently has more than 200 certification programs for fitness professionals. Figure 15-14 presents an overview of the six more successful and well-known certification programs for professionals in the health/fitness club industry.

It is important to note that it is the responsibility of club operators to determine what educational and certification expectations and minimal standards that they want to establish for the professionals in their club. Whatever levels they establish should be based on a clear understanding of the market's requirements in this regard and the standard of care demonstrated by the industry both as a whole and in their particular area.

Organizational Alignment and Structure in Individual Health/Fitness Clubs

It is important that independent club operators utilize and understand the various types of organizational structures that can effectively sustain accountability throughout the organization. The organizational structure a club chooses to employ is critical to establishing the flow of accountability and information that is essential if it is to achieve and maintain the desired level of profitability. Toward that end, an appropriate organizational structure helps to clarify the role of each employee, both in terms of personal and team responsibility. Figures 15.15 and 15.16 illustrate two different organizational structures that an individual club could utilize. Figure 15.15 depicts an organizational structure for a purely fitness club, while Figure 15.16 portrays a structure for a multipurpose club that offers racquet sports and aquatics.

The examples in Figures 15.15 and 15.16 are representative of the most common organizational structures that are utilized by individual health/fitness clubs. It is important to consider the following three critical success factors when designing a club's organizational structure:

> An appropriate organizational structure helps to clarify the role of each employee, both in terms of personal and team responsibility.

❏ *Drive accountability close to the member by maintaining a flat organizational structure.* In other words, the number of organizational layers between the member and the manager should be kept at a minimum. In the two aforementioned organizational structures, there are instances when the customer is only two layers away from the manager (sales) and other instances where the member is three layers away (personal trainers). All factors considered, the flatter the club's organizational chart, the closer the club brings accountability to the member. To achieve this objective, the club's employees need to be fully empowered.

❏ *Limit direct reports for any supervisor.* Research in organizational management has determined that supervisors can be most effective if they have no more than six direct reports and preferably less. If the club has a

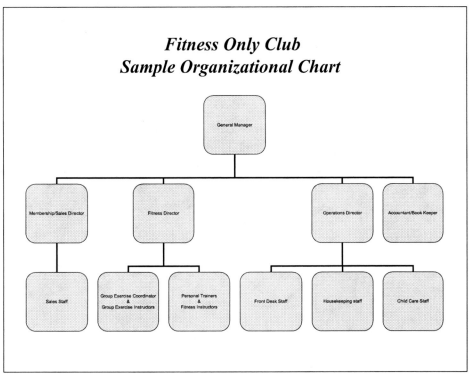

Figure 15.15. A sample fitness-club organization chart

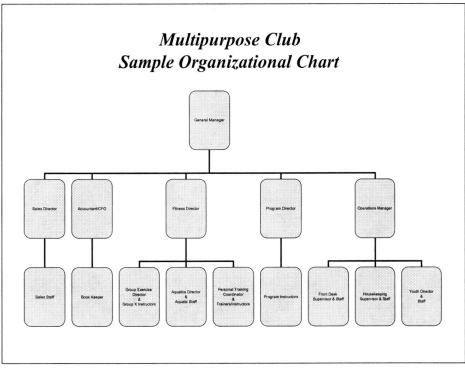

Figure 15.16. A sample multipurpose-club organization chart

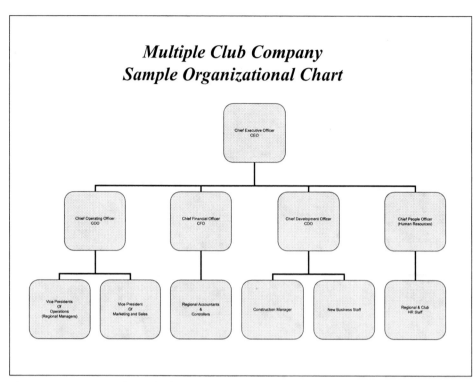

Figure 15.17. A sample multiple-club organizational chart.

structure that requires leaders/supervisors to have too many direct reports, then it will find that these leaders/supervisors are far less effective in creating a high-performing, empowered environment for their direct reports.

❑ *Don't create titles; create accountabilities.* All too often, club management creates organizational positions to provide reward and recognition for employees. While this practice might seem like a good idea, an organizational structure should be built around the roles and the accountabilities needed to drive the club's success. As a result, all factors considered, it is often better to create fewer positions rather than more.

All factors considered, it is often better to create fewer positions rather than more.

If club operators take the aforementioned three factors into consideration, they will find it easier to create an organizational structure that supports their business objectives, without placing excessive financial and communicative strain on the organization.

Organizational Alignment and Structure in a Multiple Club Operation

For multiple-club operations, the alignment of organizational accountabilities and positions is a sensitive issue. Since the cost of offsite overhead in a multiple-club operation can place a significant strain on club earnings (between three-and-eight percent of revenues), a need exists to create an organizational structure that brings accountability as close to the club employees as possible and at the lowest possible cost, while also providing the logistical and strategic resources that are essential to support the operations of each club. The three critical success factors previously detailed for establishing the organizational structure for a single club also apply to the organizational structure of a multiple-club operation. Figure 15.17 provides an example of a multiple-club organization chart. This sample organizational chart is representative of a typical multiple-club operation, with only the number of direct reports varying, depending upon the size of the company. A multiple-club operator, such as Western Athletic Clubs, that has 10 clubs, will have a smaller and flatter organizational chart than either a company like Lifetime Fitness, that has over 40 clubs or a much larger company like 24 Hour Fitness, that has over 300 clubs. It is important to note that as the number of clubs within the organization grows, the more organizational layers tend to appear. Accordingly, while the Western Athletic Clubs may only have one or two regional operational managers, 24 Hour Fitness might need as many as 15 to 20.

It is important to note that as the number of clubs within the organization grows, the more organizational layers tend to appear.

16

Building and Leading a Successful Health/Fitness Club Team

Chapter Objectives

In order to be better prepared to build a great team, it is essential for club managers to be aware of and sensitive to the key factors attendant to the four "E's": expectations, equipping, encouragement, and evaluation.

According to the article, the "Service Profit Chain," written by Leonard Schlessinger, profit is driven by great service to the customer, which, in turn, is driven by a great employee team that is the recipient of great internal service from management. In that regard, this chapter examines the process of creating an exceptional health/fitness club team. Initially, the four "E's" of developing an extraordinary team are discussed. Next, the role of recruiting and selecting team players is reviewed. Then, the underlying principles and concepts attendant to effective leadership are detailed. Finally, the chapter addresses two very important issues: determining job descriptions and developing compensation agreements that provide an incentive for high-performing team players.

The Four "E's" of Building a Great Team

The process of building a great employee team is one of the most important responsibilities that management has. The process of team development is neither an easy undertaking nor a short one. Rather, it is a task that requires an understanding of the critical stepping-stones that need to be laid in order to build a strong team foundation and provide the basic roots that are needed for a continual evolution and empowerment of the team. The four "E's" is a relatively easy-to-remember tool that outlines the four key steps in the team-building process. In order to be better prepared to build a great team, it is essential for club managers to be aware of and sensitive to the key factors attendant to the four "E's": expectations, equipping, encouragement, and evaluation.

❏ *Expectations—Setting the Course for the Team.* The club's first step in building its team of employees is to establish clear expectations for both individual and team performance. Without clear expectations, individuals and teams will not have the direction that they need to be successful. Among the components that are essential for creating clear expectations in that regard are the following:

- *Provide each team member with an introduction to the club's core values and philosophies*. These values and philosophies serve as the core foundation of the decision-making process. Families, relationships, cultures, and businesses should have a set of common values that each member respects and lives by. If the club wants its team to be strong, it must ensure that the team is values-oriented.

- *Provide each team member with a job model, a copy of the club's organizational chart, and a listing of each individual's personal annual performance goals*. The job model should detail the specific accountabilities of the employee's position, as well as the manner in which that position interacts with the other members of the team. In addition, all employees should be given a copy of their personal performance goals that are updated on at least a six-month cycle. Collectively, these documents should help eliminate any confusion or misunderstandings concerning each person's accountabilities as either an individual or a team member. The organization chart should help clarify each team player's role and how the team members should interact with each other and work as a single, functioning unit.

- *Have a clear set of employee policies and rules*. While policies and rules can be relatively brief in scope, they play an essential role as a means of helping communicate the expectations of the business concerning employee and team behavior. Together with the club's core values, they set the framework for the behavior of the team.

- *Provide each employee with a personal development plan*. The personal development plan is a relatively simple tool that helps an employee establish a path for professional development. By helping each employee set a course for such growth, the club is facilitating the team's overall development and, at the same time, creating a succession plan that will have team members ready to take on new roles when and if needed.

- *Have regular meetings of the team*. Team meetings are critical to setting and supporting the club's expectations. These meetings should be viewed as an opportunity to reinforce expectations, share achievements, and create new directions. They are also a time to build team trust.

- *Develop new tools to share the club's expectations with the team*. Newsletters, videos, weekly line-ups, and web pages for employees are all methods that can be employed to share the expectations and the performance achievements of a team with its members.

All employees should be given a copy of their personal performance goals that are updated on at least a six-month cycle.

One of the biggest mistakes that club operators can make is to set expectations for their team and then not provide the tools that their employees need to get the job done.

❑ *Equipping the Team Through Education and Growth*. The second step in building a great team is to provide an environment that equips the members of the team to successfully undertake and fulfill the club's expectations. Too many businesses mistakenly assume that once their expectations have been defined, their employees will proceed to successfully achieve them. In reality, the process is not automatic. Rather, club owners and operators should provide the members of their teams with the resources that they need to meet both theirs and the team's expectations. This process is commonly referred to as "equipping the team" and includes the following:

• *Institute an internal formal-education system for all employees*. In this instance, a formal educational program refers to a standardized program that educates all of a club's employees on its values, philosophies, policies, traditions, and basic operating systems. Every new employee and even the tenured employees should go through a formal education system that constantly updates the employee's knowledge of the club's business and expectations. At ClubCorp, this system was called Star Education. All employees were expected to complete the Star Education Program and become certified in their assigned specific area of responsibility.

• *Establish an external continuing-education program for the enhancement of each team member's technical, sales, and people skills*. Beyond its own education system, the club should develop and implement a system that affords its employees the opportunity to pursue continuing education that can help them advance their technical skills, sales skills, and people skills. For fitness employees, this process could involve several measures, such as bringing in outside speakers to discuss technical topics, offering scholarships or shared funds that would enable the fitness professional to attend industry-sponsored workshops, etc. For employees in other areas of interest, this undertaking could involve such steps as bringing in sales trainers or individuals to speak on customer service. The key point to note in this regard is that educational efforts, such as these, can play an important role in developing a strong team.

• *Provide the tools that employees need to do their jobs*. One of the biggest mistakes that club operators can make is to set expectations for their team and then not provide the tools that their employees need to get the job done. In this instance, tools refer to the assets/resources that are essential to completing a particular task. For example, if a piece of equipment is needed to do a job, that resource is provided. By the same token, if a job requires access to certain information, then that information is made available. All factors considered, the most powerful and valuable tool that a team can have is information. Accordingly, the club should ensure that its employees are able to access the information that they need to be able to do their job.

- *Open the communication lines*. Club management should make sure that the club has an open communication process that allows its employees to ask questions of management and share comments with management. The process should also make it relatively easy for management to share ideas, results, and feedback with its employees. As a rule, the greater the degree to which these lines of communication are opened up, the better the flow of information and resources will be between the team and management.

- *Walk the talk*. The axiom that leaders should act in a manner that is consistent with what they espouse has been around for a long time. Many club employees feel that one of the most important tools that the club has to equip them to perform their duties is to know that management is willing to perform those same responsibilities.

❑ *Encouragement—The Fuel of Champions*. The next step in building a great team is to create an environment that encourages employees to take ownership in their own and their team's performance. Such an environment should also reward the club's employees when certain process and outcome goals are achieved. Encouragement is normally a blend of strategies, including:

- *Have a formal employee-recognition program*. Formal recognition programs are an effective method for fostering an environment of reward and encouragement. The focus of a formal employee-recognition program should be to reward employees for performing in a manner that is consistent with the club's core values and delivering upon the team's expectations. At ClubCorp, this program was called Star Recognition, and they rewarded employees on the basis of how well they delivered on the company's values and philosophies. Other clubs undertake efforts that attempt to provide a similar level of recognition, for example employee-of-the-month programs, employee-of-the-week programs, etc. Some key elements of an employee-recognition program include:

    ✓ The program should focus on objective measures so that it is consistent from one employee to the other.

    ✓ The program should be designed to encourage employees to deliver on the values and standards of the business.

    ✓ The program should have employee ownership, such as an employee committee that oversees its conduct.

    ✓ The rewards provided by the program should be relevant to the employees, not merely what management feels that the employees would value.

    ✓ The delivery of the program should be consistent.

> **The focus of a formal employee-recognition program should be to reward employees for performing in a manner that is consistent with the club's core values and delivering upon the team's expectations.**

- *Leaders must be cheerleaders.* According to Ken Blanchard, in his best-selling book, *The One-Minute Manager*, management should catch employees doing things right. As a rule, the best encouragement that employees can receive is the personal recognition that comes from a leader recognizing their efforts and providing them with a thank you and job well done. When employees talk about encouraging environments, they often speak about the personal recognition that they receive from their managers/leaders. Accordingly, leaders should make it a habit to walk the club, looking for employees who are doing great things and then letting those employees know how much their efforts are appreciated. Another key factor is to make sure that other employees see the encouragement provided by management.

- *Have recognition meetings.* Another valuable tool that the club can utilize to provide encouragement is to hold open meetings with its employees, during which the results of the club's performance are shared and discussed. Sharing the results in an open setting and letting the employees know how much the club values their efforts creates an open and honest team environment, which is a critical factor in encouraging employees to do their best.

- *Avoid finger pointing.* One of the easiest approaches to creating an environment of encouragement is to foster a workplace that does not condone finger pointing and blaming. Instead, it fosters a workplace focus on solutions. In that regard, leadership should cultivate an environment where employees are not afraid to make mistakes. Rather, employees should be willing to take risks and should have a sense of ownership toward addressing key issues, because they realize that no blame will be placed as long as they act in a professional manner.

❑ *Evaluate the Expected.* The final step in the four "E's" is evaluation. If the club wants its employees to succeed both individually and collectively, it needs to establish an evaluation system that measures what is expected of its employees and provides constructive feedback for their continuous growth. Among the key evaluation tools that a club should consider in this regard are the following:

If the club wants its employees to succeed both individually and collectively, it needs to establish an evaluation system that measures what is expected of its employees and provides constructive feedback for their continuous growth.

- *Create objective performance evaluations for each employee.* Each employee should have a performance evaluation that is tailored to the specific performance goals set forth in their job model. The evaluation tool should be specific to each employee and include the measurement of both the personal goals and team goals in which the individual employee has a role.

- *Evaluate at least twice a year.* Performance evaluations are most effective if they are done at least twice annually. The longer the club waits between performance evaluations, the less likely it will be able to create a link in the employee's mind between what the club expects and what feedback is being provided to each employee.

- *Make it a habit to evaluate daily.* Leaders need to actively engage in the evaluation process by walking around the club. If they observe behavior that warrants their feedback, the best time to provide comments of any kind is to do so immediately.

- *Create a business scorecard.* To help facilitate the team's performance, leaders should develop a club business scorecard that every employee can understand. This scorecard should be to help assess team performance, as well as communicate recognition and education. The scorecard can be incorporated as part of every meeting to either recognize the team or educate it. The scorecard should be more than a financial tool. Rather, it should help evaluate the performance of the club's employees against the core values and standards of operation of the business.

- *Never let performance go without recognition, education, and follow-up.* If the club's managerial staff sees good performance, they should make sure that the individual or team is recognized and rewarded. By the same token, if they see performance that falls below their expectations, they should acknowledge it, educate the employee involved about how to improve it, and then follow-up to make sure that the individual's performance has changed appropriately.

One of the biggest challenges in any business, and in particular the club industry, is building a great team.

Recruiting and Selecting the Club's Team

One of the biggest challenges in any business, and in particular the club industry, is building a great team. Before the aforementioned four steps to building a great team can be undertaken, however, the club needs to have the right people as employees. The easiest way to build a great team is to hire great employees, a practice approach that requires a systematic approach to recruiting and selecting the best available employees to serve on the team. In this regard, the following factors apply:

Recruitment

❑ *Develop a Hiring Model and Posting for Each Position.* The first step in recruiting is to create a model of what the employee profile should be. A hiring model is a shortened version of the job model that identifies the values, attitudes, and skills expected for each position.

❑ *Place the Postings/Models in the Appropriate Areas.* When the club is ready to recruit, the club should make sure that it places its hiring models/posting with the right lead sources, including:

- Local two-year and four-year colleges can be excellent sources of employees. If the club is looking for fitness staff, it should contact the college's kinesiology department. On the other hand, if it is looking to hire swim instructors, it should get in touch with the coach of the college's swim team.

- The ad seeking new employees should be posted on the appropriate career-center websites for the respective specialty areas. For example, when the club is seeking to hire fitness staff, the websites of ACSM, ACE, NSCA, and IHRSA would be excellent sources. If massage and spa employees were wanted, the club should contact any institution/entity that might be aware of individuals who would accommodate the club's needs, such as the local massage schools, the American Massage Therapy Association, etc.

- The club should consider creating its own career center website. Companies, such as Tennis Corporation of America, ClubCorp, Wellbridge, Lifetime Fitness, etc., have developed their own recruitment sites.

> **The first step that a club should take when deciding whom to hire is to compare every application and resume, via a checklist, with its hiring model.**

❑ *Develop Internship Programs with Colleges.* Possibly the best recruiting tool is to develop an internship program with local colleges and high schools. By creating internships, the club can provide learning opportunities for those students who have an interest in fitness and health and, at the same time, give the club a chance to evaluate each intern's potential as a future employee. In fact, many of the top club companies in the industry offer internships. These companies report finding that their best employees often are those individuals who have previously served in internships.

❑ *Recruit from Other Service Industries.* If a club is seeking people who have a servant's heart and understand how to work within a hospitality/service business, it should consider recruiting from similar businesses. The recruiter should carry business cards and, if and when they observe a worker whose performance aligns with the club's culture, hand the worker a card and invite that individual to visit the club.

Selection

❑ *Compare Applications and Resumes to the Hiring Model.* The first step that a club should take when deciding whom to hire is to compare every application and resume, via a checklist, with its hiring model. Clubs can subsequently rank the applications and resumes by how closely they align with the hiring model. Performing this step allows the club to limit the number of candidates it takes to the next step of the selection process. Clubs can employ this method to identify those applicants who most closely reflect their hiring model.

❑ *Use Multiple Interviews.* Every candidate under consideration should go through a series of interviews. The first interview should be conducted by the immediate supervisor and should focus on uncovering the basic values, beliefs, attitudes, and skills of the applicant. This first interview can be conducted using a structured interview format and checklist. The goal of the interview should be to evaluate the candidate against a specific model. If the candidate meets the expectations of the first interview, then a second interview should be conducted with multiple members of the team, using a structured format. The second interview should be more detailed than the first and should focus on role-play situations, based on predetermined questions that are designed to be value indicators of success in the club business. If the candidate gets through the second interview successfully, then the third interview should be conducted in a team format with several members of the team present. This interview can be more free-flowing than the other two, because its primary focus is to determine if an appropriate fit exists between the team and the applicant.

❑ *Consider an Industry Profile.* Many club operators employ personality and job-profile surveys that are designed to help compare the candidate's personal profile against the known attitudes and attributes of a successful employee. These profiles are usually available through human-resource organizations and private companies that are focused on profiling new employees. As a rule, these profiles measure such key attributes as leadership, communication, teamwork, work ethic, relationship skills, etc. By comparing the profile of a candidate with the standardized profile of a top-performing employee, the club can obtain a better reading of the candidate's potential for success.

❑ *Only Hire from the Top of the List.* After completing all of the aforementioned steps, the club should develop a list of potential candidates, with the best candidate placed at the top and the others ranked in a priority order. Leaders should make an effort to let their team help compile the rankings. Once the rankings are completed, they should initiate the selection process by contacting the candidate at the top of the list.

Leadership

Leadership has been a topic of discussion for decades. In both large business organizations and small businesses, one of the most common concerns is their perception that they don't have enough good leadership. In fact, this issue is often ranked as the number one perceived weakness in most organizations. Over the years, teachers, scholars, and philosophers have attempted to provide a variety of definitions for leadership and have put forth a seemingly endless abundance of theories on what it takes to be an effective leader. One factor

Over the years, teachers, scholars, and philosophers have attempted to provide a variety of definitions for leadership and have put forth a seemingly endless abundance of theories on what it takes to be an effective leader.

that seems to be a common thread among all the definitions and theories on leadership is that organizations that want to be successful need leaders at all levels of the organization. This section is not intended to provide a detailed description of leadership or any particular style of leadership. Rather, its primary goal is to present an overview of what leadership is, how leadership impacts the club business, and how every employee of a club, from fitness instructors to managers, can develop the basic attributes of leadership.

❑ *The Role of Leaders.* The primary responsibility of leaders is to determine the culture and goals of the business and help establish an environment in which every employee takes ownership in living the culture and achieving the goals. Realistically, an effective leader might be defined as an individual who is able to influence the passion, vision, and commitment of others in order to channel the efforts and talents of individuals who are going separate directions into a cohesive team of employees who are functioning as a single unit. Among the roles that leaders most often assume in an organization, such as a health/fitness club, are the following:

- To establish a vision and culture for the business. This role is most often assumed by the primary club leader (e.g., owner or manager). The vision and the culture serve as the foundation for the success that the business achieves.

- To communicate the culture and vision of the club every day. This role should not just involve the club's top leader, but also every employee who interacts with and has responsibility for the behavior of another employee.

- To develop a team of employees who will take ownership in a common vision and goal by seeing how working together benefits both the individual and the team.

- To demonstrate trust in their team and, in return, gain the respect of their team.

- To build consensus when appropriate, but also to make tough decisions when they are needed.

- To see themselves as servants for their team by providing a vision, the support, and the resources that their team needs to achieve the club's vision and goals.

- To set the course, provide guidance along the way, remove barriers, build bridges, leverage talent, recognize the need for change, and hold people and teams accountable for their actions.

- Challenge the status quo by seeking to identify and execute business strategies that can enhance the efficiency and quality of their business.

Within every club, these roles should be assumed by those employees who are entrusted to work with other employees.

> The primary responsibility of leaders is to determine the culture and goals of the business and help establish an environment in which every employee takes ownership in living the culture and achieving the goals.

❑ *The Qualities of Leaders.* Great leaders who can take on the aforementioned roles and successfully execute them often exhibit certain basic qualities, including:

- *Dare to be different.* Daring to be different involves capitalizing on whatever is unique about the individual in such a way that it positively impacts the business. Having attributes (e.g., passion, creativity, vision, imagination, etc.) that can be leveraged to the advantage of the business are an important trait of all leaders.

- *Emotional intelligence.* Great leaders have the ability to sense what is occurring in the business environment around them. This instinct does not emanate from the ability to analyze the impact of relevant numbers on the situation. Rather, it involves having the ability to sense the soft data and the emotions of the people and then being able to interpret that information to the benefit of the organization. Leaders with emotional intelligence are sensitive to the emotions of their staff members and are able to openly discuss these emotions with these individuals as they relate to the work environment. Emotional intelligence also requires the ability to listen without prejudice, to hear what is actually being communicated.

- *Empathy with strength.* Great leaders have the ability to communicate through their actions to their employees that they care about them. Empathetic leaders demonstrate genuine care about the members of the team and are legitimately interested in the work that their employees do. This empathy evolves not only from respect and trust, but also from the ability to deal with each employee in an honest and ethical manner.

- *Reveal their weaknesses.* Great leaders realize that all other factors being equal, they can enhance the level of trust in the organization by being willing to show their weaknesses to other individuals in the organization. Revealing weakness involves the ability to let their team know that they are willing to take accountability for their actions and behaviors, rather than hiding them. Exposing their own personal limitations also enables leaders to surround themselves with people whose strengths can counterbalance the weaknesses exhibited by the leaders. In other words, leaders who are willing to lay bare their weaknesses are not threatened by the strengths of others. Instead, they are able and prefer to utilize the strengths of others to strengthen the team.

- *Manage systems, not people.* Leaders understand that people manage themselves. Leaders understand that their job is to create and support systems that enable people not only to manage themselves, but also to achieve the expectations set forth for them by the business. A leader ensures that systems are in place that will allow the goals of the

Leaders understand that people manage themselves. Leaders understand that their job is to create and support systems that enable people not only to manage themselves, but also to achieve the expectations set forth for them by the business.

business to be accomplished and then empowers employees to leverage those systems for the benefit of the organization.

- *Let the people lead.* Leaders understand that if figuratively they get out of the way and let the members of the team lead, then everyone will be successful. In other words, effective leaders are able to get everyone to take ownership of the business. They are also able to establish a work environment that enables the individual skill-sets of each employee to link together. In essence, each employee becomes a leader of the team's other employees, with each person headed in the same direction. As such, the process involves creating leadership disciples.

Great managers always seem to know their facility's numbers.

❑ *Characteristics of Great Managers.* Great managers build great teams and produce great results. As a rule, great managers in the health/fitness club industry possess the following characteristics:

- *They plan for success.* One attribute that all great managers have is that they have a plan for success at their club. In other words, they develop a comprehensive plan that identifies specific objectives for their business, including quantitative benchmarks for such areas as membership growth, revenue growth, expense control, people development, marketing, community development, and facility enhancement. Each objective is stated in relatively simple terms with clearly definable, measurable targets and is subsequently communicated to all members of that person's team. The plan includes a detailed financial budget that delineates specific financial targets for each aspect of the business. As such, great managers leave nothing to chance.

- *They know their numbers.* Great managers always seem to know their facility's numbers. In other words, they know what the budgeted targets are for every possible area of importance in their club and are aware of how well their facility is doing with regard to these key parameters on a daily, weekly, and monthly basis. Want to know what their club's membership retention level is—just ask them. Want to know what their facility's payroll percentage is—just ask them.

- *They are coaches and educators.* One of the most notable characteristics of great managers is how much time that they spend with their "people." The employees of great managers tend to speak very highly of them, particularly how they have helped them grow both professionally and personally. These manager-coaches make sure that all of their employees know the club's business plan, ensure that employees know they care about them, and expend substantial time teaching and counseling their employees. Great managers educate, motivate, and inspire their employees.

- *They get their hands dirty*. Great managers are someone who will do any job in the club, whether it is working the front desk, teaching a class, or cleaning the locker room. They do not see themselves as being above the fray. Whatever the situation, they are willing to "get their hands dirty." It is not that they spend a lot of time performing a particular task, rather that they do the job when it is needed, the way it should be done. In the process, they set the perfect example for their staff.

- *They have great relationships with the members*. When members stop by the manager's office or approach that person on the floor to converse, that manager probably has a positive relationship with the club's members. Great managers tend to make it a practice of getting close to the membership and building trust between the club's management and its members. In that regard, they try to learn (and remember) the members' names and get somewhat knowledgeable about the members' families. They express sincere interest in the members—particularly how each member is doing in the club, how well the facility is treating the person, etc.

- *They have an open door*. Individuals who want to know if the club has a great manager should just go to the manager's office. Great managers have an open-door policy in which they maintain an environment that encourages employees and members alike to approach them about their concerns—good or bad. Those managers who try to hide behind their office door have neither the courage nor the wisdom to fulfill their assigned role. Confident, successful managers, on the other hand, do not set such barriers. Rather, they make every effort to ensure that their club's members and employees know that they are there to support them and assist them.

- *They are sponges for learning*. Great managers make it a habit to continually expand their horizons. They are aware of the need for lifelong learning. They make a commitment to establish an organization with a suitable environment for group learning. They accept the value of critical thinking. They understand that learning is reciprocal. They exhibit a number of characteristics, including a thirst for relevant knowledge concerning the organization, a desire to learn, and a willingness to be teachable.

- *They are sales people*. Great managers seem to have an affinity for selling—not the hard-core approach to selling, but rather the understanding that every relationship is an opportunity for selling. These managers build upon their relationships with other people to identify opportunities to make their members aware of the fact that the facility has offerings (services, programs, and products) that they may need. Managers who are sales people are able to create an environment that encourages every employee to see themselves as a

> Great managers seem to have an affinity for selling—not the hard-core approach to selling, but rather the understanding that every relationship is an opportunity for selling.

"sales person." Great managers emphasize the point that sales is about identifying the needs of the members and then providing a service that fulfills that need.

- *They are passionate.* Anything worth doing is seldom achieved without passion. In that regard, great managers are incredibly passionate about the health/fitness club business. In a very real sense, passion is the lubricant of their success. They have the ability to exercise sound judgment, control their emotions, be passionate about what they do, and be aware of the tremendous value of a physically active lifestyle.

- *They know the competitors.* Great managers know their competition. They know everything about them, from their facilities to the way that they program their clubs. They subscribe to one of the basic principles highlighted in Sun Tzu's *Art of War*, which essentially states, "Keep your allies close and your enemies even closer." A tendency exists among some managers to criticize and belittle their competitors. Rather, they should learn from them and take advantage of their good ideas.

❑ *The Situational Leadership Model.* For the first-time supervisor or manager, the responsibility of leadership can be overwhelming. While the attributes detailed in the previous sections are essential to great leadership, a person who is new to the responsibilities of leadership cannot develop and refine all of those qualities overnight. For those novice leaders, the model of situation leadership, as presented in Ken Blanchard's best-selling book, *The One Minute Manager and Leadership*, can be an excellent tool. Blanchard's model of leadership reviews the following four styles of leadership and how they can be applied with different employee populations:

- *Directive leadership.* This style of leadership is most effective when employed with new employees and other employees whose knowledge of the job (skill level/technical expertise of job) and its expectations are relatively low and their desire to achieve is high. The leader needs to provide direction to these individuals concerning how the job should be performed. This direction might be presented in several formats, including checklists, regular meetings, teaching, goal setting, etc.

- *Coaching leadership.* This style of leadership is most effective when utilized with those employees who have garnered a stronger understanding of the job and whose level of desire or passion may have waned slightly. As a rule, these individuals are usually more tenured employees who have yet to achieve an empowered status, as an outgrowth of their skill, passion, and understanding of the job. With these employees, the leader should listen to the employee, be supportive of the employee's efforts, and if needed, provide the direction or goals for the job to get done.

A tendency exists among some managers to criticize and belittle their competitors. Rather, they should learn from them and take advantage of their good ideas.

- *Supportive leadership.* This style of leadership is usually employed with employees and teams of employees who have the knowledge, experience, and an understanding of what needs to occur in the workplace. With these employees, the leader must listen, support, and facilitate change. This style is not about giving direction; rather, it involves facilitating interaction and supporting the employees, and only stepping in if needed.

- *Delegating leadership.* This style of leadership is appropriate for use with employees and teams who are knowledgeable, experienced, focused, and passionate. With these employees, the leader is focused on providing an environment of trust and handing over the reigns of leadership. This type of leadership involves fully empowering employees and letting them lead.

It is important to understand that each style of leadership is applicable to every employee. While it might appear that the needs of each employee would dictate that a specific style of leadership be employed, it is far more likely that each employee will require each of these styles at different times. Occasions will arise when an employee or team needs to be directed, while at other times those same individuals will need to be coached, supported, or delegated. It is the role of the leader to know which style to use and when to use it. This responsibility can involve several factors, including emotional intelligence, empathy, and being open to and in touch with the work environment.

Developing Job Descriptions and Compensation Agreements for Employees

As previously discussed, one of the keys to building the team is providing each employee with a job description (model) and a compensation agreement. These two documents are two of the most critical tools in establishing expectations, offering encouragement, and providing evaluation. In reality, the job description and compensation agreement are not documents, as much as they are living roadmaps for the employee.

❑ *Building the Job Model.* The job model is a roadmap for the employee, because it establishes for them the expectations that the club has for their job and details how their job interacts with the other members of the team. Building a job model involves the following steps:

- *Begin with the job overview.* The first part of the job model is a simple paragraph that summarizes the primary responsibilities and accountabilities of the job. This narration should be clear and direct.

- *Identify whether the position is exempt or non-exempt.* The job model should detail how the various positions in the club are to be categorized. For example, a fitness director would be an exempt position, while a personal trainer would be a non-exempt position.

> The job model is a roadmap for the employee, because it establishes for them the expectations that the club has for their job and details how their job interacts with the other members of the team.

Every employee should receive a written compensation agreement, in addition to a copy of the job model for the position.

- *List the essential accountabilities of the job.* The essential accountabilities of the position involve the top five behaviors/areas for which the employee will be held accountable. Collectively, these factors should reflect the big picture. For example, employees might be held accountable for their department achieving its annual budget target for revenues.

- *List the secondary accountabilities.* Secondary accountabilities involve those areas/behaviors over and beyond the aforementioned essential accountabilities for which the club will hold the employee accountable. These areas are not tasks; rather, they are areas of accountability. For example, employees might be held accountable for completing their work schedule each week.

- *Identify the reporting lines.* This factor involves clarifying whom employees report directly to, whom the employees have indirect reporting responsibility to, and whom they supervise. For example, an employee might report to the operations manager, but is expected to work with the fitness director when needed, and is responsible for the personal trainers.

- *Identify the physical requirements of the job.* This stipulation is an OSHA requirement. It involves identifying the specific physical tasks, such as lifting, walking, etc., that are required by a particular job.

- *Identify the educational expectations for the position.* This measure refers to the fact that the club should provide a listing of any educational requirements for the position, such as certifications, licenses, etc.

The appendix presents several examples of job models that are employed in the health/fitness club industry, which help illustrate what a completed job model might look like.

❑ *Building the Compensation Agreement.* Every employee should receive a written compensation agreement, in addition to a copy of the job model for the position. A compensation agreement is a non-binding understanding of the compensation that will be provided for performing the duties expected of a specific position and not a contract for employment. The compensation agreement should be consistent with the accountabilities of the job and spell out in detail for the employees exactly how they derive their personal earnings. Building a compensation agreement can involve several critical elements, including:

- *Non-exempt hourly employees:*

  ✓ Identify their hourly wage and share with them the changes in that rate for overtime and holiday work.

  ✓ Identify what benefits they are eligible for as a non-exempt employee.

✓If employees are being paid by commission only, make sure the commission structure is outlined completely and provide an example template so that they can see how it works.

✓For employees paid by commission, also include a second hourly rate that can be applied for holidays and vacations.

• *Exempt employees*:

✓Identify their base salary. This step should be communicated in terms of the club's standard pay period and also reflected in an annualized amount. For example, the employee will receive a base salary of $2,000 every two weeks equal to $52,000 annually.

✓Identify any incentive or variable pay, based on performance. Make sure that employees must understand clearly how their variable or incentive pay is given. For example, the employee has the potential to earn $10,000 at year-end if they achieve 100% of their revenue goal and will receive a percentage of the $10,000 in proportion to the percentage of the revenue goal they achieve (i.e., $5,000 for reaching 50% of the assigned goal, etc.).

✓Identify all benefits provided, including vacation, education allowances, medical, profit-sharing, etc.

Employees must understand clearly how their variable or incentive pay is given.

(Note: To help visualize what a compensation agreement might look like, several sample compensation templates are provided in the appendices.)

FACILITIES AND EQUIPMENT IN THE HEALTH/FITNESS CLUB INDUSTRY

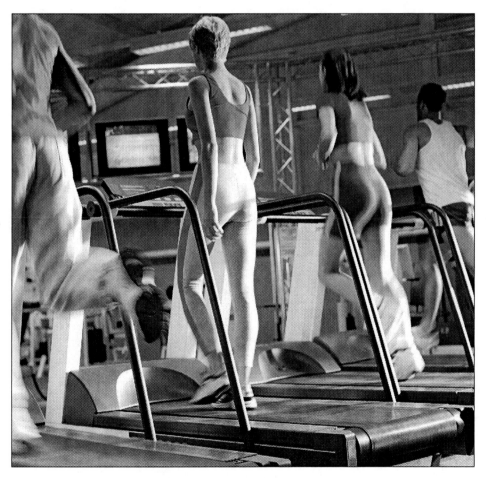

Part Six

- Chapter 17: Health/Fitness Club Facilities
- Chapter 18: Fitness Equipment for the Health/Fitness Club Industry

17

Health/Fitness Club Facilities

Chapter Objectives

The health/fitness industry is heavily dependent upon its facilities for driving business profitability. This chapter presents an overview of the facilities that make up the majority of health/fitness clubs. The chapter initially reviews the various types of facilities. The chapter then discusses the areas that typically are found in these types. Finally the chapter concludes by examining the design and construction process for health/fitness club facilities, including providing examples of cost guidelines for construction.

Types of Health/Fitness Club Facilities

The International Health, Racquet, and Sportclub Association in its 2004 industry data survey, *Profiles of Success*, separates facilities into two basic types: fitness-only and multipurpose. While these categories enable the various kinds of facilities to be grouped into two primary types of facilities, each of these major categories can be separated into even greater detail, based on the actual business operated in the facility:

❑ *Fitness-Only Facilities*. Fitness-only facilities are defined as those clubs that have facilities that provide space specifically for the pursuit of fitness activities. These facilities typically consist of activity-specific areas for cardiovascular equipment, resistance-circuit equipment, free-weight equipment, and group-exercise studios, as well as common areas, such as locker rooms and reception areas. According to IHRSA's survey, the average fitness-only facility is 36,400 square feet, with the lower 25% of fitness-only clubs averaging approximately 12,000 square feet and the upper 25% averaging about 35,000 square feet. Based on the average membership for a fitness-only club, these facilities provide approximately 12 square feet per

The average fitness-only facility is 36,400 square feet, with the lower 25% of fitness-only clubs averaging approximately 12,000 square feet and the upper 25% averaging about 35,000 square feet.

The average multipurpose facility is 75,196 square feet, with the lower 25% of multipurpose facilities averaging 31,750 square feet and the upper 25% of facilities averaging 93,869 square feet.

membership. Several fitness-only clubs exist, such as facilities operated by 24 Hour Fitness, LA Fitness, and Bally's, that provide as little as five square feet per membership. In reality, the majority of fitness-only clubs normally fall between 10,000 and 30,000 square feet in size.

Fitness-only facilities can be further broken down into more specialized units with sub-categories, such as exercise studios, free-weight gyms, personal-training studios, and express facilities, such as Curves for Women. Exercise studios normally have one or two group-exercise studios, a reception area, and locker rooms. Free-weight gyms usually provide a relatively large free-weight area, a reception area, and locker rooms. Personal-training studios are composed primarily of resistance, cardiovascular, and stretching areas. Some might have reception desks and locker rooms or changing rooms. Facilities, such as Curves for Women and Cuts (a men's-only fitness chain), typically have a relatively small open area for equipment, a small reception area, and in some cases, changing facilities. These smaller fitness-only facilities tend to occupy less than 3,000 square feet of space.

Fitness-only facilities are commonly found in strip malls, office buildings, residential buildings, and corporate wellness and fitness programs. Some U.S. companies, such as 24 Hour Fitness, LA Fitness, Club One, and Town Sports International, have a significant percentage of their clubs as fitness-only facilities.

❑ *Multipurpose Facilities.* Multipurpose facilities are defined as clubs that offer fitness facilities and one or more recreational spaces, such as racquet courts, pools, gymnasiums, spas, and outdoor recreational areas. According to the aforementioned IHRSA survey, the average multipurpose facility is 75,196 square feet, with the lower 25% of multipurpose facilities averaging 31,750 square feet and the upper 25% of facilities averaging 93,869 square feet. Based on average membership numbers, the average multipurpose club provides approximately 27 square feet per membership, over double the space allocation seen in fitness-only clubs. Similar to what occurs in the fitness-only market, some multipurpose clubs, such as those operated by Lifetime Fitness, provide as little as 10-to-15 square feet per membership. The largest commercial multipurpose clubs in the industry include the East Bank Club in Chicago, Illinois at over 450,000 square feet, the Michigan Athletic Club in East Lansing, Michigan at over 250,000 square feet, the Rochester Athletic Club in Rochester, Minnesota at over 200,000 square feet, and the Lakeshore Athletic Club in Chicago, Illinois at over 175,000 square feet. The majority of multipurpose facilities range in size from 40,000 to 100,000 square feet.

Several sub-categories of multipurpose clubs exist, including racquet courts only, pools only, gymnasiums only, clubs with tennis courts, and clubs with a blend of each type of activity area. The majority of multipurpose clubs have fitness facilities, racquet courts, and gymnasiums, with pools and tennis courts being less common features for most multipurpose clubs. Some multipurpose facilities also have outdoor facilities, such as outdoor pools, ball fields, and even team-building venues. The largest multipurpose clubs tend to be those with tennis facilities, gymnasiums, and outdoor facilities.

Multipurpose facilities are typically located in suburban settings, due to their space demands and the lower cost of land. On the other hand, the largest multipurpose facilities, such as the East Bank Club in Chicago, the Reebok Club in Manhattan, and the Michigan Athletic Club in East Lansing, Michigan, are found in downtown markets. A few companies, such as Lifetime Fitness, based in Minnesota, and Sports Club/LA and Western Athletic Clubs, based in California, are the leading operators of the larger multipurpose clubs in the industry. For example, most of the clubs that are operated by Lifetime Fitness are over 100,000 square feet, as is also the case for the clubs that were formerly and operated by Sports Club/LA.

The Spaces Within a Health/Fitness Club Facility

This section presents a brief overview of the most common spaces found in health/fitness clubs (fitness-only and multipurpose). A description is provided of each area's function, space requirements, and any critical design or construction requirements. For ease and clarity of understanding, the discussion of the areas is separated into physical-activity areas and service areas.

Primary Physical-Activity Areas

❑ *Aquatic Areas (36% of clubs offer).* The aquatic areas of a facility can serve multiple functions, ranging from lap swimming and exercise classes to full-scale aquatic entertainment and recreation centers. A number of aquatic spaces are commonly found in clubs, including lap pools, therapy pools, and recreational pools:

   • *Lap pools.* Lap pools are designed primarily for individuals who want to swim laps, but can also be used for other activities, such as water-exercise classes and swim lessons. The typical lap pool in clubs will be 25 yards long (75 feet) and 15 yards wide (45 feet and six lanes) and will be four-to-five feet deep at its deepest. Lap pools that are going to be used for swim meets must have a depth of at least seven feet at one end of the pool to accommodate surface diving. In fact, many of the lap pools that were built before 1980 have depths of 10-to-12 feet and can be used for board diving. The trend in lap pools is to build them between 60 and 75 feet in length and provide only three or four lanes for lap swimming. The larger multipurpose clubs often install regulation short-course competitive pools in their facilities that are

The aquatic areas of a facility can serve multiple functions, ranging from lap swimming and exercise classes to full-scale aquatic entertainment and recreation centers.

either 25 meters (international) or 25 yards (domestic) in length and have eight lanes. Most lap pools are built with gunite or stainless steel, though fiberglass structures also exist. The surface of these pools is plaster, stainless steel, or tile. Most clubs keep the water temperature in their pools between 78 degrees and 86 degrees Fahrenheit.

- *Therapy pools.* Therapy pools are designed primarily for group classes and therapeutic exercise. These pools may be as small as 20-feet wide by 20-feet long or as large as 40-feet wide by 60-feet long. The average size of therapy pools in the club industry is approximately 1,500 square feet. With a depth that typically ranges from 2.5-to-five feet, these pools are designed to be handicap accessible. The materials used to construct these pools are similar to those employed with lap pools. The water temperature in most therapy pools is kept between 84 degrees and 92 degrees Fahrenheit.

- *Recreational pools.* Recreational pools are the newest trend for indoor multipurpose facilities. These pools are designed to accommodate various types of recreational activities (wading, swimming, sliding, etc.). The most common features of recreational pools are zero-depth entry (sloping from deck level to the desired depth), water slides, water features (sprays, fountains, and similar), lazy river features, and non-traditional shapes. These pools can have two-to-three times the area of a typical lap pool. In fact, a few clubs in the industry have recreational pools that occupy as much as 10,000 square feet of pool surface area. Most of these pools have starting depths of zero feet and normally go no deeper than four feet, unless the pool has water slides, in which case, additional depth levels are usually required by local codes. The water temperature in most recreational pools is kept between 82 degrees and 86 degrees Fahrenheit.

Many of the newer multipurpose facilities, such as those of Lifetime Fitness, headquartered in Minnesota, the Michigan Athletic Club in East Lansing, Michigan, and the Maryland Athletic Club in Timonium, Maryland have aquatic environments that include two or more of these aquatic spaces.

❑ *Fitness Areas.* The fitness areas in most clubs include four primary spaces to house the fitness and exercise equipment of the club. As a rule, these spaces involve the cardiovascular area, the resistance-circuit area, the free-weight area, and the stretching area:

- *Cardiovascular area (86% of clubs offer).* The cardiovascular area houses the club's cardiovascular equipment, including treadmills, elliptical machines, mechanical stairclimbers, and stationary bicycles. Cardiovascular areas normally allocate between 40 and 50 square feet of space per piece of exercise equipment (the typical manufacturer space recommendation for a piece of equipment). On average, the

> **Cardiovascular areas normally allocate between 40 and 50 square feet of space per piece of exercise equipment .**

club's cardiovascular area occupies between 1,000 and 5,000 square feet. These areas are typically located in relatively open spaces, with fluorescent lighting and durable floor surfaces. Usually, the floor surface in this area is either carpet or rubber (e.g., Everlast, Mondo, or Softpave). Many of the clubs provide an entertainment system as part of their cardiovascular area, such as the systems manufactured by Broadcast Vision or Cardio Theater. One of the newest industry trends in this regard is to provide individual viewing screens for each piece of cardiovascular equipment. As a rule, the club's cardiovascular areas require sufficient airflow (measured in cubic feet a minute—CFMs) to maintain a temperature range of 68-to-72 degrees farenheit and a relative humidity level of under 50%, based on the expected head load.

- *Resistance-circuit area (51% of clubs offer)*. The resistance-circuit area in a club normally holds the selectorized-resistance machines, such as those manufactured by companies such as Cybex, Free Motion, Life Fitness, or Precor. As a rule, these areas allocate between 40-and-50 square feet of space per machine, based on the manufacturer's requirements. The average health/fitness club has one or two resistance circuits, each of which has 10-to-12 machines per circuit and occupies approximately 1,000 square feet per circuit. It is a common practice in the industry for a club to have one circuit dedicated to those members who wish to follow a dedicated circuit and another circuit that is devoted to the serious weight-training members. Some of the larger clubs, such as the Gainesville Health and Fitness Center, located in Gainesville, Florida, and Lifetime Fitness, provide more than three circuits of resistance equipment.

  Most resistance-training areas are commonly located in wide-open spaces, with a rubberized floor surface. A few club operators use carpet or wood, instead of a rubber surface. Most of the newer facilities also provide some form of audiovisual entertainment in this area. Most resistance circuit areas also have at least one wall with mirrors so that members can check on their posture and mechanics while exercising. These areas require sufficient air circulation (CFMs) to maintain a temperature range of 68-to-72 degrees and a relative humidity level of under 50%.

- *Free-weight area (95% of clubs offer)*. This area of the club houses the free weights and the plate-loaded weight machines. The free-weight area is similar to the resistance-circuit area, in that it requires 40-to-50 square feet per piece of equipment and a rubber floor surface. The size of this area varies from club to club, depending upon the amount of equipment provided. Some clubs only devote a few hundred square feet to this area, while others allocate over 5,000 square feet of space to it (e.g., LA Fitness, Sports Club/LA, Red's, East Bank Club, etc.). It is a common industry practice for the free-weight areas to have one or more mirrored walls so that members can

The average health/fitness club has one or two resistance circuits, each of which has 10-to-12 machines per circuit and occupies approximately 1,000 square feet per circuit.

monitor their mechanics and posture while training. These areas require sufficient CFMs to maintain a temperature range of 68-to-72 degrees and a relative humidity level of under 50%.

- *Stretching area (22% of clubs offer).* Over the past decade, a number of clubs have made stretching areas an integral part of their physical-activity space. While no specific design parameters currently exist for stretching areas, it is a common practice for facilities to allocate between 200-and-800 square feet to these areas. The stretching area is usually a quiet area that utilizes exercise mats for a floor surface. The temperature for this area is normally the same as for the other fitness spaces, although in an ideal environment, it should be slightly warmer to facilitate the dynamics of stretching.

While the aforementioned four spaces are typical of most fitness areas, since 2000, a growing trend has existed in the club industry to include an additional space for functional-fitness training, featuring accessory equipment, such as medicine balls, tubes, balance boards, exercise balls, steps, cones, and plyometric implements. With regard to air circulation and floor surface, these spaces are similar to the other fitness areas in the club. Some clubs dedicate a specific room for these functional fitness areas, while others devote an open area for the same purpose.

❑ *Group-Exercise Studios (85% of clubs offer).* The group-exercise area is a space designed to provide a suitable environment for offering group-exercise and fitness activities (note: these areas were formerly called aerobic-exercise studios). The group-exercise space in a club can be as small as one multipurpose studio or as extensive as four or five studios with dedicated functions. The most common group-exercise studio spaces are multipurpose, group cycling, Pilates, and yoga:

- *Multipurpose studio.* The multipurpose studio provides space to offer the majority of group-exercise activities, such as step classes, sculpt classes, resistance classes, stretch classes, yoga, and group cycling. Because such studios serve multiple activities, their design must accommodate the variety of activities performed in the allotted space. As a rule of thumb, these studios should allocate between 40-and-60 square feet of space per user, with an average of 50 square feet per user being the norm. These rooms most commonly have a cushioned wood floor (i.e., a floor with a shock-absorbing sub-layer, plywood underlayment, and solid wood surface). Two of the leading manufacturers of these floors are Conner Flooring and Robbins Sports Surfaces.

Another typical requirement for a multipurpose studio is to have mirrors on at least two adjacent walls. The multipurpose studio should also have its own thermostat to control airflow and temperature, with

The group-exercise space in a club can be as small as one multipurpose studio or as extensive as four or five studios with dedicated functions.

the temperature range during class set between 68-and-72 degrees and a relative humidity of less than 50%. When these classes are not in session, these rooms may seem cold. The multipurpose room should also have lighting as standard equipment that can be adjusted to different levels, depending upon the needs of the class.

- *Group-cycling studio.* The group-cycling studio is designed for the specific demands of group cycling. As a rule, this room requires 50 square feet per cycle, although some clubs offer far less space. The ideal floor surface for this studio is either wood or rubber, with maple and bamboo floors being the most common. Some clubs carpet the area, but this practice is not recommended because of the high level of perspiration that is generated in these studios. These studios should have at least one wall with a mirror, normally the wall behind the instructor. These studios should also have adjustable lighting as well, since many instructors like to vary the lighting levels to establish certain mood states during class. The group cycling studio should have its own thermostat to control airflow and temperature, with the temperature range during class set between 68-and-72 degrees and a relative humidity of less than 50%. When classes are not in session, these rooms may sometimes seem cold. The industry trend in the past few years has been to combine the group-cycling studio with the multipurpose studio, rather than devoting a separate space to this activity.

- *Pilates studio.* The Pilates studio, a relatively new addition to the group-exercise area of most clubs, should be designed to accommodate the unique requirements of group and private Pilates training. This room requires approximately 50-to-60 square feet per user, primarily due to the equipment that is used. These rooms may have a wood, rubber, or even carpeted floor surface. Instructors like to have a studio with at least two mirrored walls. Like the other group-exercise studios, this room requires adjustable lighting and a separate thermostat for temperature control. The Pilates room normally has a higher temperature range than either the group-cycling or the multipurpose studio. As a rule, most Pilates exercisers prefer to work out in rooms in which the temperature is over 70 degrees. Normally, the temperature is set in most Pilates studios between 72-and-76 degrees Fahrenheit.

Yoga, along with Pilates, has been one of the two fastest growing forms of group exercise over the past decade.

- *Yoga studio.* Yoga, along with Pilates, has been one of the two fastest growing forms of group exercise over the past decade. In some clubs, yoga comprises over 50% of all class offerings. Because of the unusual space demands of yoga, a separate studio is often required. Many of the newest club facilities in the industry have standard yoga studios. The yoga studio requires between 50-and-75 square feet per user. The floor surface for the yoga studio can be wood, rubber, or carpet. Regardless of what material is used for the floor of the yoga studio, the surface must be firm and level to accommodate the postures and movements of yoga. Most yoga studios require adjustable lighting, similar to the other studios. Like the other studios, at least one wall should be mirrored. The yoga room normally has a higher temperature range than the other studios, with most users preferring temperatures over 70 degrees. Typically, the temperature in most yoga studios is somewhere between 72-and-80 degrees Fahrenheit. The practitioners of Bikram style yoga (hot yoga) often turn the temperature in the studio as high as 105 degrees Fahrenheit (note: all factors considered, this is not a healthy environment for exercise). Some yoga studios also have special built-in wall units that allow selected exercises to be performed against the walls.

❑ *Racquet Courts.* Racquet courts are as varied in their design and function as are the games that are played on them. The types of racquet courts that are most frequently found in health/fitness clubs are racquetball courts, squash courts, and tennis courts. In addition to these court areas, some clubs also have some of the less-commonly used court areas, such as court tennis, paddle tennis, and platform tennis.

- *Racquetball courts (37% of clubs offer).* In the past two decades, racquetball has been far less popular than it was when it achieved its pinnacle of participation in the 1970s and early 1980s. A racquetball court is typically used for racquetball, although it can also be utilized for activities such as handball and walleyball. A regulation racquetball court is 20-feet wide by 40-feet long (800 square feet) and 20-feet high.

  Racquetball courts usually have a suspended wood floor and walls composed of panels of a compressed wood material, unlike the courts that were built in the early days of the sport's infancy, which were often constructed with plaster walls or wood-panel walls. The typical racquetball court floor should be refinished on a regular basis. Most racquetball courts have a back wall that is composed of glass, although some clubs have courts that are fully enclosed by compressed panels or plaster, with only a rear door providing visibility within. Racquetball courts require separate air circulation control due to the volume of the space and the temperature and humidity requirements for that space. Under normal conditions, the court temperature should be between 60 degrees and 68 degrees Fahrenheit. One common mistake that is often made in the construction of racquetball courts is failing to allow the wood-floor materials to acclimate to the indoor environment before laying them (e.g., a seven-to-10 day acclimation period is recommended). The lighting of a racquetball court should allow for at least 40-to-50 foot candles at floor level.

- *Squash courts (17% of clubs offer).* Over the past 10-to-15 years, squash has grown in popularity to the point it has overtaken racquetball as an indoor racquet activity in many clubs. Squash courts originally could be grouped into two categories—North American courts and International

Racquet courts are as varied in their design and function as are the games that are played on them.

courts. The North American courts were the primary playing surface in United States, while the International courts were the primary playing surface throughout the rest of the world. Since the early 1990s, the International game has been adopted as the accepted version of squash. As a result, the North American courts are no longer built.

The International court is 21-feet wide by 32-feet long (672 square feet), with a ceiling height of 20 feet. The court surface in an International court is unfinished hardwood. The walls and ceilings can be a compressed-wood panel system, plaster, wood, or a sand-filled, panel wall system. At the present time, most courts developed in recent years employ the compressed-wood panel system, although the sand-filled panel system is the surface of choice for serious squash players. Squash courts are similar to racquetball courts in their lighting and air circulation requirements. In that regard, they need a temperature range of 60-to-68 degrees and lighting levels of at least 40-foot candles.

Tennis is the most popular court sport, with over 22 million participants.

While the International court is the preferred court area for squash, many clubs still have either North American courts or converted racquetball courts as their squash-court area. The North American court, which is 18.5-feet wide and 32-feet long, requires a completely different game and ball and offers a somewhat less-than-satisfactory-playing space for the game of squash.

- *Tennis courts (14% of clubs have indoor courts, while 18% have outdoor courts).* Tennis is the most popular court sport, with over 22 million participants. Tennis is somewhat different than the other racquet-court games, because it offers players multiple playing surface options, as well as variable playing environments—ranging from outdoors to indoor-climate controlled to somewhere in between. A regulation tennis court requires a total square footage of 7,200 square feet, with the court area being 120-feet long by 60-feet wide. The actual court area (where the ball is in play) is 36-feet wide (doubles area) and 78-feet long, with a court surface that extends 12 feet to either side of the playing area and 21 feet to either end of the playing surface (note: a singles court is only 27 feet wide). If the playing area is an indoor court, it requires a ceiling height of at least 24 feet, preferably 30 feet high.

A tennis court surface can be grass, clay, or hard-court. Grass is predominately an outdoor playing surface and is not very common in North America. Grass surfaces require considerable care and produce a relatively faster game of tennis. Clay is also a predominately outdoor playing surface, although it can be used on indoor courts. The Mayfair Racquet and Fitness Clubs in Toronto, Canada, for example, have indoor clay surfaces. A clay surface can be red clay or green clay. The brand name of the most common type of clay is Har Tru. Clay courts

Since the primary function of a gymnasium is normally for basketball, most facilities design and build their gymnasiums to accommodate the space requirements of basketball, which has parameters that are more than sufficient for activities such as volleyball and badminton.

require constant care, including watering, raking, taping, and resurfacing. Clay courts offer an outstanding playing surface for older adults because they tend to place less physical strain on the player's joints and slow the game down. Hard-court is the most common playing surface in the United States and is best suited for indoor courts. Hard courts can be either blacktop or a synthetic surface that has been laid over a concrete foundation, which is the most common type of hard court. Tennis courts can also have surfaces that use either carpet or artificial turf. In reality, neither material is utilized as a court surface, as a rule, in North America, although indoor courts in Europe (primarily in England) employ such coverings.

The ideal lighting environment for tennis is to provide at least 50-foot candles of light at the net surface, using one of the following light sources: metal halide, halogen, or even fluorescent. If the courts are indoors in a climate-controlled environment (i.e., heating and cooling provided), then the air temperature of the area should be maintained between 60-and-68 degrees Fahrenheit.

❑ *Gymnasiums (18% of clubs offer)*. The gymnasium is a multipurpose area in which a host of recreational sports can be conducted. The most common activities offered in the gymnasium are basketball, volleyball, badminton, group-exercise classes, and youth-oriented activities. Depending upon the club and the market in which it is located, a variety of less common activities can also be programmed in the gymnasium, including such activities as roller hockey, roller skating, and indoor soccer. Since the primary function of a gymnasium is normally for basketball, most facilities design and build their gymnasiums to accommodate the space requirements of basketball, which has parameters that are more than sufficient for activities such as volleyball and badminton.

The standard practice for clubs that desire to offer a full array of activities in the gymnasium is to build the space in accordance with the American collegiate-sized court, which is 94-feet long and 50-feet wide, with a recommended 10-foot perimeter around the playing area of the court (7,980 square feet). Another option is to build the gymnasium to North American high-school dimensions, which are 84-feet long by 50-feet wide, with a 10-foot perimeter around the playing area of the court (7,280 square feet). On the other hand, because of the aforementioned relatively large space requirements, some clubs develop courts that are comparatively smaller, usually 60-feet long by 40-feet wide, with a minimum perimeter distance of three feet (3,036 square feet). These smaller courts are primarily used for basketball and volleyball.

The gymnasium typically has a suspended wood floor that is comprised of a cushioned or suspended sub-floor structure, with a hardwood floor surface (maple, beech, etc.) Clubs also have the option of installing a rubber-floor surface on the floor of the gymnasium court, which is less expensive than wood-floor systems.

When a gymnasium is built, the standard practice is to mark the floor surface for basketball and volleyball, and sometimes for badminton. Most gymnasiums have six basketball hoops, so that games can be played either full-court or half-court. The recommended lighting levels in the basketball area are similar to indoor tennis courts, with somewhere in the neighborhood of 40-to-50 foot candles at the floor surface.

Service Areas

While the main spaces found in health/fitness clubs are physical-activity areas, service areas are also essential. Service areas are those physical spaces that are used by members for non-physical activity. It is critical that a club provides an appropriate number of mix of service areas. The most common types of service spaces in a club are locker rooms, child-care areas, day spa/massage areas, and reception-and-greeting areas.

❑ *Locker Rooms*. The most heavily used area in most facilities, locker rooms are provided in over 90% of health/fitness clubs. It is estimated that on average, members may spend as much as 30%-to-50% of their time in the locker rooms. Locker rooms can serve several purposes, including providing an area for members to relax, network, and change their clothes before and after working out. Most clubs offer lockers, wet areas, rest-room facilities, and relaxation amenities in this area.

   • *Lockers*. In the health/fitness club industry, two distinct approaches exist concerning providing locker facilities. Some clubs have day-use lockers that members can access at no charge; others offer lockers that can only be rented, and finally, some clubs offer a blend of both alternatives. The most common scenario for a club is to provide day-use lockers. The most desirable feature of this practice involves the fact that the club only needs to provide a sufficient number of lockers to accommodate the expected number of users during any given time period. For example, a club might have 4,000 members, and might expect that approximately 1,000 members a day will utilize the club. In all likelihood no more than 35% of those members will be present in the club during any given two-hour time period. In other words, because no more than 350 members would need lockers, the club would only require 350 day-use lockers in the facility. Most lower-priced clubs and even many of the higher-priced clubs prefer this approach. Clubs operated by companies such as 24 Hour Fitness, LA Fitness, and Town Sports International utilize this approach for providing lockers.

      Renting lockers is a practice that higher-priced clubs, serving a more affluent member base, employ. These clubs build lockers and offer members the opportunity to rent the lockers on a monthly, semi-annual,

It is estimated that on average, members may spend as much as 30%-to-50% of their time in the locker rooms.

or annual basis. As a rule, this scenario involves having the club provide enough lockers to accommodate at least 70% of the expected membership. For example, if the club has 2,000 members, it needs to provide approximately 1,400 lockers. The Houstonian in Houston, Texas and the ClubCorp sports clubs are examples of health/fitness companies that utilize this particular approach to providing lockers. On the other hand, some facilities offer both day-use locker areas and rentable locker areas. The recent trend is to create "executive-locker areas," which are separate areas in the club with full-size rentable lockers (e.g., Sports Clubs/LA).

The actual lockers are offered in a variety of sizes. The most common size for day-use lockers is 36-inches tall, 12-inches wide, and 20-inches deep, while the size of rentable lockers can vary from simple 12 inches-by-12 inches-by-20-inches locker spaces to full-size 72 inches-by-15 inches-by-21-inches lockers. The dimensions of lockers are influenced by cost, the space available, and the type of market being served. Most lockers are composed of solid wood, wood laminate, or a polyvinyl material.

- *Wet areas*. The wet areas encompass both the showers and the wet-amenity spaces, such as the sauna, steam, and whirlpools. The number of showers that a club needs depends on the number of users that it expects to have. Some clubs have as few as one shower per locker room, while others have as many as two dozen per locker room. While no standard quantitative measure exists for determining the number of showers that a club should have, a basic guideline is to provide one shower in each locker room for every 250 to 500 members. For example, if a club has 2,000 members, it should have at least four-to-eight showers per locker room. The typical shower is at least nine square feet and is constructed with a surface of tile or other solid material.

> **While no standard quantitative measure exists for determining the number of showers that a club should have, a basic guideline is to provide one shower in each locker room for every 250 to 500 members.**

The amenities normally offered in the wet area include a sauna (64% of clubs offer), steam room (47% of clubs offer), and whirlpools (50% of clubs offer). The sauna is the most popular feature because of its popularity among both men and women and its relatively low installation cost. The typical sauna occupies approximately 80-to-150 square feet and is constructed of wood. A steam room, on the other hand, is more popular among men than women. A standard steam room takes up between 80-and-150 square feet and is built similar to a shower. The whirlpool requires considerable space and dollars to install, which are the primary reasons for whirlpools not being seen in a higher percentage of clubs. As a rule, whirlpools are constructed of fiberglass, stainless steel, or concrete. It is important to note that both men and women prefer these wet amenities only in their own locker rooms. Industry-compiled data indicate that individuals do not like or use coed wet-amenity spaces very often.

- *Relaxation areas.* A number of health/fitness facilities include relaxation areas as part of their locker-room offerings. Among the more popular relaxation areas are lounges, nap rooms, and massage rooms. Lounges are usually found in locker rooms that provide rental lockers, because they serve as an area for members to relax in before heading out. Nap rooms exist in many of the higher-end club facilities that cater to a high demographic. Massage rooms are the most common relaxation-area amenity, since most clubs do not have separate spa facilities.

- *Rest-room facilities.* Every locker room has rest-room facilities. As a rule, the quantity of rest rooms in a particular area or club is normally determined by the existing building codes and the occupancy levels expected in the space.

The quantity of rest rooms in a particular area or club is normally determined by the existing building codes and the occupancy levels expected in the space.

❑ *Child-Care and Children's-Service Areas (47% of clubs offer nurseries and eight percent offer dedicated kid's space).* Traditionally, facilities that offered nurseries and dedicated children's centers were not the norm. At the present time, however, such spaces are becoming an integral part of many clubs. A nursery is an area that is dedicated space for providing basic children sitting or care—not licensed day care. In most states, specific guidelines exist for these spaces. In that regard, two of the most common regulatory stipulations are children cannot be left in these areas for more than a couple of hours and their parents/guardians must be on the club's premises. These rooms may be as small as 80 square feet or as large as 5,000 square feet. In most instances, these spaces include a small area for cribs and playpens, an area for games and activity, and an area for television. In some clubs, these spaces are separated by age group, in an effort to provide dedicated space to specific age categories.

A dedicated children's area is a space where services and activities (beyond offering just nursery services) are provided, such as arts and crafts, recreational games, nap-and-rest areas, and even birthday parties. The Pacific Athletic Club in Redwood City, CA, for example, has over 10,000 square feet in its children's area, including a small gymnasium, arts and crafts area, game area, and nursery area. Lifetime Fitness offers over 15,000 square feet in many of its clubs specifically to a children's area. The Belair Athletic Club, in Belair, Maryland, operated by Wellbridge of Denver, Colorado, has a separate building just for children's services, while the Boston Sports Club in Wellesley, Massachusetts has a dedicated children's area of over 5,000 square feet. In all of these facilities, the focus is on providing a space that is safe for young people. As a rule, these spaces typically have rubber flooring, no edges, no mirrors, and no breakable materials that could harm a child. Finally, most state laws require a separate children's rest room that is handicap accessible.

❏ *Spa and Massage Facilities (59% of clubs offer massage space and 11 percent offer day spa space).* Massage has grown increasing popular over the past decade, as have day spas, in the health/fitness club environment. The space allocated to either massage or spa services ranges drastically in the health/fitness club industry. Some clubs offer one room for massage, while other clubs, such as the Houstonian in Houston, Texas or the Village Gainey Health Club and Spa that is operated by DMB Sports in Phoenix, Arizona, have full-blown spas that are over 15,000 square feet. Many of the larger club chains, such as Sports Club/LA and Lifetime Fitness, offer a branded spa facility in each of their clubs. The most common spaces in a day spa include:

- *Massage rooms.* The standard massage room is at least 90 square feet, preferably 100 square feet. A massage room will normally have a wood floor or other floor surface that is attractive and easily cleaned (a carpet is not a good choice). These rooms typically have indirect lighting on dimmer switches to control the light levels and are constructed with soundproofing to reduce noise from entering the room. As a rule, most massage rooms also have both a sink and a storage space.

- *Facial rooms.* Typically, the facial room (a room for providing facial and basic skin care services) shares space with the massage room, since both involve the same basic design and construction.

- *Wet-treatment rooms.* Wet-treatment rooms are areas that are normally used for body scrubs and body wraps. As such, these activities involve considerable moisture. The room should be at least 100 square feet, have floors and walls that are impervious to water, and have a shower and sink. On occasion, these rooms are utilized for Vichy Showers, hydrotherapy treatments, and related water treatments, all of which require additional plumbing.

- *Pedicure space.* The typical pedicure space requires an operational area of between 50-and-60 square feet. This space should have a floor that is impervious to water (e.g., be constructed of tile or a similar material) and have drainage that accommodates the small footbaths that commonly are a part of the newest pedicure stations.

- *Manicure space.* The manicure space requires an operational space of between 25-and-50 square feet. This space should be open, rather than enclosed, like the other treatment rooms. Preferably, the floors of this room should be either wood or another hard surface that is easily cleaned, although they could also be carpeted.

In addition to the aforementioned facility spaces in a spa area, the spa facilities in many clubs also include a relaxation area that allows customers to sit and relax before and after receiving a treatment. In fact, many of the larger spas also offer reception areas and have separate relaxation areas for men and women. Ideally, a club-based

Massage has grown increasing popular over the past decade, as have day spas, in the health/fitness club environment.

day spa is between 1,400-and-2,000 square feet, a space that would accommodate a relaxation area, four-to-eight treatment rooms, two-to-three manicure and pedicure stations, and a small retail area.

❑ *Reception-and-Greeting Areas.* The reception-and-greeting area is one of the most important spaces in the club. This area is the first internal space in the club that members see when they arrive and the last space that they see when they leave. Accordingly, this space should be designed and constructed to provide a positive impression and to facilitate the immediate needs of the members who are entering and leaving the facility. In most clubs, the reception area (the front-desk area) serves as the entry point for the club and is designed to accommodate such essential functions as security, member greeting, appointment scheduling, phone answering, and information dissemination. Some larger clubs often have a separate area that is dedicated to scheduling appointments and answering the phones. The reception area normally occupies 400-to-1,000 square feet and includes a desk and a small lounge space. As a rule, this area often has some of the most aesthetically pleasing features in the club, including stone or wood floors, wood or solid surface desks, and attractive low lighting.

Storage space is often the area that receives the least amount of attention in the design phase of developing the club and the most needed area when the facility finally opens.

Other Facility Areas

Besides activity and service areas, most clubs also have operational spaces that are used to support the operational and administrative functions of the business. Examples of such spaces include offices for the key staff, the laundry room, and storage area(s). In most clubs, the amount of space allocated to offices is 80-to-100 square feet per office, with the typical facility providing offices for accounting, membership sales people, the manager of a club, and the key department heads. In most facilities, the total space that is allocated to offices does not exceed 1,000-to-1,500 square feet. The typical laundry (two washers, two dryers, and circulation space) ranges in size from 150-to-200 square feet. Storage space is often the area that receives the least amount of attention in the design phase of developing the club and the most needed area when the facility finally opens. Since the typical club design allocates 10%-to-15% of the facility's total space to circulation, at least 25% of that area should be allocated to storage.

The Design and Construction Process

Whether the endeavor involves building a new health/fitness facility, expanding an existing facility, or just renovating some space, it is important to understand the basics of the design and construction process. Understanding this process can help club owners/operators avoid many of the pitfalls and expenses that often occur during these processes.

❏ *The Design Process.* The design process occurs in several stages, which if carried out in their proper sequence, will help ensure that the facility is properly designed. One of the first steps that every club operator should take is to hire a licensed architect to design any facility additions, expansions, or renovations. In most cases, an architectural firm will charge a fee ranging from as low as six percent to as high as 10% of the total construction costs for the design work. The average rate is seven-to-nine percent. With small jobs, some architectural firms will charge their clients a higher rate than normal because certain services are required on all jobs. It is recommended that owners enter into one of the standard agreement forms between an architect and owner, as provided by the Architectural Institute of America (AIA). As a rule, the design process involves several phases, including:

The design process occurs in several stages, which if carried out in their proper sequence, will help ensure that the facility is properly designed.

- *Programming phase.* The programming phase is primarily an internal process in which the club team identifies its specific program and activity needs for the spaces they want in the facility. Most architects will ask to meet with the team and conduct a review of the club's program plan so that they have a clear understanding of what the team believes is needed in the space that will be designed. This phase is usually part of the schematic design phase for architects. The key for the club team is to be as specific as possible concerning what their needs will be with regard to facility space.

- *Schematic-design phase.* This phase of the design process involves the architect taking the programming information and combining it with the field work of the architect that has been undertaken to that point to identify a preliminary floor plan and "appearance" for the facility space. During this phase, the architect normally takes pictures of existing spaces, performs field measurements, asks for existing plans, and meets with local authorities about special regulations and zoning issues. The architect uses this information to prepare a preliminary floor plan and some elevations (vertical representations of the design) that are then shared with the club team. This process normally can take from two-to-six weeks, depending upon the size of the project. The cost for this phase normally ranges from 10%-to-15% of the overall design costs.

- *The design-development stage.* During this stage, the architect, using feedback from the club team on the schematic design, prepares a more complete set of plans. During this phase, the architect utilizes the services of structural, electrical, and mechanical engineers, as well as those of soil engineers and surveyors, if needed. The goal of this stage is to provide the owner with a set of plans that offers substantial detail on each space, including the basic electrical, plumbing, mechanical, and structural work. During this stage, the architect also provides the owner with additional details on the space dimensions and elevations of the facility. Upon the completion of this stage, it is essential that the club owner/operator reviews the plans and provides input. Once this stage has been concluded, many architects then obtain initial cost estimates for the work that is to be performed so that they can get an initial estimate of the approximate cost of the planned project. The cost of this phase can range from 15%-to-25% of the overall design costs.

- *Construction-document stage.* During this stage, the architect takes the design development plans and the feedback that has been received from the club and local authorities to prepare a full set of construction documents. Most top architectural firms usually meet at least once during this phase with the owner to give the club owner an additional opportunity to review the plans, which are usually at 90% of completion at that point. During this phase, the architect completes a full set of construction documents, which contain details on all aspects of the project. The architect also works closely with the local authorities at this point in the process to address all use and permit requirements so that finished plans can be submitted for building permits. At the completion of this stage, the architect and club owner normally meet one final time to make sure all plans are correct. At the end of this stage, the architect, at the owner's direction, then forwards the design plans to at least three general contractors for bidding documents. The bidding process normally takes approximately 30-to-45 days to complete, at which time the owner should receive three cost estimates (bids) from the general contractors. The cost for this phase is the balance of the design costs already paid subracted from 85% of the total estimated design cost.

- *Construction-administration stage.* This phase includes the architect's involvement in the bidding process and the selection of the general contractor (which is typically undertaken with the club owner), as well as the architect's efforts during the construction process. During construction, the architect reviews and approves all general contractor submittals for work, approves all changes recommended by the contractor, reviews pay applications, and checks the progress of work through inspections at each phase of construction. Subsequently, in concert with the owner, the architect completes the final punch list and approves the final conditions of the construction. The cost for this phase of services is normally 15% of the overall design work.

❑ *The Construction Process.* The construction process begins once a general contractor has been selected and hired. The selection of the contractor should be based on several factors, including bid price, references, and experience with similar projects. It is important to note that accepting the lowest contractor's bid does not always lead to the best work or even the lowest price once the project has been completed. Once the decision has been made to hire a particular contractor, the club owner should consider and be sensitive to the following factors, all of which can impact the job:

It is important to note that accepting the lowest contractor's bid does not always lead to the best work or even the lowest price once the project has been completed.

- *Be aware of the fact that contractors have a fudge factor in their price.* General contractors base their submitted bid on cost estimates that they have received from sub-contractors. Most sub-contractors double their costs in order to arrive at their bid price. In turn, the general contractor applies a 20%-to-100% profit margin to each sub's bid price. Furthermore, the general contractor includes a line item for general conditions in their bid, which consists of their cost to supervise the job, along with another line item for profit and overhead that normally runs from five-to-15% of the total cost from all bids. In other words, the final bid price that the club owner receives from the contractor usually has another 15%-to-25% of wiggle room for price negotiation.

- *Get a contract.* Club owners should utilize one of the standard agreements from the American Institute of Architects (AIA), such as a lump-sum agreement, with the contractor. These agreements provide considerable protection for the owner. Such an agreement should address all details of the project, including the payment schedule, change orders, pay applications, liability insurance, performance criteria, etc. The owner should consider including deadlines and penalties in the agreement to cover situations in which the contractor fails to finish a particular part of the project on time, as well as for cost overruns. It is critical that the contract stipulate that between five-and-10% of the contract price is held out of each payment until after the final punch-list work is completed. The contract should also require the contractor to provide evidence of liability insurance (e.g., the owner should be listed on the contractor's insurance as co-insured) and, if the contractor is from a relatively small company, evidence of bonding.

> **The final bid price that the club owner receives from the contractor usually has another 15%-to-25% of wiggle room for price negotiation.**

- *Limit change orders.* Change orders occur when a contractor has to perform work that is not reflected in the original construction documents. As a rule, contractors charge a premium for change orders. Once a change order has been received, the contractor obtains a bid from a sub-contractor for the work involved in the change order and adds a premium of at least 10 percent to the bid (note: the degree of mark-up that is permissible can be specified in the contract). Change orders occur most often because owners want to make changes during the construction phase or the architect and owner have not clarified the plan documents. As a result, it is critical that the plans are reviewed by all parties involved so that no misunderstandings exist and that the owner is aware of the fact that any changes to the plan once construction begins will involve additional costs. Finally, all change orders should be submitted to the architect for approval before any work mandated by the change order can begin or be paid for.

- *Review all pay applications in detail.* Contractors submit a pay application for work performed each month. The pay application provides a detailed listing of all divisions of work and the percentage of work completed for each category. The amount to be paid is based on the work completed. On each application, the contractor lists the contract price, the amount paid to date, the balance, the amount due, and the retainage held out. The pay application should be reviewed and approved by the architect first and then by the owner to ensure that the work that has actually been completed corresponds with the figures shown on the pay application and that no extra costs are included.

- *Conduct regular meetings with the contractor.* The owner and architect should meet regularly with the contractor during the course of construction. In most cases, these meetings are held once a month, but on smaller jobs, they might be scheduled once a week. These meetings should focus on a review of all work, change orders, and pay applications. These meetings should also include an inspection of the job site.

- *Get partial and full lien waivers.* A lien waiver is a form that says that the contractor has received payment for the work completed and that all subcontractors and parties have been paid for their work. When a contractor submits a pay application, lien waivers should be turned in at the same time that equal the amount of work completed and the amount of the work paid for by the club owner. This process ensures that a lien is not placed on the business if a sub-contractor claims that they have not been paid for work they performed. The final lien waiver should be submitted when all of the work has been completed.

- *Conduct a punch list.* After the contractor completes the job, the owner, architect, and contractor should walk through the job and complete a punch list. The punch list identifies any work that either has been performed in an unsatisfactory manner or work still to be done. The punch list ensures that the work is completed to the satisfaction of the owner. Once the punch list is completed, the contractor is paid the retainage fees that have been held out during the course of each pay application.

- *Obtain the warranties and owner's manuals.* At the completion of a construction project, the contractor is obligated to provide the owner with an operator's manual on each product that was utilized in the project (e.g., carpet, HVAC, lighting, floor surfaces, etc.). The operator's manual provides the owner with resources that might be useful with any product-related problems that might subsequently arise with the construction. The standard practice for contractors and their sub-contractors is to provide a one-year guarantee on all work and products, commencing from the time the project is completed. Before making a final payment to the contractor, the owner should obtain these warranties from the contractor.

- *Be aware of the fact that under certain circumstances, the contractor can be removed from the job.* If the owner uses a standard AIA agreement, that agreement includes a section that spells out the

The standard practice for contractors and their sub-contractors is to provide a one-year guarantee on all work and products, commencing from the time the project is completed.

owner's right to remove the contractor, select another contractor, and let the new contractor finish the job, using the original contractor's equipment. This stipulation can be important, because some small contractors start out relatively strong and then fade as the project moves forward.

Costs Associated with Design and Construction

Some general cost guidelines for design and construction exist that can be useful in determining the scope of a project, including:

❑ *Design Costs.* As discussed previously, an architect's costs can run from as low as six percent to as high as 10% of total construction costs. The fees of structural engineers, mechanical engineers, and electrical engineers are all included in this expense. Among the expenses that are not included in the architect's fees are the costs attendant to landscape design, civil engineering, acoustical engineering, surveys, and other specialty work. Collectively, the total cost for all design work can run as high as 12% of the overall construction costs.

❑ *Construction Costs.* Most construction is priced on a unit basis, either as linear feet, square feet, or some other basic unit of measurement.

> **Collectively, the total cost for all design work can run as high as 12% of the overall construction costs.**

- *Overall construction costs.* The cost per square foot can vary considerably, depending on the facility's level of finish. The average cost for building a shell (i.e., site work, foundations, bringing in utilities, and building a frame) normally run approximately $20-to-$100 a foot, depending on the region of the country. The national average would be in the neighborhood of $35-to-$50, depending on the local conditions. The balance of construction after the shell has been completed is considered finish work (i.e., plumbing, electrical, HVAC, surfaces, etc.). The range of cost for this stage varies considerably, based on finish levels, with costs as low as $30 a square foot to as high as $200-to-$400 a square foot in some markets. The national average for this kind of work would be in the neighborhood of $50-to-$75 a square foot. For example, if a freestanding facility was being constructed in a state like Florida or Texas, it might cost from $80-to-$130 a square foot, whereas the cost of that same facility in California or New York might be between $200-and-$300 a square foot.

- *Area cost averages.* The price that club owners can expect to pay for selected areas and floor surfaces in a facility varies from project to project and region to region. Figure 17.1 illustrates the average cost across the country for building and installing selected facility areas and surfaces. The specific costs in a particular region will vary, depending on the level of work, the region of the country, and the local regulations that impact the work.

Facility Area or Surface	Unit	Cost per Unit
Sauna	Unit	$8,000 to $12,000
Steam room	Unit	$10,000 to $25,000
Whirlpool	Unit	$30,000 to $50,000
Squash court	Unit	$30,000 to $50,000
Tennis court	Unit	$40,000 to $60,000
Wood floor (group exercise or gym)	Square foot	$10 to $15
Tile floor/walls (ceramic or porcelain)	Square foot	$7 to $12
Stone Floor (e.g., granite, etc.)	Square foot	$10 to $15
Painting	Square foot	$2 to $3
Sprinkler systems	Square foot	$2 to $3
HVAC	Square foot	$12 to $16
Plumbing	Square foot	$8 to $10
Electrical	Square foot	$8 to $10
Ceiling tiles	Square foot	$2 to $4
Carpet	Square foot	$2 to $3
Pool (standard 25-yard pool with all mechanical systems)	Unit	$250,000 to $400,000
Showers (mud and tile)	Unit	$2,500 to $5,000
FF&E	Square foot	$15 to $25

Figure 17.1. Average total cost (construction and installation) for various types of facility areas and surfaces

18

Fitness Equipment for the Health/Fitness Club Industry

Chapter Objectives

The health/fitness club industry is capital-intensive, with facilities and equipment encompassing the majority of that capital outlay. According to industry research, as reflected in IHRSA's publication, *Guide to Lenders and Investors*, most newly built clubs expend approximately $15-to-$25 a square foot on equipment. This initial investment in equipment is compounded by the need for club owners to reinvest in equipment on an annual basis to stay current with equipment trends in the industry and to deal with the depreciation and wear on existing equipment. This chapter reviews the basic categories of fitness equipment in the industry, the leading equipment manufacturers, and the costs associated with the equipment, including a brief discussion of the pros and cons of purchasing versus leasing. The chapter is not intended to delve into great depth on this subject; rather, it is designed to provide a basic overview of the key factors attendant to the equipment end of the industry. As such, the information is grouped and reviewed according to the major equipment categories in the industry, including cardiovascular equipment, resistance-circuit equipment, free-weight equipment, cardiovascular-entertainment equipment, and other types of equipment that are frequently required in the health/fitness club industry.

Most newly built clubs expend approximately $15-to-$25 a square foot on equipment.

Cardiovascular Equipment

Cardiovascular equipment exists in 86% of health/fitness clubs and is second only to free-weight equipment in terms of its availability in the industry. According to IHRSA's 2004 survey report, *Profiles of Success*, cardiovascular equipment areas are the number one expansion priority for club operators heading into the new year. Although cardiovascular equipment has been around as long as the club industry, it has only been since the 1970s that it has been accorded such a prominent role in the marketing and programming of clubs.

❑ *Historical Overview*. The first pieces of cardiovascular equipment that were utilized in the club industry were stationary cycles (e.g., Monarch, Tunturi, Bodyguard), rowing machines, and self-propelled treadmills. The earliest clubs offered rowing machines with actual oars, small treadmills on rollers that were propelled by the person's actual motion, and stationary bicycles, including the Exercycle created in 1932. The first commercial treadmills were relatively large machines that were developed by Robert Bruce (who is possibly best known for the Bruce protocol) and Wayne Quinton in 1952, and almost two decades later by Trotter in the early 1970s.

In the 1970s, the Lifecycle indoor cycle was introduced. As the first mass-produced electronic piece of cardiovascular equipment, designed specifically for the health/fitness club industry, it subsequently became the benchmark for all future developments in the industry. The Lifecycle established itself as one of those brands that become virtually synonymous with the product type. Like it or not, all indoor cycles, at one time or another, have been called Lifecycles. The Lifecycle gave rise to other early brands of indoor cycles, such as Biocycle and Universal. During the late 70s, treadmills began to have a presence in the health/fitness club market through models built and sold by companies such as Quinton, Marquette, and Trotter. Since then, treadmills have blossomed into the largest segment of cardiovascular equipment in the industry, a segment that is dominated by companies such as Cybex, Life, Fitness, Precor, and Star Trac.

The next landmark type of cardiovascular equipment to hit the industry was the development of StairMaster machines in the mid-1980s. To many industry observers, StairMaster evolved into the industry equivalent of the Lifecycle of the 80s and early 90s. The developmental evolution of cardiovascular equipment continued in the mid-1990s when Precor introduced the first elliptical machine. Subsequently, the Precor EFX became the StairMaster of the previous decade.

During the 1980s, a number of other types of cardiovascular equipment were also popular, including the Nordic Track cross-country ski machine, the Cybex upper body ergometer, and the Concept II Rower (originally introduced in 1976). The late 1980s and early 1990s also witnessed industry efforts to expand the types and features of "cardio" equipment. Some of these machines, such as the Reebok Sky Walker, had an early, but not lasting, impact on the industry. At the present time, cardiovascular equipment continues to evolve, as manufacturers incorporate new technology and improved mechanics and as the public looks for even better/newer exercise tools.

❑ *Categories*. Cardiovascular equipment can be grouped into the following major categories: elliptical machines, stairclimbers, recumbent and upright bicycles, and treadmills. In addition to these major categories, a few, less-prominent categories exist, such as rowing machines, upper-body ergometers, and cross-country ski machines.

The first commercial treadmills were relatively large machines that were developed by Robert Bruce (who is possibly best known for the Bruce protocol) and Wayne Quinton in 1952, and almost two decades later by Trotter in the early 1970s.

• *Elliptical machines.* Elliptical machines encompass the fastest growing category of equipment since their introduction in the mid-1990s. Elliptical machines reflect an evolution in how the industry looks at cardiovascular exercise. These machines exert load forces on the body similar to those imposed on an individual's musculoskeletal system while walking and running, but with significantly less impact. These machines also feature technology that allows for integrated upper-body movement with lower-body movement. At the present time, elliptical machines are available both with and without upper-body movement arms. The industry leader in this type of equipment is the Precor EFX. Companies, such as Life Fitness, Star Trac, Matrix, Cybex (Arc Trainer), Sport Art, and Technogym also manufacture well-received models of elliptical machines. Most of the elliptical machines that are currently available in the market offer heart-rate technology, integrated entertainment technology, and accessories for holding items such as water bottles and reading materials. The average retail cost of a commercial-grade elliptical machine ranges from $3,000-to-$5,000 per machine.

Elliptical machines encompass the fastest growing category of equipment since their introduction in the mid-1990s.

• *Stairclimbers.* Mechanical stairclimbers have lost much of their market share since the introduction of the elliptical trainers. Once the highest volume seller in the industry, stairclimbers currently rank behind treadmills, elliptical machines, and bicycles in terms of their popularity among health/fitness club users. StairMaster Sports/Medical Products, Inc. (a company that is part of the Nautilus Group), which developed and manufactured the first mechanical stairclimbing machine, remains the industry leader in this equipment category. Several other companies, such as Life Fitness, Star Trac, Precor, Technogym, and Cybex, also produce stairclimbing machines that are popular in the industry. The first model of a stairclimbing machine that Stairmaster produced, which featured a series of stairs that actually rotated, is often still the piece of cardiovascular equipment of choice among those individuals who either would like to engage in a particularly intense workout or see a direct correlation between the exercise afforded by revolving stairs and a personal activity interest (e.g., outdoor climbing). The technology involved in mechanical stairclimbing has not changed all that much since these machines were first introduced. Some of the newer stairclimbing machines feature heart-rate monitor technology and entertainment technology, as well as offer soft pedals and accessories to hold water bottles and reading materials. The average retail price for a commercial-grade stairclimber ranges from $2,000-to-$3,000.

• *Recumbent and upright bicycles.* Upright bicycles were the first type of cardiovascular equipment that was introduced to the club market. Within the industry, they remain popular among club users. Recumbent bicycles, the more popular of the two types of bicycles (recumbent and upright), were introduced in the industry in the late 1980s and early

1990s, to ostensibly serve an older demographic. Bicycles are third in popularity, behind treadmills and elliptical machines, among current facility users. The current trend in the technology for both types of bicycles is to provide lower starting workloads, heart-rate feedback, fully adjustable seats and pedals, self-adjusting workloads based on heart-rate response, and integrated entertainment technology. The leading manufacturers of bicycles include Life Fitness, Star Trac, Precor, and Technogym. The average retail price for either a recumbent or upright bicycle ranges from $1,500-to-$3,000.

- *Treadmills.* Treadmills are the single most popular piece of cardiovascular equipment in the industry and involve the largest expenditure for cardiovascular equipment by clubs. As previously discussed, the first treadmills offered to the club industry were models developed by Quinton, Marquette, and Trotter, each of which was relatively large and cumbersome to use. Over the years, treadmills have become the cardiovascular modality of choice for many club members. Much of their popularity can be attributed to the evolution of technology, often based on research into the mechanics of human motion, which is featured in most treadmills. For example, almost every treadmill offers some form of soft deck (shock-absorbing surface), programmable features, controllable speed that ranges from less than one mph-to-10 mph (some as high as 15 mph), adjustable grades (negative-degree grade to as high as a positive 50-degree grade), contact and remote heart-rate monitoring, integrated audiovisual entertainment, accessories for holding items, such as water bottles and reading materials, and, on occasion, fans for "cooling" the individual who is using the machine. The leading manufacturers of commercial-grade treadmills are Star Trac, Life Fitness, Precor, Cybex, Technogym, and Woodway. Some smaller companies, such as True, Matrix, and Sport Art, also produce treadmills. Two of the newest innovations in treadmills are built-in fans, introduced initially by Star Trac, and LCD entertainment, introduced initially by Life Fitness. The average retail price of a quality commercial-grade treadmill ranges from $3,500-to-$6,500.

Selectorized/Variable Resistance Equipment

According to *IHRSA's 2004 Profiles of Success*, selectorized/variable-resistance equipment is found in a majority of all facilities. In reality, almost all clubs offer some form of variable-resistance equipment. Variable-resistance or selectorized-resistance equipment encompasses strength-training equipment that utilizes weight stacks and pulley mechanisms to provide resistance to movement, while the user typically assumes (and maintains) a set position. The primary advantage of this type of resistance exercise is that it provides a safe and efficient strength-training modality, while reducing the level of exercise anxiety and the perceived need for demonstrable fitness prowess that some individuals experience.

Treadmills are the single most popular piece of cardiovascular equipment in the industry and involve the largest expenditure for cardiovascular equipment by clubs.

❑ *Historical Overview.* Resistance-training machines, in one form or another, have been in existence for more than a century. The first such machines consisted of wall-pulley systems that involved weight stacks, pulleys, and ropes. In the early 1900s, the most common types of resistance-training equipment were rudimentary leg press, leg extension, and overhead press machines. The selectorized resistance machines that currently exist in the club industry originated in the late 1950s, as a result of the efforts of Harold Zinkin, Sr. to develop the first Universal machine. Zinkin's equipment featured a single-training unit that had multiple-exercise stations, each with its own weight stack. Paramount Fitness also introduced resistance-training equipment in the 1950s. These early machines employed a system of levers to move the weight stack and provide resistance (Universal called it dynamic-variable resistance). As a rule, the machines offered an uneven distribution of the resistance load at different points in the range of motion. Until the mid-1970s, however, Universal and Paramount were the preferred choices of the industry where it involved the purchase of resistance-training machines.

In 1970, Arthur Jones revolutionized the equipment manufacturing and club industries with the introduction of Nautilus machines. Nautilus machines featured variable resistance, made possible by the use of a cam that controlled the level of resistance afforded to the user. The cam allowed the resistance offered by the machine to vary based on the fulcrum's (mechanical movement arm) position on the cam while the machine was being used. Concurrently, the concept of "strength curves" was introduced into the mindset of many club members. According to Nautilus, one of the most desirable features of its equipment was the machine's capacity to provide resistance to the user that is applied in a manner that is consistent with the normal strength curve of the user's muscles. Another selling point for Nautilus machines was their ability to isolate specific muscle groups while exercising. Nautilus also featured mechanisms that allowed users to adjust their seat position and body position while exercising, which is designed to enhance both the mechanical efficiency and effectiveness of their exercise bout. Nautilus advocates adhered to a prescription and training concept that involved performing one set of each exercise to near muscular fatigue, doing each repetition in relatively slow motion (e.g., four-to-six seconds each), and placing equal or greater emphasis on the eccentric portion of the exercise movement (versus the concentric phase).

Eventually, Nautilus was followed by a new group of equipment manufacturers, such as Eagle (later to become Cybex), Body Masters, and Icarian, among others, who led the effort to expand the technology involved in variable-resistance machines. For example, by the early 1980s, Eagle had entered into the market for variable-resistance machines and captured much of the demand for such equipment. Cybex and many of the resistance equipment companies that followed improved on the original Nautilus design by creating lighter machines that required less space, employed airplane cable or Kevlar belts instead of chains, offered additional color options, and were aggressively marketed at a lower-price point to the industry.

While the number of variable-resistance equipment manufacturers grew over the years, no new innovations hit the industry until later in the 1980s, with the introduction of Keiser pneumatic machines. The Keiser machines involved a new, innovative concept—the use of air pressure to create resistance. This feature provided exercisers with greater flexibility in adjusting either the level of resistance or speed. Subsequently, companies, such as Hydra Fit, introduced a line of resistance-training machines that were powered by pneumatic cylinders, while others developed machines that employed water as a means to adjust the level of resistance. At the present time, Keiser is one of the only companies that manufactures resistance machines that do not employ a weight stack.

The next stage in the evolution of resistance-training machines occurred in the early 1990s, when several manufacturers introduced computerized-resistance training (e.g., Powercise, Life Circuit) machines. These machines employed electromagnetic forces (controlled through computer chips) to produce resistance. The most noteworthy feature of these machines was their ability to adjust the resistance level, based on the user's strength that day, as well as memory of how the user had performed on the previous workout. This approach to resistance training did not catch on with consumers and disappeared from the industry within a few years.

While the number of variable-resistance equipment manufacturers grew over the years, no new innovations hit the industry until later in the 1980s, with the introduction of Keiser pneumatic machines.

At the end of the 1990s, Ground Zero, later renamed Free Motion, developed a line of functional resistance-training equipment, featuring pulleys, that enable users to exercise in a variety of positions and planes. The efforts of Free Motion have since given rise to an entire manufacturing segment in the industry attempt to design and produce functional resistance-training machines.

❑ *Categories*. Variable-resistance equipment can be grouped into three distinct categories: fixed-position weight stack, functional fitness-based weight stack, and alternative resistance.

• *Fixed-position weight stack*. This category encompasses over 80% of the market for variable-resistance equipment. This type of machine provides resistance through the use of cams or other pulley-based systems that are attached to weight stacks. These machines enable users to perform a specific exercise movement in a fixed position that isolates one or two muscle groups. The basic design of these machines provides a high degree of user safety since most of the postural and mechanical alignment errors that can occur in more functional exercise are eliminated. Another benefit category of variable-resistance equipment is the ability to set up circuits of the machines that allow a user to perform movements for each of the major muscle groups by exercising on eight-to-12 machines that have been arranged in a circuit. Most of these machines also allow personalized position adjustments to accommodate multiple body types, as well as feature more aesthetically pleasing designs. A host of manufacturers of this type of equipment exists in the industry, including Life Fitness, Cybex, Technogym, Nautilus, Body Masters, Icarian (a company that is now owned by Precor), Paramount, Flex, and relative newcomers such as Matrix. The average retail price for a complete circuit of 12 machines is approximately $30,000, with each piece ranging from $1,750-to-$4,500 in price.

- *Functional fitness-based weight stack.* This category of variable-resistance equipment has evolved from having a relatively small role in the club industry to being a major focus of variable-resistance equipment manufacturers. At the present time, all of the leading manufacturers of variable-resistance equipment offer machines in this category. This type of equipment is based on the two primary concepts. First, muscles don't contract in isolation. Rather, a synergy of contraction occurs during exercise, involving agonist, antagonist, and stabilizer muscle groups. Second, the body does not function in an isolated or a fixed position. Instead, the functional performance of movement requires both balance and posture. Accordingly, the design of these machines features pulley and cable systems that allow users to adjust their position and angle of movement, as desired. Furthermore, these machines often require that users perform the movement in a standing or similar position—where the body is not fixed in a set position, thus incorporating an element of balance in the exercise. The manufacturing leader in this area is Free Motion Fitness, although additional companies, such as Life Fitness, Cybex, Icarian, and Matrix, among others, have developed their own models of this equipment. These machines range in cost of approximately $2,500-to-$5,000 each, with a complete circuit of 12 machines retailing in the neighborhood of $30,000-to-$40,000.

- *Alternative resistance.* Alternative-resistance machines are similar to the fixed-position, weight-stack equipment, except that they utilize a resistance source other than weight stacks. These machines operate on the same basic principles as the other two basic categories of variable-resistance equipment (i.e., most of these machines provide isolated movements, with the user set in a fixed position). The leader in this category is Keiser, which manufactures a line of equipment that uses air resistance. Keiser has been able to attract a relatively strong following in some segments of the industry, based on the ability of air resistance to allow for loads light enough for the weakest individual and loads in excess of what the strongest human could lift. Keiser has also capitalized on the fact that its equipment nearly eliminates placing undue load forces on the joints, which makes it a very suitable

The body does not function in an isolated or a fixed position. Instead, the functional performance of movement requires both balance and posture.

resistance-training modality for older adults. Other manufacturers exist that use alternative forms of resistance, such as water, air, and hydraulics. On average, these machines retail for between $2,500-and-$4,000 per machine and for approximately $30,000-to-$40,000 for a complete 12-station circuit.

Free-Weight Equipment

Free-weight equipment has been around longer than any other form of exercise equipment. According to IHRSA's *2004 Profiles of Success*, 95% of all clubs indicate that they offer free-weight equipment, thereby making it the most popular type of exercise equipment in the health/fitness club industry.

❑ *Historical Overview.* Free-weight equipment has been around for well over two hundred years. In the early part of the twentieth century, free weights were primarily used by strongmen and bodybuilders to train, mostly in the form of barbells and kettle bells (which are currently becoming popular again). Milo barbells, introduced in 1902, were the first commercially made free-weight sets. These early free weights allowed the user to perform functional movements using weighted objects, such as kettle bells and barbells. During the early years of the health/fitness club industry in the late 1940s, most free-weight equipment consisted of barbells, dumbbells, and benches built by individuals for their gyms. The free-weight equipment industry underwent its first major thrust in popularity with the introduction of the York barbell in the 1950s. Developed by the legendary Bob Hoffman, the York Company created an entire market for barbells, dumbbells, and free-weight benches. In fact, until the late 1980s, York was one of only a few companies that made free-weight equipment,.

> Free-weight equipment has been around longer than any other form of exercise equipment.

The popularity of free-weight equipment received a substantial boost in popularity in the late 1980s and early 1990s, when research began to document and reinforce the enumerable benefits of strength training for all segments of the population. As a result of the impetus for resistance training that was provided by this research, companies began to expand into the free-weight market. Among the manufacturing companies that were at the forefront of this effort were Cybex, Icarian, and Body Master. By the mid 1990s, a number of companies offered full lines of free-weight plates, benches, and accessories.

One of the biggest developments in the history of the free-weight industry occurred in the 1990s, when Hammer developed plate-loaded resistance equipment. Hammer machines featured the functional advantages of free-weight movements, combined with the advantages of variable-resistance, weight-stack equipment. Initially, Hammer developed a significant following in both colleges and professional sports, before gaining in popularity in the club industry. Hammer's prime engineer was none other than Gary Jones, son of Arthur Jones, the creator of Nautilus.

The most recent attempt at innovation in free-weight technology has been the introduction of weight plates with holes for easier grasping. Free-weight equipment has evolved from an exercise tool primarily targeted at bodybuilders to the resistance-training modality of choice for many average consumers.

❑ *Categories.* Free-weight equipment can be grouped into three primary categories: barbells and dumbbells, benches and support machines, and plate-loaded equipment.

- *Barbells and dumbbells.* Barbells and dumbbells have evolved very little since they were first introduced. At the present time, most barbells involve old Olympic-style bars and plates that have ball-bearing sleeves that allow the weights to revolve around the end of the bar. The most innovative change in barbells in recent years has been the introduction of plates (technology first introduced by Iron Grip) that have holes that allow the user to more easily grasp the plates.

  Dumbbells have also not evolved very much over the last century. Two changes that have occurred in dumbbells are rubber plate coatings that have been put on the plates to protect them and more ergonomic handles that have been developed. Another change has been the use of kettle bells, which have become popular in the past few years. First used by old-time strongmen, kettle bells are large metal balls with a fixed handle on top. The leading manufacturers of barbells and dumbbells are Ivanko and Iron Grip. The retail cost of barbells varies, with most commercial grade bars retailing for between $150-and-$300 dollars, while plates cost between $.30-and-one dollar per pound. The cost of solid dumbbells ranges from less than $.30 a pound to over $1.00 a pound, depending on the actual weight (e.g., heavy dumbbells cost less per pound).

- *Benches and support machines.* Benches and support machines comprise the largest segment of the free-weight product line. These products range from simple Olympic style flat benches for performing bench presses to power racks and Smith machines. Each bench and accessory is designed to be used with barbells and dumbbells. The variety of products in this category is substantial and includes such items as adjustable incline benches, flat benches, decline benches, leg-press machines, Smith machines, power racks, cable-crossover machines, curling benches, T-bar rowing machines, calf machines, 45-degree back benches, and abdominal benches. The leading manufacturers of this product segment include Life Fitness, Cybex, Technogym, Icarian, Body Master, Flex (Star Trac), Nautilus, and Matrix. These benches and machines have wide-ranging retail prices. For example, most benches retail for between $400-and-$900 each, while larger machines, such as power racks and Smith machines, cost in the range of $1,000-and-$3,000 each.

Free-weight equipment has evolved from an exercise tool primarily targeted at bodybuilders to the resistance-training modality of choice for many average consumers.

- *Plate-loaded machines.* Plate-loaded equipment is the most recently developed type of free-weight equipment, having only been around since the early 1990s. Plate-loaded machines involve a hybrid piece of equipment that allows the average health/fitness club user to experience some of the benefits of free weights, while simultaneously receiving the advantages that variable-resistance equipment can provide, such as enhanced safety and the ability to exercise isolated muscles. Plate-loaded equipment enables users to perform a variety of fixed-position (isolated exercise movements) and functional based movements (exercises that involve closed-chain movements). The leading manufacturer of this type of free-weight equipment is Hammer (owned by Life Fitness), although other companies, such as Cybex, Icarian, Nautilus, and Body Master also offer plate-loaded machines. The majority of plate-loaded machines retail for between $1,000-and-$2,000, with only a few pieces ever exceeding $2,000 in cost.

Cardiovascular Entertainment Equipment

Cardiovascular entertainment equipment involves a system of apparatus that is employed in concert with aerobic-exercise equipment (e.g., indoor cycles, treadmills, elliptical machines, stairclimbers, etc.) that allows individuals to watch televised images while they work out. Such a system can accomplish several goals, including: enable individuals to disassociate from the perceived effort to exercise, help mask general feelings of fatigue, enliven the workout, make the exercise bout more interesting, etc.

❏ *Historical Overview.* Assumptions concerning how to "entertain" individuals while they are exercising changed substantially when Tony DeLeede introduced Cardio Theater to the health/fitness club industry in the 1980s. Before Cardio Theater, the entertainment efforts of most clubs were strictly limited to background music systems that played soundtracks from either licensed programs, such as Musak, or from radio stations. Prior to Cardio Theater, a few clubs set up televisions in their cardiovascular areas and tuned them to established stations so that members could watch and listen to television while they trained. The constraints of these various efforts became quite apparent when Cardio Theater developed a system that allowed users to tune into the television or music station of their choice through a special control that is mounted on the equipment on which the individual is exercising. The popularity of Cardio Theater led to the development of other audiovisual entertainment systems, including one produced by Broadcast Vision. The effort was further advanced when two companies, E Zone and Net Pulse, developed personal viewing systems that were attached to each piece of equipment. Net Pulse created individual kiosks for each piece of equipment that allowed users to surf the net or tune into their favorite television station. E Zone established a system, featuring small viewing screens, that could be mounted in front of

Plate-loaded equipment is the most recently developed type of free-weight equipment, having only been around since the early 1990s. Plate-loaded machines involve a hybrid piece of equipment that allows the average health/fitness club user to experience some of the benefits of free weights, while simultaneously receiving the advantages that variable-resistance equipment can provide, such as enhanced safety and the ability to exercise isolated muscles.

each piece of equipment and allowed users to view television stations, listen to CDs, or listen to music stations. E Zone also introduced personal headsets that enabled users to navigate throughout the club and continue listening to the station to which they were tuned. In recent years, however, both E Zone and Net Pulse experienced problems with their business models and basically disappeared from the cardio-entertainment industry. Subsequently, both Broadcast Vision and Cardio Theater have developed personal viewing systems that have been incorporated into their offerings.

Categories

Cardio-entertainment systems are offered in three distinct categories: personal viewing systems, interconnected audiovisual systems, and personal tuner audiovisual systems.

❑ *Personal Viewing Systems (PVS).* Personal viewing systems involve individual LCD screens (13 inches to 15 inches) that are mounted in front of each piece of equipment and are connected to an integrated audiovisual network. Each user is able to dial into the station to which they want to watch or listen, using a control module that is mounted on the equipment. As a result, users have their own personal entertainment system while exercising. In a few instances, some manufacturers of cardiovascular equipment have made their machines compatible with these systems so that the control module is part of the equipment's control panel. Cardio Theater and Broadcast Vision are the leading manufacturers of the PVS. Recently, companies such as Life Fitness and Star Trac have begun placing PVS within the control panel of their cardiovascular equipment. The price of PVS ranges between $1,000-and-$1,300 per station if each station is part of an overall system. When PVS is incorporated into the control panel of a piece of cardiovascular equipment, $600-to-$800 is normally added to the cost of the equipment.

> **Personal viewing systems involve individual LCD screens (13 inches to 15 inches) that are mounted in front of each piece of equipment and are connected to an integrated audiovisual network. Each user is able to dial into the station to which they want to watch or listen, using a control module that is mounted on the equipment.**

❑ *Interconnected Audiovisual Entertainment Systems.* These systems integrate wall/ceiling-mounted televisions with audio and video channels that are connected through a transmitter and equipment-mounted control boxes. Users can utilize the control box to select a channel that corresponds to either a television station or audio channel. These systems have four channels, eight channels, or 16 channels that allow users to select from a variety of audiovisual options. These systems feature headsets that users connect to the equipment-mounted control boxes. Most of the systems are wireless, but a few clubs employ hard-wired systems. The leading manufacturers of these systems are Broadcast Vision and Cardio Theater.

The cost of these systems varies, based on the number of televisions, the number of channels on the system receiver, the number of control boxes needed, whether a DVD or video deck is provided, and whether wiring is needed. The control boxes retail for between $140-and-$175 each, while an 8-channel receiver ranges in price between $1,300-and-$1,500. A club that has 50 pieces of cardiovascular equipment might expect to spend in the range of $20,000-to-$30,000 for a full system. One of the biggest challenges facing clubs that have these systems is the constant need to replace headphone jacks that are damaged through the constant placement and removal of user headsets.

❑ *Personal Tuner Audiovisual Systems*. These systems are similar to the aforementioned integrated systems, except that they do not involve having control boxes on the equipment. These systems require that all televisions are set to specific unused FM frequencies. This step enables users to bring their own personal audio machine to their workout and tune into the frequency that corresponds to the television station they want to watch. Users can also tune into their favorite radio station. Many clubs prefer these systems because they involve less upfront expense and do not cost as much to operate because they don't include equipment-mounted control boxes.

Other Frequently Required Equipment for the Health/Fitness Club Industry

As discussed previously, the health/fitness club industry is a capital-intensive business, especially from an equipment perspective. The majority of the capital spent on equipment is expended in one of the aforementioned four categories. Nonetheless, some relatively smaller categories also exist that can play an important role in the delivery of the health/fitness club experience, including:

❑ *Pilates Equipment*. Pilates equipment has slowly evolved into a significant equipment category with the growth of Pilates programs. Pilates equipment consists of reformers, trapezes, barrels, ladders, and some additional accessory equipment. The majority of Pilates equipment purchased by clubs falls into the category of personal reformers (e.g., a single-user reformer that can be used in an individual or group setting), which is the primary piece of equipment employed in both personal-Pilates training and group-Pilates training. The leading manufacturers of Pilates equipment are Balanced Body, Peak, and Stott. The cost of Pilates equipment varies from item to item, brand to brand, and model to model. For example, the average retail price for reformers ranges between $2,500-and-$3,000 each, with the classroom-designed reformers, such as Balanced Body's "Allegro Reformer" retailing for around $2,200. Another popular piece of Pilates equipment, the Cadillac (which is also referred to as the "Trapeze") ranges in price from $2,700-to-$4,000, depending on the accessories purchased with it. (Note: The Cadillac is a Pilates table with a series of attached overhead implements.)

> The majority of Pilates equipment purchased by clubs falls into the category of personal reformers (e.g., a single-user reformer that can be used in an individual or group setting), which is the primary piece of equipment employed in both personal-Pilates training and group-Pilates training.

❑ *Spa Equipment.* As day spas have evolved into a noteworthy profit center for many clubs in the health/fitness industry, the market for the equipment utilized in day spas has grown substantially. An incredible variety of equipment is needed to operate a successful spa, including:

- *Massage tables.* Massage tables range from fixed tables to adjustable tables, including hydraulic-driven adjustable tables. The price of a massage table ranges from $800-to-$1,200 if it is self-adjusting and closer to $2,000-to-$3,000 if it is hydraulic.

- *Facial tables.* Facial tables are similar to massage tables, except that they also have armrests and backs that enable users to be elevated so that they can be placed in a partially seated position. The cost of these tables ranges from $1,300-to-$4,000, depending on the features desired.

- *Manicure tables.* The typical manicure table includes all the storage for the manicure products. A high-quality manicure table retails for between $900-and-$1,500.

- *Pedicure stations.* The most popular pedicure stations include features such as a custom chair with armrests and a separate footbath/whirlpool. These stations retail for between $4,000-and-$6,000. Some pedicure stations are also available that employ portable footbaths and chairs, rather than the more first-rate features. These stations cost approximately $2,000 less than the more upscale models.

- *Facial Stations.* A facial station encompasses a variety of devices necessary for performing basic facials, such as a magnifying light and rotary brush. A quality system retails for around $2,500-to-$3,000.

  Examples of other equipment that is often employed in spas include hot wax units, paraffin baths, thermal heaters for hot packs, Vichy shower units, hydrotherapy tubs, scotch hoses, massage chairs, wet tables, and aromatherapy diffusers.

❑ *Sources.* Purchasing spa equipment can be a somewhat difficult task because no one manufacturer makes all of the items needed to operate a day spa. Some companies, such as Living Earth Crafts and Golden Ratio, provide a variety of tables and accessories, but not the full line of spa equipment. A few companies, such as Universal and Takara Belmont, distribute spa equipment from a variety of different suppliers.

Because the equipment industry is an ever-changing, fast-evolving enterprise, health/fitness professionals need to stay abreast of the changes that occur if they want to be knowledgeable about essential equipment-related factors. IHRSA annually produces a publication, *FIT (Fitness Industry Technology)*, that provides an overview of the various equipment categories and a listing of the various equipment suppliers. Several industry-related magazines, including *Fitness Management, Athletic Business, Club Industry, and Recreation Management* also produce annual

IHRSA annually produces a publication, *FIT (Fitness Industry Technology)*, that provides an overview of the various equipment categories and a listing of the various equipment suppliers.

publications on equipment that is utilized in the health/fitness club industry. (Note: A list of the leading manufacturers of health/fitness equipment in the industry is included in the appendices.)

Purchase or Lease Equipment

As previously stated, outfitting a health/fitness facility with new equipment can range from $10-to-$25 a square foot. As a result, a typical health/fitness facility might have to spend $300,000 to as much as $1,000,000 for equipment. This expense can often represent a significant financial hurdle for owners, and as a result, leasing becomes a viable alternative to acquisition and later depreciation. Many of the most successful club operators choose to lease their equipment rather than purchase it and thereby save the initial investment that would be required if they had purchased it. The following list provides a brief overview of the pros and cons associated with either leasing or purchasing equipment.

❑ *Purchasing Equipment*
- Pro:
  ✓ Outright ownership of the equipment
  ✓ Able to depreciate the equipment on financial statements
  ✓ Not at the mercy of leasing companies
  ✓ Causes club owners to have a greater "stake" in the business and commitment to making the business work
- Con:
  ✓ Initial up-front investment can be overwhelming
  ✓ Equipment depreciates in value as an asset
  ✓ Clubs are often less likely to invest in new equipment in coming years

❑ *Leasing Equipment*
- Pro:
  ✓ Eliminates up-front investment
  ✓ Allows cost of equipment to be spread over several years
  ✓ Provides opportunity to upgrade equipment more readily and remain current with trends
  ✓ Owners can step away from leases in the event of financial challenges
- Con:
  ✓ Increases the cost of equipment due to interest payments to leasing company
  ✓ May require club to have leases with more than one company

Many of the most successful club operators choose to lease their equipment rather than purchase it and thereby save the initial investment that would be required if they had purchased it.

OPERATIONAL PRACTICES IN THE HEALTH/FITNESS CLUB INDUSTRY

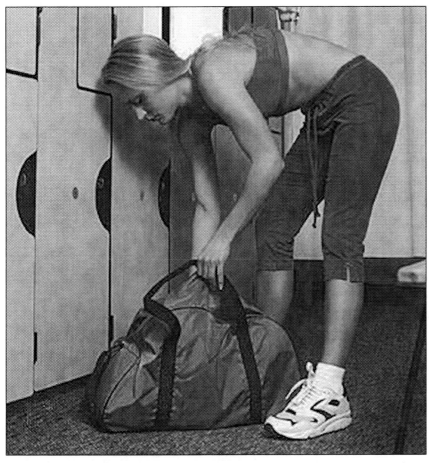

Part Seven

19

Risk Management

Chapter Objectives

Risk management refers to the practices and systems that businesses put in place to help reduce and/or eliminate their exposure to liability and financial loss. In the health/fitness club industry, risk management refers to the practices, procedures, and systems by which the club reduces its risk of an employee or member experiencing an event that could result in harm to the individual (employee or customer) or the business itself. This chapter reviews the most critical risk-management practices and factors that clubs should address in order to provide an environment that presents the lowest possible risk to the employees, members, and business.

Risk Management Practices to Reduce Employee and Business Risk

There are a number of key practices, policies, and systems that clubs should consider when managing their business risk as it applies to their employees, and ultimately to their members, including:

❑ *Background Checks for Specific Employee Populations.* Most of the employees in the health/fitness club industry are actively involved in providing personalized experiences that can expose not only themselves, but also the club, to considerable risk. Numerous club personnel, such as personal trainers, massage therapists, fitness instructors, and swim instructors, among others, typically work closely with members in a one-on-one environment, where the chance of a risk-related situation occurring exists. Some club employees, such as child-care workers, swim instructors, summer camp instructors, tennis instructors, etc., are in even more potentially risk-vulnerable positions, because they work closely with young adults and children. The key point that should be emphasized is that clubs should seriously consider doing background checks on every employee

Clubs should seriously consider doing background checks on every employee who comes into personal contact with the members to ensure that each individual member of the staff has no prior record of unsavory behavior that might expose other employees, members, or guests to harm.

who comes into personal contact with the members to ensure that each individual member of the staff has no prior record of unsavory behavior that might expose other employees, members, or guests to harm. For example, a simple background check can be performed by an outside agency to determine whether an employee has a past criminal record. In addition to those individuals who work closely with people, any employee who is responsible for handling money on a regular basis should also be a serious candidate for a background screening.

As such, numerous businesses, including many the health/fitness club industry, conduct annual background checks of those employee populations who present the greatest risk, such as those who meet the aforementioned criteria. It is important that if a club performs background checks, it should make its employees aware of its practices, policies, and procedures in this regard.

❑ *Drug and Alcohol Pre-Employment Testing.* The use of alcohol or drugs can impair an employee's judgment, which, in turn, could ultimately expose other employees or members to harm. Accordingly, drug and alcohol pre-employment testing is recommended for individuals employed in certain positions, such as those that require the handling of dangerous equipment, working with minors, or dispensing of alcohol. Such testing can help reduce the risk of an employee being impaired while acting on behalf of the club. Clubs should also consider testing other employees, such as bartenders, servers, housekeepers, engineering staff, locker-room attendants, and even fitness instructors. By law, drug, and alcohol pre-employment screening cannot be conducted without the permission of the individual who will be tested. As such, clubs must give their employees (actual and prospective) the option of whether to participate in the testing program. Fair or not, many businesses will view the refusal of an individual to undergo testing as a negative factor with regard to that person's worthiness as an employee.

Drug and alcohol pre-employment testing is recommended for individuals employed in certain positions, such as those that require the handling of dangerous equipment, working with minors, or dispensing of alcohol.

❑ *Ensure that Employees Have the Right Credentials to Perform Their Job.* The health/fitness club industry has numerous positions that require specific licensing, registration, or certification. In that regard, clubs can limit their risk by ensuring both at the time of an individual's employment and during the course of employment that each employee's credentials are valid and current. If a person who holds a particular position that requires special education, training, registration, or licensure is found to be lacking, that club may be exposing itself to considerable financial risk. Among the positions in a club where an individual's credentials should be checked at the time of employment or contract signing and thereafter on an ongoing basis are the following:

- *Massage therapists.* In thirty-three states, massage therapists must be either licensed, registered or certified to practice. Accordingly, clubs should ask all of their massage therapists for a copy of their license, registration, or certification documents (as appropriate) at the time of their employment and ensure that these are maintained.

- *Estheticians.* Estheticians are employees/contractors who provide selected spa services, such as manicures, pedicures, facials, and hair styling. Because these employees must be licensed, similar to massage therapists, clubs should obtain evidence of licensure upon employment.

- *Dieticians/nutritionists.* Many clubs offer nutritional counseling and related dietary advice. A registered dietician is a professionally trained individual who is recognized as having the education and qualifications needed to counsel and prescribe a nutritional plan. If the employee or contractor is not a registered dietician, then the club is exposing itself to an increased risk of liability.

- *Personal trainers and instructors.* At the present time, no established national standard or law exists concerning the required qualifications for a personal trainer. Both the American College of Sports Medicine, in its highly regarded text—*ACSM's Health/Fitness Facility Standards and Guidelines*, and IHRSA, in its book, *Standards Facilitation Guide: Health and Safety, Legal, and Ethical Standards for U.S. IHRSA Clubs as of 1998*, indicate that it is essential that personal trainers and other exercise instructors have the appropriate level of education and credentials. In fact, IHRSA has indicated that, effective January 1, 2006, it would only recognize those professional certifications with third-party accreditation from a nationally recognized certifying agency [e.g., National Commission of Certifying Agencies (NCCA)]. Accordingly, personal trainers should be certified by a nationally recognized certification program, such as those offered by ACE, ACSM, and NSCA. In some state legislatures (e.g., Texas), efforts are underway to compel personal trainers to be either registered or licensed. If a personal trainer does not have the appropriate certification, the club is exposing itself to greater risk.

- *Lifeguards.* In all states, lifeguards are required to have advanced lifesaving and water safety certification. Employing lifeguards without those credentials would expose a club to a substantial risk in the event of an accident.

Besides ensuring that their employees/contract labor possess the appropriate credentials, clubs should be aware of exactly what actions these individuals are legally permitted/qualified to perform. For example, a personal trainer is not qualified or legally recognized as someone who can prescribe either supplements or rehabilitative exercises. Likewise, a personal trainer cannot diagnose a member's health status. Similarly,

Besides ensuring that their employees/ contract labor possess the appropriate credentials, clubs should be aware of exactly what actions these individuals are legally permitted/ qualified to perform.

massage therapists are not legally qualified to perform therapeutic treatments using massage, unless they have the appropriate credentials. Clubs can avoid these issues by making sure that their job descriptions and employee policies clearly clarify such matters.

❏ *Handling Hazardous Chemicals and Materials.* The health/fitness club industry is a field in which many of its employees are exposed to materials that the Occupational Safety and Health Administration (OSHA) considers dangerous. Club positions, such as housecleaners, lifeguards, locker-room attendants, and fitness staff, among others, are occasionally exposed to hazardous chemicals and materials. These chemicals and materials include items such as cleaning agents, paints, and lubricants. For example, employees who work in closed areas where air circulation is inadequate, particularly in locations where sanding, drilling, or similar activities are occurring, can suffer undue exposure to particle matters. To comply with OSHA guidelines and reduce the level of risk involving the handling of hazardous chemicals and materials to their employees, clubs should undertake the following actions:

> **Too many club operators fail to realize that even the handling of towels involves an increased risk of exposure for employees and members to the problems that can arise from handling bodily fluids.**

- Ensure that the material data sheets (MDS) for every chemical and agent used in the club are posted in a visible location for all employees to see.

- Provide an MDS binder for all employees/contractors to review. Confirm that these individuals have viewed the information and understand the issues, usually by having them sign a designated sheet.

- Store all chemicals and agents in safe locations. Make sure that these materials are stored off the floor and in an area that is off-limits to the members. These storage areas should have locks in order to prevent their access by unauthorized individuals.

- Provide regular training in the proper handling of hazardous chemicals and materials.

❏ *Handling Body Fluids.* The health/fitness club industry is a field that exposes its members and employees to various bodily fluids. In fact, almost every individual who works in the industry can come into contact with bodily fluids, thereby being exposed to the resultant risk of disease. Too many club operators fail to realize that even the handling of towels involves an increased risk of exposure for employees and members to the problems that can arise from handling bodily fluids. As a result, an increased risk to the business itself exists in such circumstances. Among the key steps that every club can take to minimize their risk in this area are the following:

- Provide training for employees. Make sure that employees are taught how to handle bodily fluids. In this regard, OSHA provides training materials, as do many other organizations.

- Provide literature for employees on the handling of bodily fluids.

- Make sure employees who are handling towels, cleaning, or picking up papers wear gloves (surgical-style gloves). Employees who have to handle bar soap or razors should be provided with latex or similar type of gloves.

- Have a system within the club for the disposal of items that contain bodily fluids. If the club provides razors for members' use, it should have a biowaste container for their disposal. If the club washes the towels that are utilized in the facility, it should use bleach, which will help kill most of the pathogens that are carried in bodily fluids.

- If blood is visible, clean it immediately with bleach or similar agent, and do not let employees or contractors handle it.

Many of the costs and liabilities incurred by clubs result from not having a safety program in place that provides the proper education to employees about the risks of each job and how to prevent them.

❑ *Have an Employee Safety Program.* Clubs that want to reduce their level of risk involving their practices, policies, and procedures and the costs associated with those faactors need to provide worker safety programs that address the key safety issues inherent in each job. Many of the costs and liabilities incurred by clubs result from not having a safety program in place that provides the proper education to employees about the risks of each job and how to prevent them. For example, massage therapists, tennis instructors, and group-exercise instructors experience more work-related injuries than any other positions in the health/fitness club industry. The key point that should be emphasized in this regard is that a club must establish clear guidelines concerning certain positions and job responsibilities, for example, setting limits on the time a therapist can perform massage during a given schedule or placing strict boundaries on the number of classes that instructors are allowed to teach. A sound employee-safety program addresses several factors, including:

- Making sure that every job description identifies the tasks and activities of that job that may expose an employee to an increased risk of being injured. Having the employees sign-off that they are aware of those job-related parameters and risks.

- Providing ongoing educational programs on worker safety.

- Establishing a reward program for safety that recognizes actions that increase the safety level of the work environment.

- Making sure that all accidents or incidents are immediately reported and documented and that appropriate action is taken to deal with the incident.

> Clubs should maintain the appropriate types and the proper amounts of insurance in order to minimize their level of risk in the work environment and help protect both the physical and intellectual assets of their business.

❑ *Have the Appropriate Insurance Policies.* Clubs should maintain the appropriate types and the proper amounts of insurance in order to minimize their level of risk in the work environment and help protect both the physical and intellectual assets of their business. In this regard, club operators should carry the following types of insurance:

- *General liability insurance.* Every club should have a general liability insurance package that provides at least one million dollars in coverage per occurrence and up to three million dollars of total coverage. General liability insurance covers most incidences of negligence or accidents.

- *Professional liability insurance.* Professional liability insurance is one key type of insurance that many clubs fail to provide. Certain positions in a club, such as personal trainers, group-exercise instructors, and massage therapists, should be covered by professional liability insurance. This insurance covers issues involving professional competency. Although most clubs do not have this type of insurance, they should. Several of the professional associations in the industry (e.g., ACE, ACSM, NSCA, etc.) offer professional liability insurance-coverage packages, which members of those associations can obtain.

- *Worker's compensation insurance.* Clubs should consider establishing a worker's compensation program for their employees, especially if they have individuals who are performing jobs that expose them to injury and loss of work. In many states (e.g., California), such a program is required.

- *Property insurance.* Although property insurance covers the physical assets of a business, this type of insurance can be another key element in managing a club's risk, particularly its risk of financial loss if something happens (damage or loss) to its property or other physical assets.

- *Business interruption.* Business interruption insurance provides clubs with insurance against revenue loss due to unforeseen circumstances. For example, if a club has to close for a month due to fire damage, this insurance would protect their revenue stream during the time they are closed.

Risk Management Practices to Reduce Member/User and Business Risk

Effectively managing the level of risk to which members are exposed is important to clubs for at least two reasons. First, having sound member risk-management practices can help provide a safer environment in the club for the members and help reduce their chances of being injured or suffering other health-related problems. Second, properly managing the risks that members encounter in a club's facility can help reduce the likelihood of litigation directed to the club that can drain the financial health of the business. In that regard, several policies, practices, and systems exist that clubs can utilize to reduce the level of risk for their members.

❑ *Pre-Activity Screening.* The first basic step in increasing member safety and reducing risk is to make sure every member and club user has completed a pre-activity screening. According to both the most recent editions of the two most highly regarded texts on the subject, *IHRSA's Standards Facilitation Guide* and *ACSM's Health/Fitness Facility Standards and Guidelines*, a club must provide pre-activity screening for its users. Pre-activity screening should involve, at the minimum, screening for certain basic health risks, particularly, coronary-risk factors. In that regard, proven tools, such as the Par-Q or a simple medical history questionnaire (samples of which are included in the Appendices), can be extremely useful.

❑ *Medical Release and Waiver of Liability.* Clubs that utilize pre-activity screening tools should also have a system by which those individuals who are identified as having an increased risk due to their health profile either are referred to a physician for physician clearance before engaging in physical activity or if they refuse to obtain a physician's release (for whatever reason), are required to sign a waiver indicating they have decided not to obtain clearance from a physician and, as a result, are releasing the club from any liability associated with their participation in any physical-activity offering of the club.

> The medical release can be as simple as a one-page document that is forwarded by the club to the member's physician or provided to the member to personally take to their physician. The medical-release form should clearly indicate that the member has been identified as being at an increased risk of incurring an injury or health-related problem if the individual participates in a physical-activity program and that by completing and signing the form, the physician is clearing the member to participate in physical activity. The release should allow physicians to provide any recommendations they may have concerning the individual's participation in physical activity. An example of a medical-release form is included in the Appendices.

The first basic step in increasing member safety and reducing risk is to make sure every member and club user has completed a pre-activity screening.

❑ *Waiver of Liability.* A waiver is a legal document that members/users sign, indicating that they are aware of the risks associated with their participation in a physical-activity program that involves the club's facilities, programs, and services and that they knowingly accept full responsibility for their decision to participate in such offerings and are releasing the club from any and all responsibility for their participation. A waiver should be prepared by an attorney and should address the following:

Having an appropriate emergency-response system is an essential factor in the effort to establish a safe environment for members and employees, as well as a sound risk-management practice.

- The facilities, programs, and services that the member has access to and might use to pursue a program of physical activity

- The risks involved in engaging in physical activity, including and up to the risk of a cardiac event or even death

- A statement that the member is aware of the risks involved, that the club has explained those risks thoroughly, and that the member is willing to accept those risks

- The member's willingness to accept all responsibility for their participation in light of the information they have been provided and that they are accepting complete responsibility for their actions and releasing the club from any and all liability associated with their decision

The use of a waiver should be standard practice for every club. Ideally, all members/users should complete and sign a waiver form upon joining a club. Both *ACSM's Health/Fitness Facility Standards and Guidelines* and *IHRSA's Standard Facilitation Guide* indicate that waivers should be a standard practice for health/fitness club operators. (Note: Some recent court rulings have upheld a plaintiff's right to legal action even when a waiver has been signed.)

❑ *Emergency-Response System*. Having an appropriate emergency-response system is an essential factor in the effort to establish a safe environment for members and employees, as well as a sound risk-management practice. In that regard, health/fitness clubs must develop emergency response systems that help ensure that their members have the highest reasonable level of safety. An emergency-response system should encompass several key elements, including:

- Local healthcare and/or medical personnel should be solicited to help develop the emergency-response system that the club utilizes. Most emergency-medical services are willing to assist a club in developing an emergency-response program. Clubs can also pay for the services of a qualified person, such as a physician, registered nurse, or certified emergency-medical technician, to help guide the development of their program.

- The club's emergency-response system should address the major emergency situations that might occur, such as heart attacks, strokes, orthopedic-related injuries, accidents, etc.

- The club's emergency-response system should detail explicit steps or directions concerning how each emergency situation should be handled, including the roles that should be played by first, second, and third responders to an emergency. In addition, the emergency-response system should specify the locations of all emergency equipment and all emergency exists.

- The emergency-response system should be fully documented and kept in an area that can be easily accessed by the club's staff. In addition, the emergency-response system should be reviewed with each employee on a regular basis.

- The emergency-response system should be physically rehearsed by everyone involved at least once annually and preferably once every quarter.

- The emergency-response system should incorporate the use of an automated external defibrillator (AED) and cardiopulmonary resuscitation equipment (both of which are covered in greater detail in a later section of this chapter).

- The emergency-response system should address the availability and location of first-aid kits within the club.

- The emergency-response system should identify an on-site coordinator for the program (the employee who is responsible for the club's overall emergency readiness).

❑ *Signage.* Clubs can reduce their level of business risk and, at the same time, help create a safer physical activity environment for their members by developing signage that is then posted in appropriate locations that communicates to its members those areas of the club that involve a potentially substantial risk to an individual's health and safety. This signage should indicate the risks involved and include information that can lessen the member's risk if they respond appropriately to the information provided to them. Detailed information on developing proper signage for the health/fitness club industry is available in the American Society for Testing and Materials' article, *ASTM's Standard Specifications for Fitness Equipment and Fitness Facility Safety Signage and Labels.* The key areas of a health/fitness facility that should have signage include:

- *Sauna, steam room, and whirlpool.* Due to exposure to high heat and humidity, these areas present an elevated risk to both apparently healthy and at-risk users. As a result, clubs should post signage that provides users with the basic warnings and information concerning these areas that can help them make a more-informed decision about whether to utilize these facilities. Signage in each of these areas should include:

  ✓ Information about the temperature range to which the user will be exposed

  ✓ A warning about the increased risk of hyperthermia if too much time is spent in any of these facilities

  ✓ A warning about specific populations that should avoid exposure to these areas unless they have their physician's approval, such as

Clubs can reduce their level of business risk and, at the same time, help create a safer physical activity environment for their members by developing signage that is then posted in appropriate locations that communicates to its members those areas of the club that involve a potentially substantial risk to an individual's health and safety.

those individuals with either high blood pressure or coronary artery disease, women who are pregnant, members on vasodilator medications, etc.

✓ A warning to cool down after exercise before entering these areas

✓ Guidelines on what constitutes a reasonably safe time period for individuals to utilize these areas

- *Aquatic areas.* Most state and local health departments require certain signage be posted in the pool areas. These signage requirements are designed to protect users from exposure to risky behavior. Among the key elements that are normally indicated in pool signage are the following:

    ✓ A warning about not running or playing on the pool deck

    ✓ A warning about deck surfaces being slippery when wet

    ✓ A warning about no diving

    ✓ Information about food not being allowed around the pool

    ✓ Information that no supervision or lifeguard is present (if the pool is not required by law to have lifeguards)

    ✓ Information about not entering the pool immediately after eating

    ✓ Information about showering before entering the pool

    With regard to signage for aquatic areas, club operators should be familiar with the local laws and regulations to ensure that their facilities are in full compliance with all the legally required signage expectations.

- *Enclosed racquet courts (e.g., handball, racquetball, and squash).* Clubs should provide signage that indicates that individuals should wear appropriate eye protection when using the courts.

- *Fitness areas.* Certain risks exist in the fitness areas of a club with which many users might not be familiar. In those circumstances, the use of relatively simple signage can help rectify the situation. Examples of signage in these areas might include:

    ✓ Recommendation to have a spotter when performing certain free-weight exercises (free-weight area)

    ✓ Recommendation to get instruction or guidance from a professional before embarking on a fitness program

    ✓ Recommendation to stop exercising if the individual experiences dizziness, pain, or unusual discomfort

    ✓ Instructional signage that helps enhance the safety level of a particular piece of equipment

    ✓ Signage indicating when a piece of equipment is out of order

Certain risks exist in the fitness areas of a club with which many users might not be familiar. In those circumstances, the use of relatively simple signage can help rectify the situation.

In addition to signage in the fitness areas that focuses on the aforementioned information and warnings, clubs should also provide either perceived-exertion charts or target heart-rate charts so that members/users can monitor their level of exertion while exercising.

- *Hazardous conditions signage.* Hazardous conditions signage is general signage that warns members/users of any unusual risk attendant to a particular physical condition or practice at the club. For example, these signs should be used in situations such as:

  ✓ When equipment is out of order, and the club wants to make its members aware that the equipment is out of use

  ✓ When floors are being wet, and the club wants to make its members/users aware of slippery conditions

  ✓ When a condition exists, such as damaged walking surfaces, loose impediment, or a related condition that would increase the risk to the club's members/users exists

  ✓ When repairs or construction are being performed and the club wants to warn its members/users of specific dangers or locations to avoid

❏ *Preventative Maintenance Schedules and Audits.* One of the best practices that clubs can adopt for increasing member/user safety and reducing their business risk is to implement preventative maintenance procedures that are audited on a daily or weekly basis. The majority of accidents in the health/fitness club environment occur because club operators fail to execute basic preventative maintenance procedures and provide the necessary inspection of these procedures. Among the core practices that a club can execute in this regard are the following:

- Employ cleaning and preventative maintenance checklists for all fitness equipment. Clubs should ensure that its equipment is maintained on a daily, weekly, and monthly basis. This endeavor should include checking all bolts, checking all cables, checking for loose parts, cleaning surfaces, etc.

- Adhere to daily, weekly, and monthly schedules for cleaning all areas of the club

- Utilize checklists for performing preventative maintenance of lights, plumbing, and HVAC

The most critical factor is to have a system in place to verify compliance with the aforementioned, prescribed checklists. Many club operators employ supervisors to conduct regular audits of their maintenance procedures and practices. When audits are conducted, it is important to make sure the audit is documented, and the results are kept on file.

One of the best practices that clubs can adopt for increasing member/user safety and reducing their business risk is to implement preventative maintenance procedures that are audited on a daily or weekly basis.

❑ *Incident Reports.* Incident reports are standard forms that a business completes whenever an accident or incident occurs on its property. For health/fitness clubs, it should be standard practice to complete an incident report each time an accident or safety-related event occurs at the club. The purpose of the incident report is to obtain all of the information attendant to a particular event, such as the nature of the event, time of the event, witnesses, extent of any injury resulting from the event, response of the club to the incident, etc. This information can be extremely important for situations involving insurance, litigation, and responding medical agencies.

Automated External Defibrillators (AEDs)

❑ Overview. AEDs are sophisticated, computerized machines that are simple to operate and enable a layperson, with minimal training, to administer a potentially lifesaving intervention to individuals who experience cardiac arrest. AEDs are devices that can be employed in an emergency situation to detect a life-threatening cardiac arrhythmia and then to administer an electrical shock that can help restore the normal sinus rhythm. AEDs represent the third step in the American Heart Association's (AHA's) renowned "chain of survival"—after calling 911 and administering CPR.

> For health/fitness clubs, it should be standard practice to complete an incident report each time an accident or safety-related event occurs at the club.

The AHA reports that research shows that the delivery speed of defibrillation, as provided by an AED, is the major determinant of success in resuscitative attempts for ventricular fibrillation (VF) cardiac arrest (the most common type of cardiac arrest). Survival rates after VF decrease seven-to-10% with every minute delay in defibrillation. A survival rate as high as 90% has been reported when defibrillation is administered within the first minute of collapse, but decreases to 50% at five minutes, 30% at seven minutes, 10% at nine-to-11 minutes and two-to-five percent after 12 minutes.

Those communities that have incorporated AEDs into their emergency systems have achieved significant improvements in the survival rates for those individuals who have experienced cardiac events. In Washington state, for example, the survival rate increased from seven-to-26%, whereas, in Iowa, the survival rate increased from three-to-19%. Some public programs have reported survival rates as high as 49% with prompt administration of an AED. The American Heart Association is a strong proponent of having AEDs as accessible to the public as possible. The use and application of AEDs in a public setting is detailed in the American Heart Association's 2000 book, *Guidelines for Emergency Cardiac Care.* A revised version of the Guidelines is scheduled to be released in early 2006.

At the present time, the use of AEDs in the health/fitness club industry is a somewhat controversial issue. In 2003, IHRSA released a position statement on AEDs that indicated that although the Association felt that clubs should consider the installation of an AED, it did not believe that clubs should be mandated to install AEDs. Since that time, five states have passed legislation that would require health/fitness clubs to have AEDs in their facilities: Arkansas, Louisiana, Illinois, New York, and Rhode Island. In addition, as of July 2005, seven other states have legislation pending with regard to mandating AEDs in health/fitness clubs. Quite likely, more (if not all) states will pass legislation in the future that requires health/fitness clubs to provide on-site access to AEDs. Many of the premier health/fitness club operators in the industry have already made AEDs an integral part of their emergency-response system, including ClubCorp, Dallas, Texas; Fitcorp, Boston, Massachusetts; Sport and Health, Washington, D.C.; Tennis Corporation of America, Chicago, Illinois; Western Athletic Clubs, San Francisco, California; and Wellbridge, Denver, Colorado.

❑ *Guidelines for Implementing an AED Program in a Health/Fitness Club*:

- Every site with an AED should make an effort to get the response time from collapse to defibrillation to less than four minutes.

- AEDs that are located in the club facility should ideally be within a 1.5-minute walk of a potential collapse site. A responder should be able to reach an AED within a 1.5-minute walk time.

- The FDA requires that a physician must prescribe an AED before it can be purchased. The AHA strongly recommends that a physician, licensed to practice medicine in the community, should provide the oversight of the facility's emergency system and the role of AEDs in that system. In most cases, the company from which the AED is purchased will assist the club with identifying a physician to provide these services. Physician oversight refers to:

  ✓Prescribing the AED

  ✓Reviewing and signing off on the emergency plan

  ✓Witnessing at least one rehearsal of the emergency plan and providing a written report of such events

  ✓Providing standing orders for the use of the AED

  ✓Reviewing documentation of any instances when the emergency plan is initiated and the AED is used

- A club's emergency plan and AED plan should be coordinated with the local emergency medical services (EMS) provider (the product provider normally does this). Coordinating with the local EMS provider refers to:

  ✓Informing its local EMS provider that the club has an AED or AEDs

  ✓Informing its local EMS provider of the location of each AED in the club's facility

Quite likely, more (if not all) states will pass legislation in the future that requires health/fitness clubs to provide on-site access to AEDs.

All employees who are likely to be involved in a situation where they might have to administer an AED should complete a program in Basic Cardiac Life Support (BCLS) and AED usage from an accredited training organization.

✓ Working with the local EMS provider in providing ongoing training of the club's staff in the use of the AED

✓ Working with the local EMS provider to provide monitoring and review of AED events

- The AHA's Emergency Cardiac Care Committee and international experts encourage a skills review and practice sessions with the AED at least every six months. Regular practice drills every three-to-six months are recommended.

- The AED should be monitored and maintained to the manufacturer's specifications on a daily, weekly, and monthly basis. All results from those efforts should be recorded. AEDs currently on the market provide this capability through an automated process.

- All incidences involving the administration of an AED must be recorded and then reported to the physician who is providing oversight. It should be noted that the HIPPA (Health Insurance Portability and Protection Act) does not allow medically sensitive information to be released to anyone other than the medical director.

- Each club should have an AED program coordinator who is responsible for all aspects of the facility's emergency-response plan and the use of the AED, as outlined in *ACSM's Health/Fitness Facility Standards and Guidelines.*

- All employees who are likely to be involved in a situation where they might have to administer an AED should complete a program in Basic Cardiac Life Support (BCLS) and AED usage from an accredited training organization. Currently, ACE, AHA, and the American Red Cross (ARC) provide AED Basic Life Support training and certification. These programs involve a minimum of four hours of direct-contact training. Because training and certification lasts for two years, all employees should be required to complete such training on an every-other-year basis.

- A club should have at least one employee on duty at all times who is currently trained and certified in BCLS and AED administration. Ideally, more than one such trained and certified employee should be on duty at all times.

- Four special situations exist involving the use and application of an AED that the club should be familiar with and which should be reviewed during the initial AED training of the club's employees:

   ✓ AEDs should not be used in or around water. Because electricity takes the path of least resistance, it should not be used in or near puddles of water (shower, steam room, whirlpool, etc.) or in the rain. If necessary, the patient should be moved and dried off before attaching the AED.

✓The American Heart Association currently recommends that AEDs should not be used on children who are less than eight years old (it should be noted that this guideline may change with the release of newer guidelines).

✓External factors, such as clothing, jewelry, medication patches, and too much hair on the chest, could interfere with the AED effectiveness, and as a result, these items should be removed. The prep kit is normally included with the AED and can assist in the removal of these items.

✓Some individuals may have implanted internal devices, such as pacemakers and defibrillators. These devices create a small prominence under the skin. If such devices are detected, the individual using the AED should make sure that the pads are not placed directly over these devices because they may block the flow of energy.

❑ *Guidelines for Locating AEDs in a Health/Fitness Facility:*

- A critical step in the standard of care for use of an AED is the need to locate the AED where it can easily and rapidly be accessed in the event of a cardiac event. According to the AHA, this factor refers to the fact that an AED must be reachable within 1.5 minutes by a responder and must be applied in under four minutes from the time of a cardiac event. Accordingly, the club must consider these two time-related factors, when determining how many AEDs are needed and where they should be located in the facility.

- Clubs should determine which locations in the facility could be most easily accessed with a 1.5-minute walk. The average person who is walking at four mph can cover a distance of approximately 350 feet a minute, which translates to a distance of approximately 525 feet (175 yards) in 1.5 minutes.

- For clubs that have tennis facilities, the most suitable location in the tennis area for an AED would be the reception or reservation desk. If the desk cannot be reached in 1.5 minutes from some courts, then a second AED may be required and located at a second site. In most cases, a club with fewer than 20 courts will probably need only one AED, whereas a club with more than 20 courts might consider two AEDs. The highest risk areas in a health/fitness facility are normally the courts, the steam, sauna and whirlpool areas, and the locker rooms.

- For clubs that offer fitness facilities, the most suitable location to locate an AED would be the front desk. If any portion of the fitness facility cannot be accessed from the desk in 1.5 minutes, then at least one additional AED may be required and located at another site. Clubs that

A critical step in the standard of care for use of an AED is the need to locate the AED where it can easily and rapidly be accessed in the event of a cardiac event.

Clubs that have two floors should consider positioning an AED on each floor.

have two floors should consider positioning an AED on each floor. Other than the front desk, an AED might also be located in the exercise area, pool, or locker rooms. As a rule, the highest risk areas in an athletic facility are the locker rooms (where the steam, sauna, and whirlpool areas are located), fitness center, group-exercise studios, and racquet courts.

The key point that must be emphasized when deciding where to position AEDs in a facility is to ensure that every AED can be easily accessed. In other words, the AED should be positioned in an open location that has limited traffic congestion, rather than locked or placed in a closet or other area that cannot be easily accessed.

20

Front-of-the-House Operations

Chapter Objectives

Health/fitness clubs are successful because of many factors, including their operating practices. Operating practices are those administrative policies, practices, procedures, and systems that enable a club to deliver its products and services in such as manner as to create memorable member experiences and drive financial profitability. This chapter examines the "best" industry practices involving front-of-the-house operations. These practices are particularly relevant to those departments within a club that involve direct interaction between the facility's employees and members, including the front-desk department, child-care department, fitness department, aquatics department, and racquet/tennis department. Not intended to be all-inclusive, the chapter reviews the most critical practices (i.e., the "best" practices) that club operators should address in their operations.

Defining an Operating Practice

Operating practices can be most easily defined as administrative policies, practices, procedures, and systems that enable and empower employees to deliver the club's products and services to its members as consistently as possible. Operating practices range from the policies governing scheduling appointments to the practice of conducting new member orientations. The more formalized these operating practices are, the easier it is for the club to consistently deliver its products and services. The health/fitness club industry has numerous well-thought-out and proven operating practices. As a result, no one best method for operating a club exists. Instead, there are benchmarks or best practices that can help clearly define what health/fitness club operators should do in order to run their business successfully. The most successful club operators divide operations into two important components: standards and

No one best method for operating a club exists. Instead, there are benchmarks or best practices that can help clearly define what health/fitness club operators should do in order to run their business successfully.

systems. The operating standards are the minimum expectations that a club has for the delivery of a practice. These expectations provide a basic action framework for the staff. The systems are the tools that the staff can employ to meet the established standards or expectations.

Front-Desk Department

The front-desk department at the majority of health/fitness clubs in the industry has four primary responsibilities: greeting members and guests, scheduling appointments, answering phones, and disseminating club information. The degree to which the club is successful at each of these responsibilities is dependent to a great extent on the operating practices it has implemented.

❑ *Greeting Members.* The practice of greeting members is especially important in the club business because it sets the tone for each member's or guest's overall experience in the club. Successfully greeting members and guests depends on several factors, such as being able to make contact with each member/guest and calling them by name. It also requires being aware of their arrival and monitoring their access to the club. As a result, most club operators establish baseline policies and practices that are designed to drive the greeting process. Examples of some of the most effective operating practices or systems include:

> The practice of greeting members is especially important in the club business because it sets the tone for each member's or guest's overall experience in the club.

- *Membership identification system.* The majority of clubs require members to show their membership card upon entry to the club. Not only does requiring members to present their card enable the staff to ensure that each visitor to the club is a member, more importantly, it provides a means for personally identifying and greeting each guest by name. Some clubs ask their members to show their card to front-desk staff, while others require members to swipe their card through a card reader. The card reader system usually drives a screen on the front-desk computer that displays basic information on the member, including the individual's name, the last time the person visited the club, the individual's activity interests, etc. A recent trend is to use fingerprint or eye scan technology to indentify members. If the visitor is an invited guest, clubs require the presentation of an authorized guest pass that identifies the name of the guest, the dates the guest pass is valid for, and the name of the club member or staff person who authorized the guest pass.

  The most important policy for clubs with regard to greeting members is to have standards concerning their expectations on how members should be greeted. At ClubCorp, for example, one basic standard is to greet each member by name within 10 seconds of their arrival. Another standard is to stand and smile when greeting a member or guest. On one hand, ClubCorp's standards set the framework for its employees, while, on the other hand, the actual systems for performing standard-related tasks, such as collecting cards, swiping cards, etc., are the practices that allow the standard to be met at ClubCorp.

- *System for monitoring member and guest access.* Monitoring the access of members and guests is different than greeting them. Monitoring refers not only to being able to identify who is using the club, but also making sure that whoever is using the club is not exposing the club to any undue liability. The most critical step in monitoring access to the club is identifying if the visitor is a member or guest and whether that person is authorized to have access privileges. The majority of clubs utilize special technology to accomplish this step. Numerous software applications (e.g., Check Free, Aphelion, Innovatech, and CSI are examples of the many vendors that provide such software) enable staff to verify a member or guest's status, using existing databases that are stored on the software.

  The most critical step in monitoring access to the club is identifying if the visitor is a member or guest and whether that person is authorized to have access privileges.

  The monitoring process is important for several reasons. For example, it helps make sure that the club's facilities are made available to only those individuals who have paid for the privilege. It also provides a means to know who is in the club at any given time. In addition, it enables the club to determine overall club usage, information that can later be used to make other operating decisions. Knowing who is in the club can become extremely valuable in the event of an emergency or if someone needs to contact that individual. For those clubs that do not use software, the next best practice is to employ a sign-in log. A sign-in log involves having each visitor, member, or guest sign their name and list the time of their entry to the club.

  Another operating practice involved in monitoring is to ensure that each non-member/guest has completed a pre-activity screening instrument and has signed a waiver (if appropriate) within the past 12 months. According to *ACSM's Health/Fitness Facility Standards and Guidelines*, all club users must undergo pre-activity screening. Completing this requirement at the time of a person's entry to the club makes the most sense. At ClubCorp, the standard is to require each visitor, member, or guest to sign-in when they enter the facility and to have guests complete a pre-activity screening instrument at the same time and sign a waiver (if necessary).

❏ *Scheduling Appointments.* In most health/fitness clubs, the front-desk staff has the responsibility of making all reservations and appointments, including court reservations, appointments for personal training or massage sessions, class registrations, and event sign-ups. In some of the larger clubs, these functions are often handled by a separate reservation desk (e.g., East Bank Club, Chicago; Western Athletic Clubs, California; and

It is critical that clubs establish a standard concerning what information should be obtained when scheduling an appointment or reservation.

Lifetime Fitness, Eden Prairie, Minnesota). Regardless of which personnel in the club are assigned responsibility for handling reservations and making appointments, standards and practices for performing those duties should be established.

- *Scheduling Standards.* To ensure that the scheduling of appointments and reservations is handled properly, basic standards need to be established concerning what constitutes an appropriate reservation. In that regard, some of the key standards might include:

  ✓*Having a set restriction concerning how far in advance appointments can be scheduled.* In most clubs, this standard can range from one day to as far as a month in advance. Within the industry, for example, some tennis clubs limit their reservations to seven days in advance, while others allow reservations to be made only one day in advance. The key is for the club to identify the appropriate time limit during which its membership can schedule appointments in advance.

  ✓*Having a cancellation/no-show policy.* The most successful club operators establish clear cancellation and no-show policies concerning reservations and appointments. Such policies help establish clear value for the club's services and also help provide flexibility to accommodate other members and guests. A common practice in the industry is to have a 12-hour cancellation policy. In other words, those appointments that are cancelled more than 12 hours in advance result in no charge, while those that are terminated with less than 12 hours notice involve some form of penalty charge. A no-show policy involves establishing some type of consequence if an appointment does not show. For example, the club might charge a $10 fee for no-shows.

  ✓*Specifying the information to be collected.* It is critical that clubs establish a standard concerning what information should be obtained when scheduling an appointment or reservation. For example, at ClubCorp, when an appointment is made for a tennis court, the staff must get the member's name, the member's membership number, the time and date of the appointment, the court the reservation is for, and the staff person who made the appointment. In addition, the ClubCorp staff person who made the reservation/appointment must initial the reservation.

  ✓*Having a procedure that confirms appointments and reservations.* Another essential standard is to develop and adhere to a firm practice of confirming all appointments. Some club operators require their staff to send a confirmation e-mail 24 hours in advance of the appointment, while others have one of their employees reconfirm the appoint by calling the individual who made the appointment.

✓*Scheduling systems and practices*. Most clubs employ a paper reservation and scheduling system. These systems utilize pre-designed appointment books or reservation sheets that enable the necessary appointment information to be documented for each reservation and appointment. A few larger clubs have adopted electronic scheduling systems. Such systems allow the club's staff to make reservations, using custom-designed software. Not only do these software systems allow appointments to be made more quickly, they also have the capability of printing out daily appointment and reservation sheets. The most recent industry trend in scheduling is to use web-based scheduling systems that enable members to go online and make reservations and appointments through the web. Some clubs also permit their staff to make reservations on the club's computers. Supplier companies, such as Bookings Plus, CSI, and Xpiron have all developed good web-based, scheduling software. While no documented studies have been published regarding the frequency of using the web-based programs, empirical evidence exists that indicates between 10%-and-20% of members schedule appointments through web-based programs.

> **Clubs should identify a standard way in which the phone should be answered by every staff person.**

❑ *Answering Phones*. For most independent club operators, the front desk is the location where all phones are answered and information from those calls are processed. Many larger clubs have a separate department that is dedicated to answering the phone. The most recent trend in the club industry has been to automate the phone answering system so that callers never speak to a staff person; instead, calls are handled through a voicemail system. Those clubs that still view answering the phone as a primary responsibility of the front desk should establish standard practices for answering the phone. Examples of the more critical standards in this area include:

- *Specifying the number of rings before answering the phone*. At ClubCorp, for example, all phones must be answered within five rings. The key is for each club operator to establish a standard for this issue that is appropriate to the club.

- *Specifying the greeting*. Clubs should identify a standard way in which the phone should be answered by every staff person, for example, 'Hello, this is the Racquet Club, Mary speaking, how may I assist you?" Customer research indicates that it is very important for a business to answer the phone in an appropriate manner. Accordingly, clubs must establish clear standards concerning how the phone will be answered.

- *Specifying how callers should be put on hold or forwarded and, if necessary, messages should be taken*. Every club should have a standard practice concerning how calls should be forwarded and how

Clubs should establish standards and practices for handling the dissemination of information at the front desk.

callers should be put on hold. For example, at ClubCorp, callers are never left on hold for more than 30 seconds, before being given the opportunity to speak with a staff person. In this instance, the primary goal is to make sure that callers know that their needs are being taken care of in a prompt manner. With regard to forwarding calls, clubs should also have a set policy concerning this practice. As such, the club standard might involve requiring the staff person who answered the phone to contact the requested staff person to notify that individual of the phone call before forwarding the call. If the staff person is not in, the outside caller should be informed and asked if that person wants to leave a message. Each club can establish its own policies concerning how to handle phone calls. However, if the club wants to provide great service, it should establish clear standards in this regard. Similar to forwarding calls and putting the caller on hold, when it comes to taking messages, clubs should ensure that they have a standard format for taking messages. At ClubCorp, the front-desk staff is expected to get the name of the caller, the time and date of the call, the name of the person the call is for, and to initial the message.

❏ *Disseminating Club Information.* Another key responsibility of the front-desk staff is to disseminate information about the club. Front-desk staff are often expected to share important information about the club, either over the phone or in person. Accordingly, clubs should establish standards and practices for handling the dissemination of information at the front desk. Examples of basic standards and practices in this regard include:

- *Establishing what information can be disseminated.* Most clubs like to have their front-desk staff provide information about club programs and events. On the other hand, front-desk staff should never be required to give out membership information or employee/member information. Accordingly, club operators should develop a clear set of standards and/or practices that clarify the information that can be provided through the front desk.

- *Making the information accessible.* Once the club has established what information may be distributed through the front desk, it then becomes the club's responsibility to make that information easily accessible. For example, at some clubs, the front-desk staff are provided with binders that include information on:

  ✓Quarterly events and program calendar

  ✓Monthly newsletters

  ✓Group-exercise class schedules

  ✓Basic club information (e.g., the location, operating hours, and general description of the club's facilities, programs, and services)

  ✓Daily information (e.g., what is scheduled to occur that day at the club)

✓Club phone numbers

✓Names of department heads

✓Emergency procedures and information

✓Club policies and rules

Child-Care Department

In most health/fitness clubs, the child-care department provides what could reasonably be considered as short-term "babysitting" for parents who are participating in activities at the club. These "babysitting" activities differ from both licensed day care, which requires state licensure, and youth programming, which involves the delivery of organized and structured activity programs for children. Several policies and practices are very critical to the safe and successful operation of a child-care department, including:

❑ *Hours of Operation*. Clubs should inform their members when the child-care services will be available. Within the industry, these schedules can vary from club to club. For example, in some urban clubs, the hours that child-care services are available are scheduled around specific programs or times of the day, while in many of the suburban clubs that target the family market, these services are provided during the entire day.

❑ *Age Groups*. Clubs should make it crystal clear what age groups can be handled by the child-care department. Most clubs don't normally permit children below the age of six months or above the age of eight years to participate in their child-care programs. Many family-oriented clubs offer separate child-care areas for different age groups, such as a room for children who range in age from six months to 18 months, another for those from 19 months to three years, yet another for kids from three years to five years, and one for those from six years to eight years old. Every club should establish clear policies in this area. Many clubs also develop activity areas within the facility that are designed specifically for those children who are over the age of eight, but who are not yet teenagers (individuals who are often referred to as "tweeners").

Definitive guidelines concerning drop-off and time-limit stipulations are among the most important child-care policies and practices that a club can establish.

❑ *Drop-Off and Time-Limit Policies*. Definitive guidelines concerning drop-off and time-limit stipulations are among the most important child-care policies and practices that a club can establish. Since most states have strict restrictions governing the amount of time and extent of child-care services, clubs must be aware of the relevant regulations involving those matters so that they don't find themselves delivering a service that requires state licensure. For example, most states place restrictions on a club's drop-off policies if the facility offers "babysitting" services. Examples of key, specific issues that should be addressed in this regard include:

It is critical that every club spell out in detail what services are provided in the child-care area and how the children will be handled.

- *Time limit.* In most states, the maximum time a child can be left in an environment such as a child-care area in a health/fitness club is four hours, before licensing is required. To be on the safe side, many clubs limit the hours that they will "watch" a child to two-or-three hours.

- *Parent's presence.* Because of state requirements, clubs must require that parents be on the premises at all times when their children are in the child-care area. As a result, clubs should communicate this fact to their members. Furthermore, clubs should make sure that the members indicate their presence when they sign their children in.

- *Sign in and sign out.* A standard practice in most clubs is to require the parents or guardians to sign their children in and out of the child-care area. This practice usually involves having the parent/guardian sign their name, identifying their child's name, note (in writing) the time of the drop-off, and indicate which part of the club they will be in. If the parent chooses to have someone other than themselves pick the child up, when they sign in, they must provide that person's name and a means of identification for that person. At the time of signing out, the parent must present themselves, sign a sheet indicating the time they picked the child up, and note their relationship to the child.

❑ *Services Provided.* It is critical that every club spell out in detail what services are provided in the child-care area and how the children will be handled. In that regard, the following should be addressed:

- *Food.* Clubs should establish a policy concerning the provision of food for children in the child-care area. Some club operators require that parents/guardians furnish all of the food and beverages that their children consume while in the child-care area, whereas others adopt policies that indicate that they will provide water, crackers, etc. for the children. All factors considered, the prudent approach for a club is to have a policy that requires the food to be provided by the parents or guardians.

- *Rest-room practices.* Rest-room policies are a very sensitive issue for clubs and parents. With some children still in diapers, clubs must have a policy regarding the changing of diapers. The safest approach is to state that the club will not change diapers and will notify parents in the event that a diaper has to be changed. Clubs also should have a policy that clearly states what the policy will be when an older child needs to use the restroom. In these circumstances, some clubs require that the parent/guardian handle the situation. Other clubs have a policy that mandates that an adult of the same gender must accompany the child to the restroom entry and stand outside the restroom while the child is using the facility. This latter approach involves a higher level of risk from a liability perspective. Another option involves the fact that many child-care areas currently have a separate children's restroom that cannot be locked from the inside. In these facilities, a child can use the restroom, while the child-care staff maintains supervision of the child without direct contact or interference. Some clubs conduct background checks on all staff members who work in the child-care area and share the fact that these individuals have satisfactorily cleared their background checks with the parents who bring their children to the club. Another very important part of any policy concerning the child-care area is to have a sheet that the parent or guardian must sign, indicating how they want the club to deal with this issue while their child is in the club's care.

- *Activities.* Clubs should include in their policies what activities are provided for children while they are in the care of the club, for example, arts and crafts, computers, video games, nap time, etc. These activities should be spelled out very clearly for parents/guardians.

❑ *Registration and Enrollment.* Every club should have a policy regarding what information should be obtained the first time that a child is left with the child-care department. In most instances, this step would involve:

- *Obtaining medical/health information.* Clubs should obtain a basic medical background on each child, including any allergies, medical-health issues, special-handling instructions, name of the child's physician, etc.

- *Getting family-background information.* Each parent/guardian should provide certain background information, such as their names, contact information (phone, e-mail, etc.), whom to contact in an emergency, etc.

- *Waiver or release.* Each parent/guardian should sign a waiver or release indicating that they are aware of the club's policies and practices and concur with them. The waiver/release sheet should include specific space that can be used to document any special requests of the parent concerning the child.

- *Special instructions.* Each club should have a form that allows the parent/guardian to identify any special requirements or practices they want addressed with their child.

> Every club should have a policy regarding what information should be obtained the first time that a child is left with the child-care department.

❑ *Staff-to-Child Ratio.* If the club offers licensed day care, it is legally required to abide by certain child-to-staff ratios. These ratios vary, depending on the age of the children. Even though most clubs do not offer licensed day care, it is still important that all clubs have policies that address the ratio of staff-to-children in their child-care areas. While clubs should determine what is best for them concerning this factor, the following guidelines illustrate some of the practices that exist in the industry:

- Children under age two: no more than three children per adult.
- Children two-to-five: no more than five children per adult.
- Children five-to-eight: no more than six-to-seven children per adult.

❑ *Medical Situations.* It is extremely important that the club has a policy for handling any medical situations involving children in the child-care area. The two most important issues in this regard are handling children who are sick and their parents want to leave them in the child-care area and responding to a medical situation that arises while a child is under the care of the child-care department. In the case of a child being ill, clubs should have a firm policy concerning whether children who are ill can be left in the child-care area. Most clubs do not allow children who are ill to be left in the child-care area. This particular policy, while strict, helps prevent other children from catching an illness from the sick child. All factors considered, it is a well-advised policy to have in place. In the event of medical emergencies, the club should have a clear policy concerning what to do that is communicated to all staff and members. A critical part of that policy or practice should be to contact the parent or guardian immediately in the event of any emergency. Another key element of such a policy should be to have a signed form that indicates how the parent wants any emergency to be handled, if they cannot be reached immediately and the emergency requires prompt action.

> It is extremely important that the club has a policy for handling any medical situations involving children in the child-care area.

Fitness Department (Fitness and Group Exercise)

The fitness department is primarily responsible for making sure that each member and guest of the club is able to engage in a physical-activity program in a safe and effective manner. Although much of what this department does revolves around programming and risk management, there are a few operating practices that are critical to the achievement of its goals, including pre-activity screening, fitness assessment, orienting new members/guests to the fitness facilities, exercise prescription and training, on-the-floor supervision, and equipment care and maintenance.

❑ *Pre-Activity Screening.* The purpose of pre-activity screening is to identify the physical and behavioral factors that will influence the member's/user's ability to participate safely in a physical-activity program. Clubs should establish policies and practices that ensure that each member/user receives such a pre-activity screening prior to participating in a physical-activity program. The two most common pre-activity screening tools are the Par-Q (physical-activity readiness questionnaire) and the medical history questionnaire (MHQ).

- *Par-Q.* The Par-Q is a simple, one-page written instrument that screens for coronary-risk factors and identifies individuals who are at an increased risk of having a cardiovascular incident with the onset of moderate-to-vigorous physical activity due to their present coronary health status. The Par-Q was developed over 30 years ago as a basic, straightforward tool for identifying coronary heath risks. By having each member/user complete this form, a club can easily identify those individuals who will require further assessment or more careful guidance with their physical-activity program. This tool is designed to be used by both lay people and fitness professionals.

- *Medical history questionnaire (MHQ).* The MHQ is a more complete screening tool than the Par-Q and allows a club not only to identify coronary health risks, but also to uncover other health-related issues that might compromise the member's/user's ability to exercise safely. The MHQ can come in a variety of formats, ranging from a short form that seeks information on the most basic health-related issues to a form that elicits information concerning past exercise patterns and related lifestyle behaviors. The results of a MHQ should be interpreted by a qualified fitness professional.

Clubs should determine which of the screening tools will work best for them. Once a tool is identified, the club should then establish a process by which each new member of the club completes the pre-activity screening assessments.

❑ *Fitness Assessment.* Assessing the members' level of fitness is a practice that clubs should consider undertaking. All factors considered, such a fitness assessment may not be appropriate for every member. Primarily, fitness assessments should be used with those club members for whom additional information is needed to properly design their exercise program or for those members/users who want to establish benchmarks for monitoring their body's responses to physical activity. Clubs should have a system in place that provides a clear path concerning which members/users should be channeled into the fitness-assessment process. Fitness-assessment systems tend to vary considerably and can include any or all of the following elements:

- *Cardiovascular assessments.* Cardiovascular assessments can be as simple as a three-minute step test or as complex as a physician-supervised, graded exercise test. Most clubs typically employ either a step test or a sub-maximal exercise test using a bicycle ergometer to evaluate a member's level of cardiovascular fitness.

- *Muscular strength and endurance assessments.* The industry benchmarks for assessing muscular strength and endurance are component-specific tests, such as a grip-strength test, one-minute sit-up test, 1RM or 10RM test with specific exercises, or timed push-up test. On the other hand, a few clubs utilize sport-specific tests to evaluate the muscular strength and endurance levels of their members.

Fitness assessments should be used with those club members for whom additional information is needed to properly design their exercise program or for those members/users who want to establish benchmarks for monitoring their body's responses to physical activity.

> **It is essential that every club has a system in place to orient each new member to its fitness and exercise facilities.**

- *Flexibility assessments.* The most common flexibility assessment is the sit-and-reach test. A number of clubs use a goniometer to measure joint-specific ranges of flexibility for the trunk and limbs.

- *Body-fat assessment.* Body-fat assessment may be the fitness measurement that is most desired and used by members. The assessment tools for this factor range from simple circumference measurements to skin-fold measurements with calipers to underwater weighing for more exact determination of body fat. In recent years, some clubs have opted to use bioelectric-impedance devices and technologically advanced apparatuses, such as the Body Pod, to assess body-fat levels.

- *Metabolism.* With the recent focus on the nation's obesity epidemic, many clubs have started to employ more health-oriented assessments, such as those that measure an individual's overall resting metabolism and caloric expenditure. Devices such as the Body Gem, which is an indirect calorimeter, allow clubs to obtain relatively accurate measurements of a member's resting caloric expenditure. Such information can be used to provide better guidance with regard to weight-management efforts.

A club can offer other assessments to its members, depending on the level of sophistication the club wants to achieve. More detailed information on both pre-activity screening and fitness assessment is available in the most recent editions of both *ACSM's Guidelines for Exercise Testing and Prescription* and *ACE's Personal Trainer Manual*.

❑ *Fitness and Physical-Activity Orientation.* It is essential that every club has a system in place to orient each new member to its fitness and exercise facilities. The primary goal of this orientation process is to ensure that all members/users have the information and guidance that they need to safely use the club's facilities to pursue a program of physical activity. Some club operators design their orientation process to provide members/users with a brief introduction to their facilities and equipment, while other club operators view the orientation process as an opportunity to fully engage every new member into the club. Within the industry, clubs take several approaches to the orientation process, including the following:

- *Group orientations.* Many clubs schedule group orientations, which involve having new members attend a 30-to-60 minute session that is facilitated by a fitness professional. These sessions typically provide an overview of the club's equipment, a sample exercise program for working out with the equipment, and a brief explanation of how to use the equipment. Not only are these sessions designed to get new member started, they are also intended to introduce them to other services the club offers. In the higher-end clubs, these group orientations may also include an overview of other departments and an introduction to other services offered by the facility.

- *Individual orientations.* An individual orientation is a more personalized approach that is employed by some clubs. An individual orientation allows a new member to spend time one-on-one with a fitness professional who provides a more personalized introduction to the club's fitness facilities and services. In some instances, these gatherings feature a single 30-to-60 minute session, while in other clubs, they are offered as a series of 30-to-60 minute sessions. The extent of these individual sessions might range from a tour of the fitness facilities and overview of the equipment to a complete exercise prescription and multiple personal-training sessions. The trend among many of the larger club operations (e.g., 24 Hour Fitness, Town Sports International, Equinox, etc.) is to offer new members a three-session, personal-training package at an introductory rate as a means of orienting them to the club's fitness facilities.

❑ *Exercise Prescription and Personal Training.* The process of providing members with an exercise prescription and personal-training session may be the most effective approach for integrating new members into the club. Over the last decade, clubs have moved away from the tendency to provide each new member with an exercise prescription. Instead, they have focused on promoting personal training. This trend, while a positive step for those individuals who can afford to utilize personal training (five-to-15% of the membership), creates a situation where other members/users might be left without the guidance that they need to be successful with their physical-activity program. All factors considered, wise club operators should provide both of these systems for their members, given the fact that they build on and enhance each other's effectiveness and can help increase the overall level of member/user participation in the club's fitness offerings.

The process of providing members with an exercise prescription and personal-training session may be the most effective approach for integrating new members into the club.

- *Exercise prescription.* An exercise prescription is a personalized-exercise plan that is based on the needs of the individual. An exercise prescription takes into account several factors, including the member's/user's health status, level of inactivity/activity, and related lifestyle behaviors. Properly designed, it should serve as the foundation for a sound exercise and lifestyle program. Ideally, all members/users should receive a personalized exercise prescription that is documented for them on either an exercise card or software program. The exercise prescription should then be used to provide personalized fitness instruction from a qualified professional. The process of providing new members with an exercise prescription often involves having someone from the fitness staff initially take the member through the exercise program at least once or twice. After the initial sessions, the fitness staff should monitor the member's progress and, if needed, develop a revised program for the member. One of a club's primary goals should be to establish an exercise roadmap for members to follow and then to check their progress on a regular basis.

- *Personal training.* All factors considered, personal training is more of a program than an actual operating practice. Nonetheless, personal training is an important system that clubs should incorporate into their operations. In recent years, personal training has developed into one of the leading sources of incremental revenue for the health/fitness club business. The original focus of personal training was to provide members/users with the opportunity to work closely with a fitness professional who could provide them with a personalized exercise prescription and ongoing motivation. Currently, many club operators (e.g., Equinox, 24 Hour Fitness, Western Athletic Clubs, and others) have sophisticated systems for introducing new members to personal training.

❑ *Fitness-Floor Supervision.* The process of supervising the fitness floor is an operational practice that can lead to improved membership retention, enhanced level of revenue, and a safer club environment. Fitness-floor supervision refers to the process of having the club's fitness staff regularly walk the fitness floor to assist members with their exercise programs and to answer any questions members may have about their fitness programs. According to the most recent edition of *ACSM's Health/Fitness Facility Standards and Guidelines*, clubs should have at least one fitness professional on duty at all times who is dedicated to supervising the fitness floor. Accordingly, clubs should have a floor-supervision system that ensures that a fitness professional is always available to assist members on the fitness floor. The activities involved in fitness-floor supervision may include one or more of the following:

- Answering questions for members who are having problems
- Correcting members with their exercise technique, when appropriate
- Teaching new exercises to members, if appropriate, to replace ones that they are currently performing
- Checking the status of the equipment to make sure it is working
- Meeting new members
- Promoting other services and programs of the club
- Checking exercise cards and redesigning exercise programs
- Providing towels or water to the members
- Reinforcing the fact to members that they are exercising in a safe environment

> The process of supervising the fitness floor is an operational practice that can lead to improved membership retention, enhanced level of revenue, and a safer club environment.

Over the past few years, clubs have focused on offering personal training and have deemphasized the practice of maintaining a strong floor-supervision presence. One of the difficulties with this approach is that personal training reaches only five-to-15% of the membership, while supervising the fitness floor can touch the needs of far more members. It is interesting to note that one of the primary complaints of members on the fitness floor is the lack of attention they receive and the difficulty of obtaining assistance without having to pay for it. The key point that must be emphasized is that clubs that focus on establishing a process for providing supervision of the fitness floor can reap substantial rewards, in terms of both member satisfaction and membership retention.

❏ *Equipment Care and Maintenance.* Another critical operating practice that the fitness department must have is an established system for monitoring and caring for the equipment on the fitness floor. By monitoring the condition of the equipment, the fitness department can provide a safer and more convenient exercise environment. The process of monitoring and caring for the equipment should be a standard element of every fitness department's operating practices. In that regard, clubs should establish daily, weekly, monthly, and annual checklists for monitoring and caring for the equipment on the fitness floor. These checklists can serve as a means for the club to audit its equipment and ensure that all equipment is ready for use by the members. Almost without exception, all equipment manufacturers provide care and maintenance guidelines for their equipment. Figures 20.1 and 20.2 detail some of the important monitoring and care activities for fitness equipment.

Aquatics Department

The aquatics department requires strict attention to operating standards and systems. Much of this requirement stems from the fact that local health departments regulate many of the practices that are employed to operate commercial and public pools. Although not intended to cover every operating practice that is required to operate a pool environment, this section reviews the key operating practices and practices that are essential for the safe operation of an aquatics department, including:

❏ *Monitoring and Controlling Pool Chemistry and Temperature.* Maintaining the proper chemical balance in the pool is a crucial factor in member/user safety, not to mention a strict requirement of most state and local departments of public health. Some health departments mandate that pool operators monitor and record pool chemistry and temperature at least three times a day, while others only require such monitoring once daily. In addition to monitoring the chemistry and temperature levels in the pool, most health departments have established guidelines for what constitutes

Clubs that focus on establishing a process for providing supervision of the fitness floor can reap substantial rewards, in terms of both member satisfaction and membership retention.

Equipment	Daily Care	Weekly Care	Monthly Care	As Needed
Bicycles and Recumbent Bicycles	Clean off control panel with a damp cloth. Clean off seats with mild soap and water. Clean housing with mild soap and water.	Check equipment diagnostics on the control panel for any warnings or indications of problems. Check all screws and bolts and tighten as needed. If positioned on a carpet, vacuum underneath.	Remove housing covering the bike and clean out any dust or lint.	Refer to manufacturer's guidelines.
Elliptical Trainers and Stairclimbers	Clean off control panel with a damp cloth. Clean housing and pedals with mild soap and water.	Check equipment diagnostics on the control panel for any warnings or indications of problems. Check all screws and bolts and tighten as needed. If positioned on a carpet, vacuum underneath.	Remove housing covering the elliptical or stairclimber and clean out any dust or lint.	Refer to manufacturer's guidelines.
Treadmills	Clean off control panel with a damp cloth. Clean housing with mild soap and water.	Check equipment diagnostics on the control panel for any warnings or indications of problems. Check all screws and bolts and tighten as needed. If positioned on a carpet, vacuum underneath.	Clean belts using a damp cloth. Check belt/deck surface and lubricate as needed. Check rollers and adjust if they're out of alignment.	Replace belts if warranted Replace deck surfaces if diagnostics indicate. Refer to manufacturer's guidelines.

Figure 20.1. Care and maintenance guidelines for cardiovascular equipment

appropriate chemical levels. The four primary chemical levels that should be monitored and maintained are:

• *Chlorine or bromine level.* Most public/commercial pools use either chlorine or bromine as the chemical agent to prevent harmful organisms from reaching unsatisfactory levels in the pool. Chlorine, the

Equipment	Daily Care	Weekly Care	Monthly Care	As Needed
Variable-Resistance Equipment	Clean frames with mild soap and water. Clean upholstery with mild soap and water.	Check all cables and bolts and tighten as needed. Check moving parts and adjust as needed.	Lubricate the guide rods with lightweight oil.	Repair and/or replace pads. Replace cables if needed.
Free-Weight Benches and Accessories	Clean frames with mild soap and water. Clean upholstery with mild soap and water.	Check all cables and bolts and tighten as needed. Check moving parts and adjust as needed.		Repair and/or replace pads. Replace cables if needed.
Dumbbells and Bars	Clean off bars with a dry cloth.	Check all screws and bolts and tighten as needed.	Use lightweight oil on a cloth to remove any rust.	Repair and/or replace broken bars and dumbbells.

Figure 20.2. Care and maintenance guidelines for resistance equipment

most frequently used chemical, is added to the pool in one of two ways—either in tablet form (calcium or lithium) or in liquid form. In either instance, the chlorine level is controlled through automated systems that maintain the free chlorine level between one part per million (1 ppm) and three parts per million. According to the National Spa and Pool Institute (NSPI), the minimum level of free chlorine should be above 1 ppm. With regard to user safety and comfort, the level of chlorine should not exceed 3 ppm.

Because chlorine is a highly dangerous chemical, the club's staff should take considerable care whenever they handle it. While bromine is used less frequently than chlorine, many individuals consider it to be a more effective and user-friendly chemical than chlorine. Bromine is colorless and odorless and, as a result, is not as irritating to the member/user. NSPI standards indicate that bromine levels should normally be maintained between 2 ppm and 4 ppm, with the most appropriate levels being between 2 ppm and 3 ppm. Most modern pool systems monitor the chemical levels and adjust them automatically, based on the requirements established by the operator. A highly recommended practice involves having pool operators hand-monitor the chlorine and bromine levels in the pools themselves, as a back-up to the automatic monitoring systems.

Most public/ commercial pools use either chlorine or bromine as the chemical agent to prevent harmful organisms from reaching unsatisfactory levels in the pool.

According to industry practices, the temperature of the pool should be maintained within plus or minus two degrees of the temperature that is appropriate for the circumstances in the pool during the course of the day.

A third system for introducing chlorine into pools has recently found favor with club operators. This option involves using a "salt water" system that breaks down salt into free chlorine that enters the pool.

- *Total alkalinity.* The alkalinity level is another important factor that should be monitored at least once daily. The NSPI standard for the total alkalinity level is between 80-and-100 ppm when a chlorine system is employed and between 100-and-120 ppm when bromine is used.

- *Calcium hardness.* The NSPI standard for calcium hardness is that the level should be between 200-and-400 ppm, with a minimum level of 150 ppm and a maximum level of 1,000 ppm.

- *PH (percent hydrogen).* The recommended standard for pool pH is 7.4, with a range of 7.2-to-7.6 being ideal. If the pH falls below 7.2, then the pool water is becoming too acidic, and if it rises above 7.6, it is becoming too basic. Changes in a pool's pH level can be an indication that a chemical imbalance exists.

In addition to monitoring and maintaining the aforementioned chemical levels, pool operators should also monitor and control the temperature of the pool. According to industry practices, the temperature of the pool should be maintained within plus or minus two degrees of the temperature that is appropriate for the circumstances in the pool during the course of the day. The proper temperature for a pool depends on the activities that are being performed in the pool. While no universal standard exists, Figure 20.3 offers temperature guidelines that are consistent with policies and practices in the industry.

Activity	Temperature Range
Fitness and lap swimming	78-to-82 degrees Fahrenheit
Recreational swimming	82-to-86 degrees Fahrenheit
Aquatic exercise	82-to-88 degrees Fahrenheit
Children (under three years of age)	90-to-96 degrees Fahrenheit

Figure 20.3. Recommended pool temperatures, based on the activities that are being conducted in the pool

❑ *Cleaning the Pool and Filters.* Next to monitoring and maintaining the pool chemistry, cleaning the pool is the second most important day-to-day operating practice that clubs should systemize. Clubs should establish a cleaning checklist that is audited on a daily, weekly, and monthly basis to ensure that all basic cleaning functions are undertaken as scheduled. Figure 20.4 provides a general overview of the most critical cleaning practices for

Cleaning Activity	Comments
Vacuuming the pool	Pools should be vacuumed daily, using either built-in vacuums or automatic vacuum systems. The best time to perform vacuuming is at closing to allow for the appropriate interlude (at least five hours) to pass before allowing members to use the pool.
Cleaning skimmers	This practice is only required in pool systems that use skimmers. Most modern pools use gutter systems. In busy pools, this task should be done on a daily basis.
Cleaning the walls and tile	If the pool surface is paint, vinyl, or fiberglass, then the cleaning should be done with a nylon brush. This process needs to be done at least monthly and more often in pools with heavy usage. In addition, the scum line should be cleaned on a regular basis, using a soft brush or cloth.
Backwashing the filter	Backwashing needs to occur on a regular basis. In very busy pools, this step can be as often as once a day, but more likely will need to be done weekly. The frequency of backwashing normally is based on the guidelines of the filter manufacturer and type of filter employed (sand, diatomaceous earth, or cartridge). A pressure rise of 5 psi is often an indicator that a filter needs to be backwashed.

Figure 20.4. Key pool-operating practices

commercial pools, each of which should be an integral part of a club's pool-operating practices.

❑ *Emergency and Safety Preparation.* The pool facilities are among the most likely areas of a club to experience incidents that place members and guests in harm's way. As a result, clubs should implement operating systems that allow for the safest possible environment for members and users. The previous chapter presented an overview of basic emergency preparedness factors, measures that are especially important in the pool area. Beyond these basic emergency preparedness steps, clubs should also consider standardizing and executing the following pool-specific emergency and safety practices:

The pool facilities are among the most likely areas of a club to experience incidents that place members and guests in harm's way.

• *Post all appropriate signage, per local and state codes.* This signage should address several key elements, including showering before entering the pool, not running on the pool deck, no diving, notices on pool depth, communications on pool supervision or lack thereof, location of emergency/safety equipment, and information on contacting assistance.

- *Making sure that the proper safety equipment is positioned at poolside, and its location is communicated to staff and members/users.* Most local and state governments have specific requirements concerning safety equipment in the pool area. Far too often, these requirements are insufficient. The proper safety equipment for a pool includes:

  ✓ First aid kit

  ✓ Automatic electronic defibrillator (AED)

  ✓ Spinal board

  ✓ 25-foot rope attached to a ring buoy

  ✓ Shepard's crook

  ✓ Extension poles (at least one)

  ✓ Eyewash station

  ✓ Blankets or similar wrap

- *Providing the necessary supervision and oversight of the pool area.* In many states, a lifeguard is not required for pools that are less than five feet in depth. While the best operating practice is to provide a lifeguard during all hours that a pool is in operation, in those regions where one is not required, clubs should establish a monitoring system that ensures reasonable oversight of the pool area. Examples of such a system could include the following steps:

  ✓ Using video equipment and monitors

  ✓ Having staff do a walk-through of the pool every hour that the pool is open to members and guests

  ✓ Using volunteer lifeguards during peak hours

- *Conduct weekly safety audits.* Clubs should develop an audit checklist that addresses such factors as safety equipment, pool chemistry, pool cleaning, and supervision, and perform an audit, using that checklist, on a weekly basis to make sure that the appropriate safety procedures are being taken.

- *Store all pool chemicals in a safe area.* The chemicals used in pool care should be stored in a dry area and off the floor. Many of the chemicals used in pool care are highly volatile if they come in direct contact with moisture or other chemicals.

- *Have members/users sign in.* A highly recommended operating practice is to have every member/user sign in and out when using the pool. Limiting access to the pool area to authorized individuals can be a life-saving measure.

> **While the best operating practice is to provide a lifeguard during all hours that a pool is in operation, in those regions where one is not required, clubs should establish a monitoring system that ensures reasonable oversight of the pool area.**

Tennis Department

The tennis department, like the other aforementioned departments, can also benefit from having structured operating systems that can help ensure the consistent delivery of a safe and enjoyable experience. Administering the tennis department often involves many of the same operating practices that other front-of-the-house departments employ. Several operating practices exist that are somewhat specific to the circumstances attendant to the tennis department, including:

❑ *Cleaning and Maintenance Practices.* In order for members to have a relatively safe and enjoyable experience with the club's tennis facilities, certain cleaning and maintenance practices are necessary. Above and beyond the normal cleaning practices that a club conducts, these steps include:

- *Checking light levels and adjusting as needed.* The light levels at net height should be at least 40-foot candles, preferably closer to 70-foot candles. If the club has indoor courts, it should establish a practice of regularly monitoring light levels and replacing bulbs whenever the light levels fall below the minimum recommendation. Every few years, the light ballasts also need to be replaced.

- *Cleaning the courts surfaces of debris.* Cleaning the court surfaces of indoor hard courts typically involves vacuuming the courts at least once a day to remove ball fuzz. For outdoor hard courts, this task entails vacuuming or blowing off the courts on a regular basis, while for clay courts, it involves sweeping and watering the courts. Regardless of the type of court-playing surface or the method used to clean that surface, the key goal is to remove any loose impediment that could interfere with play or present a potential danger to the members/users.

- *Checking and adjusting the nets.* On a daily basis, the club staff should check the nets for damage and tension levels. Nets with holes should be repaired or replaced, and nets at the improper height should be adjusted.

- *Inspecting and repairing court surfaces.* Hard courts often crack and present a danger to the member/user. Clay courts can have low spots or areas of hardening that also present a danger. Accordingly, clubs should regularly inspect the court surfaces and make the appropriate repairs.

❑ *Scheduling Court Reservations.* Every club should establish operating policies and practices regarding the scheduling of tennis-court time. These policies and practices should be understood by the staff and clearly communicated to the club's members. Examples of reservation and scheduling practices and policies include:

> **Regardless of the type of court-playing surface or the method used to clean that surface, the key goal is to remove any loose impediment that could interfere with play or present a potential danger to the members/users.**

It is important to note that a club's practices for front-of-the-house operations are not exclusive of other club practices.

- *Establishing limits for court time.* Most indoor courts normally schedule time in one-hour blocks, while outdoor courts employ 90-minute blocks.

- *Establishing advance reservation limits.* Clubs should set limits concerning how far in advance members/users can reserve a court. Most clubs in the industry permit reservations to be made up to one week in advance.

- *Establish matchmaking services.* Many clubs establish practices that allow the club to arrange matches for members in those instances when the facilities are provided with sufficient notice.

- *Establishing a requirement for the basic information needed to reserve a court.* As a rule, this requirement involves obtaining several pieces of information, including name, member number, number of players, etc. This practice is very similar to front-desk operations.

- *Permanent court-time policies.* Some clubs provide their members with permanent court time, which refers to the practice of giving members the same reservation timeslots each week. This practice requires careful consideration to ensure that too many members of the club are not precluded from playing because of other members taking the most desirable timeslots.

❑ *Programming Functions.* Sound programming is the essence of a successful tennis program. The most successful tennis operators establish specific operating practices that govern their facility's approach to programming. In turn, these practices enable members to actively participate in those tennis programs that most interest them. Examples of operating practices often employed in the industry involving tennis programming include:

- Establishing and distributing an annual program calendar and booklet

- Having a matchmaking policy and detailed steps that should be taken for matchmaking to occur

- Having registration forms for each tennis program available in areas that members/users can easily access

- Posting the guidelines and rules pertaining to each program. This step can involve several tools, including websites, newsletters, or handbooks for members.

Key Points to Consider

It is important to note that a club's practices for front-of-the-house operations are not exclusive of other club practices, involving such diverse elements as programming, service delivery, and marketing. In many instances, what might be considered service delivery might actually be an operating practice, or what is considered programming could also be termed as operations. Accordingly, the operating practices reviewed in this chapter involve those policies, practices, and systems that were not previously detailed in other chapters.

21

Heart-of-the-House Operations

Chapter Objectives

The previous chapter presented an overview of the basic operating practices and systems that are important to front-of-the-house departments (e.g., front-desk, child-care, fitness, pool, and racquet/tennis). This chapter examines the "best" practices for "heart-of-the-house" operations. Heart-of-the-house operations encompass supporting those areas of the club that directly interact with the members and users, the functions and staff of those departments that so that they can better serve the needs of the facility's membership. "Heart-of-the-house" operations in health/fitness clubs involve several departments, including locker rooms, laundry, housecleaning, and accounting. This chapter provides a detailed review of the key operating practices and systems for each of those departments.

The operating practices involving locker rooms tend to vary from club to club.

Locker Rooms

The health/fitness club industry has a diverse array of locker-room offerings and operations. For example, some clubs have locker rooms that only offer changing areas and day-use lockers, while other facilities feature full-scale locker rooms that include such conveniences, as rental lockers, laundry services, and a full array of amenities. As a result of this diversity of offerings, the operating practices involving locker rooms tend to vary from club to club. This section on locker rooms initially presents an overview of basic locker-room operating models and then examines the key practices that clubs should adopt to facilitate operations in their locker rooms.

❏ *Types of Locker Rooms.** There are four basic types of locker rooms. The first type of operating set-up for locker rooms is the basic model that

*It should be noted that some of the information in this section is also addressed in Chapter 17.

involves a changing area with day-use lockers (users bring their own locks), shower areas, and restrooms. Locker rooms in this category offer no towel service (although some clubs provide towels for a fee) or any type of amenity, such as soap or shampoo. In most instances, this type of locker room is typically found in clubs that have a lower dues structure (e.g., normally under $40 a month), such as national chain LA Fitness.

The second type of locker room (this structure is the most common in the industry), consists of locker rooms that have changing areas with day-use lockers (the lockers have day-use access with cards, keys, or personal locks), showers, restrooms, sauna, steam and/or whirlpool (usually a combination of these), and several basic service amenities, such as towels, soap, and shampoo. This type of locker room arrangement typically exists in clubs that have monthly dues structures that range from $40-to-$100 a month, such as national chains 24 Hour Fitness and Lifetime Fitness or regional clubs, such as Town Sports International. The third type of operating structure for locker rooms, which appear mostly in high-end clubs, such as Western Athletic Clubs, Wellbridge, and Tennis Corporation of America, entails locker rooms that include changing areas with both day-use lockers and rentable lockers (a combination of card access and keyed locks), showers, restrooms, sauna, steam and/or whirlpool (usually all three are provided), a full line of amenities, such as towels, soap, and shampoo, and services, such as laundry and shoe shines.

Members see cleanliness as one of the critical factors in choosing a club.

The fourth type of locker room operating structure is available in some of the premier clubs and club companies in the industry, such as the Houstonian, ClubCorp, Sports Club/LA, and Pacific Athletic Club (operated by Western Athletic Clubs). This "executive" premier locker-room space includes premium lockers (i.e., full-height, rentable lockers), private showers, separate sauna, steam room and whirlpool, uniform and laundry service, shoe shines, lounges, coffee services, and more.

Each of the aforementioned operating structures has its advantages and disadvantages. On one end of the continuum is the simple locker-room structure that requires minimal staffing and work to maintain and brings in no incremental revenue. On the other end of the continuum is the full-service locker room that involves considerable staffing and work to maintain, but concurrently produces significant revenue streams.

❑ *Operating Practices for the Locker Room*:
   • *Cleaning and care of locker rooms.* According to research conducted by Roper Starch for IHRSA, members see cleanliness as one of the critical factors in choosing a club. This attribute becomes even more crucial when it comes to women, since they tend to see cleanliness as far more important than men when choosing to join or remain a club member. Since locker rooms typically have the most traffic of any area in the club (statistics indicate that members spend between 33%-and-

Club operators should establish a system that ensures that their facility's locker rooms are well maintained and clean at all times.

50% of their time in the locker room), the value of maintaining the locker room in tip-top condition is heightened. Accordingly, club operators should establish a system that ensures that their facility's locker rooms are well maintained and clean at all times. Figure 21.1 illustrates the most important areas of cleaning in the locker room.

- *Maintaining the sauna, steam room, and whirlpool.* It is important that clubs that offer one or more of these amenities should care and monitor these areas on a regular basis. Accordingly, clubs should establish a system of standardized practices to help maintain these areas. Examples of standardized practices for the sauna, steam room, and whirlpool include the following:

Daily Activities	Bi-monthly	Monthly/Quarterly/Annually
Remove trash and replace liners	Completely clean mirrors and glass surfaces	Refill air fresheners and dispensers (monthly)
Refill paper dispensers	Clean all hard surfaces by scrubbing with a machine or similar brush	Clean grout lines in showers (monthly.
Refill all soap and related dispensers	Clean and disinfect showers, steam room, sauna, and whirlpool completely	Clean carpets with bonnet-style cleaner (quarterly)
Dust all surfaces with a lint-free cloth	Clean and dust all HVAC grills and vents	Extraction clean carpets (annually)
Spot clean all mirrors and glass surfaces	Clean light fixtures	Wash down all walls (annually)
Spot clean locker surfaces, doors, and all exposed hardware	Empty and clean out all dispensers	
Clean and disinfect sinks, commodes, and urinals	Empty and clean out all waste repositories	
Clean and disinfect sauna, steam room, and whirlpool	Clean and polish all wood surfaces	
Vacuum carpets		
Dust-mop or sweep wood surfaces		
Wet mop and disinfect hard-floor surfaces.		

Figure 21.1. Locker room cleaning and care chart

✓ *Sauna*:

- Monitor the temperature in the sauna every couple of hours and maintain it between 160-and-170 degrees Fahrenheit.
- Make sure that a working clock and thermometer are present at all times in the sauna area.
- Clean the surfaces daily.
- Check the room every couple of hours to make sure no member is in harm's way.
- Pick up all loose papers in the room.
- Post appropriate signage regarding the precautions that members should take before entering and using the sauna (refer to the chapter on risk management for additional information).
- Have a mechanism in place to shut down the sauna if the room's temperature rises too high.

✓ *Steam room*:

- Monitor the temperature in the steam room every couple of hours and maintain it between 100-and-110 degrees Fahrenheit.
- Make sure that a working clock and thermometer are present at all times in the steam room.
- Clean and scrub the steam room's surfaces, floors, and walls daily.
- Make sure that a source of cold water is available in the steam room.
- Check the steam room every couple of hours to make sure that no member is in harm's way.
- Pick up all loose papers in the room.
- Post appropriate signage regarding the precautions that members should take before entering the steam room (refer to the chapter on risk management for additional information).
- Have a mechanism in place to shut down the steam room if the room's temperature rises too high.

✓ *Whirlpool:*

- Monitor the temperature in the whirlpool every couple of hours and maintain it between 102-and-105 degrees Fahrenheit.
- Monitor the pool chemistry (pH and chlorine levels) at least twice a day and maintain the proper balance (ph 7.2-to-7.4 and chlorine 1 ppm-to-3 ppm)

Monitor the temperature in the steam room every couple of hours and maintain it between 100-and-110 degrees Fahrenheit.

— Make sure that a working clock and thermometer are present in the area of the whirlpool at all times.

— Empty and clean the whirlpool daily, including cleaning the scum line along the top edge of the whirlpool.

— Check the whirlpool every couple of hours to make sure that no member is in harm's way.

— Remove any unwanted containers that might be adjacent to the whirlpool.

— Post appropriate signage regarding the precautions that members should take before entering the whirlpool (refer to the chapter on risk management for additional information).

— Have a mechanism in place to shut down the whirlpool if the temperature in the whirlpool rises too high.

• *Locker Assignments and Usage.* As discussed previously, lockers are handled in one of three ways in most clubs. The first method allows members/users to bring their own locks to use with available lockers. The second option permits members to use available lockers, but requires the utilization of either an access card (usually the individual's membership card), token, or key. The third approach involves renting the lockers and providing the member/user with a combination for the locker. Among the more important practices that apply to each of these systems are the following:

Lockers are handled in one of three ways in most clubs.

✓*Available lockers, with the user's padlocks:*

— Provide signage at the front-desk area, inside the locker room, and inside the lockers that indicate that the club is not responsible for items that the member leaves in the lockers.

— Have a daily system in which the staff removes padlocks that remain on lockers at closing each evening.

— Have a system in place where the staff removes any items remaining in the lockers at closing each evening.

✓*Available lockers, accessed with a card, key, or token:*

— Provide signage at the front-desk area, inside the locker room, and inside the lockers that indicate that the club is not responsible for items that the member leaves in the lockers.

— If members have to obtain the access card, key, or token from the club, have a system for requiring the user to leave personal identification or other item as collateral for the access item. The club employs this collateral to help motivate individuals to return the access tool before leaving the club.

— Have a system in place where the staff checks the lockers at closing each evening and removes any remaining items.

— Have a system in place that enables the staff to open the lockers if members lose their key or access card/token.

✓ *Rented lockers, accessed with a combination:*

— Provide signage at the front-desk area, inside the locker room, and inside the lockers that indicates that the club is not responsible for items that the member leaves in the lockers.

— Provide a system that ensures that each member registers for a locker. This step requires a process of obtaining specific information from the member, assigning a locker and combination, and initiating charges for the locker.

— Provide a system to audit/monitor the rented and un-rented lockers each month to verify occupancy and charged fees.

— Provide a system that allows members to forego their commitment to rent a locker. As part of this system, the club must have a method for ensuring that those lockers are not in use and have a process to make sure that the combination on all resigned lockers is changed before a locker is rented to another member.

— Have a system in place where the staff checks the lockers after a resignation and removes any items that remain in the locker.

— Have a system in place that enables the staff to open the lockers if members forget their combination.

- *Dispersing and handling amenities.* As discussed previously, many locker-room operational set-ups offer various amenities to club members. In this instance, the most commonly provided amenities are towel service, basic personal-care items, shoe shines, and uniform services. Clubs should establish standardized systems for each of these practices to ensure that they are handled in a consistent, appropriate manner. These operational practices can address the following key factors:

✓ *Personal-care items.* Two of the items most frequently provided by clubs are soap and shampoo. Other personal-care items that some clubs offer include conditioner, body lotion, hair spray, shaving cream, and razors. With regard to personal-care items, the following operational practices can help ensure an orderly dispensing system:

— Establish a practice of having the staff check all dispensers before each high-activity period and make sure that all dispensers are filled.

— Establish a par-stock inventory practice. This requires the club to have the staff sign out and identify the quantity of items they remove from the inventory and place in the locker rooms. This process helps ensure that clubs do not fall low on their inventory and helps control potential inventory theft.

Many locker- room operational set-ups offer various amenities to club members. In this instance, the most commonly provided amenities are towel service, basic personal-care items, shoe shines, and uniform services.

—Establish consistency in the types of personal-care items that the facility provides. Many members perceive changes in personal-care items among the most disturbing actions that clubs can take.

✓*Towels*. Towels are among the most worthwhile amenities that a club can offer its members. At the same time, if a club does not handle the disbursement of towels properly, it can present one of the greatest operating challenges that the staff might experience. The type of towels offered will depend on the dues structure and market position of the club. Clubs serving less affluent demographics and with lower price points normally offer import towels that weigh between six-and-eight pounds to the dozen, while clubs serving a more affluent demographic normally provide domestic towels that range in weight from 10-to-14 pounds to the dozen.

If a club does not handle the disbursement of towels properly, it can present one of the greatest operating challenges that the staff might experience.

—Establish a system for distributing towels. Some clubs, for example, distribute towels at the front desk and require users to pay for them, while other clubs leave the towels out in the locker rooms and allow members to use as many as they desire. The tendency for clubs that leave the towels out in the locker rooms is to charge higher dues.

—Establish a system to monitor towel usage. If the club distributes towels at the front desk, this practice can also serve as a system for monitoring or controlling towel usage. Clubs that leave towels out in the locker room, however, should perform regular weekly inventory counts to maintain better control of their towels. These clubs should consider placing an abundance of towel bins in the locker-room areas to encourage members to leave the towels that they use in the club.

—Establish a system where the staff monitors the locker rooms every few hours to pick up towels and replenish the supply of towels.

✓*Shoe shines*. In many of the higher-end clubs (e.g., ClubCorp, Tennis Corporation of America, Western Athletic Clubs, and Sports Club/LA), shoe shines are an important locker-room amenity. Some of these clubs provide shoe shines purely as a value-added service, while others see it as a source of added incremental revenue. From an operating perspective, several key practices should be developed with regard to offering a shoe-shine service, including:

—Establish a process for members/users leaving their shoes. Some clubs require that members take their shoes to a designated shoe-shine area, while others have members leave their shoes in front of their lockers, where the staff picks them up and returns them.

— Establish a fee system for the members, where the members either charge the shoe-shine service to their membership or pay the locker room staff directly. In a few facilities, the service is provided on a complimentary basis.

✓ *Uniform service.* Providing uniforms (workout shorts, shirts, socks, and supporters—if needed) in the locker room has become an increasingly popular amenity, especially in urban clubs and clubs that serve a corporate market. Two distinct approaches exist with regard to offering uniform service. In one scenario, some clubs provide and wash the uniforms of members and employees (e.g., ClubCorp and Sports Club/LA). The other option involves clubs allowing their members (and in some cases, employees) to use their own workout apparel, which the club washes and cares for them. Both of these approaches require that clubs should establish practices that help ensure that this amenity is provided (delivered) in an appropriate manner. In that regard, the following steps can facilitate the process:

— Establish a detailed delivery process if the club supplies the uniforms. Some clubs, for example leave the uniform items on shelves for members to select. In this situation, members wear the uniform and afterwards drop the used uniform in a bin to be washed. Other clubs issue each member a uniform and uniform bag. This practice involves having the member wear the uniform and afterwards place it in a bag that is left in a bin for washing. The bag is subsequently returned to the member's locker.

— If the club washes the member's/user's personal workout apparel, establish rules and processes governing this practice. In this regard, clubs should specify what workout apparel the club will wash and whether the club will assume responsibility for any lost apparel (except for very unique circumstances, clubs should not be responsible for lost apparel). The club should also develop a system for handling personal workout apparel (e.g., the club provides laundry bags for members to use).

— Establish a policy that limits the club's responsibility for replacing lost or damaged uniforms (e.g., one uniform per member per year if the club provides the uniform).

Laundry

Laundry operations exist in over 50% of health/fitness clubs in the industry. As a rule, they are standard service in those clubs that serve a more affluent

Laundry operations exist in over 50% of health/fitness clubs in the industry. As a rule, they are standard service in those clubs that serve a more affluent member demographic.

member demographic. The laundry department's sole responsibility is to handle the laundry needs of the club, ranging from washing towels only to cleaning an array of items, such as towels, uniforms, sheets, table covers, etc. Although a few clubs employ outside laundry services for their towels and related items, the cost of these services and the quality of the towels normally provided by them does not always serve the best interests of either the club or the members/users. While laundry operations are not very complicated, if the right systems are not in place, clubs will likely discover that the laundry can cause far more difficulties than expected, particularly with regard to member satisfaction. Accordingly, clubs should standardize the most basic laundry practices to ensure that difficulties do not arise. Among the key practices involving the laundry are the following:

> **Despite its importance to the consumer, the need to keep the facility clean and well-maintained is frequently neglected by club operators.**

❑ *Have the Right Equipment.* If the club is going to have a laundry, it is essential that the facility has the equipment that the staff needs to handle the laundry demands of the club, for example, commercial-grade washer extractors and dryers. Most clubs will find that they need a minimum of one 50-to-60 pound washer extractor for every 1,500 memberships and twice that (100-to-120 pounds) in dryer capacity for every 1,500 memberships if they do towels only. If the club provides laundry service for uniforms, then the aforementioned equipment requirements will apply for every 1,000 memberships. In addition to an appropriate number of washers/extractors and dryers, clubs should have automated dispensing systems (machines that mix the cleaning agents and dispense them at the right time and in the right combination in the washers). Several companies, such as Ecolab, manufacture these systems.

❑ *Establish Task-Oriented Checklists.* Many clubs assign the responsibility of handling the laundry to the housecleaning department or earmark the duties involved to all staff members. Other clubs, such as the East Bank in Chicago or the Houstonian in Houston, have dedicated laundry staff. Figure 21.2 presents a list of those operational practices that should be established (and monitored through task-oriented checklists) to effectively manage the laundry.

Housecleaning

The cleaning and care of the overall facility is often one of the most overlooked elements of club operations. According to consumer research, the cleanliness of a facility is one of the most important factors that influences a person's decision to either join or remain a club member. Despite its importance to the consumer, the need to keep the facility clean and well-maintained is frequently neglected by club operators. In fact, cleaning the facility should not occur either by accident or as an afterthought. Rather, it should be a by-product of an established system of formalized practices that are adhered to on a routine

Activity or Task	Frequency
Clean out dryer filter	After each drying cycle
Check cleaning-fluid levels for the washer	Before each load is put in
Adhere to recommended guidelines concerning specific number of items that can be placed in either the washer or dryer	Count before each load and the machine is started
Clean out behind washers and dryers	Daily
Follow cleaning and drying instructions, per manufacturer guidelines	Adhered to with each load
Fold towels and uniforms (clubs should outline their expectations)	After each load
Inventory towels	Daily, weekly, and monthly

Figure 21.2. Recommended operational practices involving the laundry

Facility Area	Cleaning Activity	Frequency
Fitness Floor	• Remove trash	Daily
	• Dust all horizontal surfaces	Daily
	• Clean and disinfect vinyl pads on equipment	Daily
	• Clean and disinfect equipment frames	Daily
	• Vacuum carpets and clean stains	Daily
	• Spot-clean mirrors	Daily
	• Wash and disinfect hard-floor surfaces, including all rubber-floor surfaces	Daily Daily
	• Clean HVAC vents	Bi-monthly
	• Clean light fixtures	Bi-monthly
	• Vacuum and clean under all equipment	Bi-monthly
	• Fully clean mirrors and glass surfaces	Bi-monthly
	• Clean carpets	Quarterly or annually
	• Clean wall surfaces thoroughly	Annually
Group-Exercise Studios	• Remove any trash	Daily
	• Dry mop wood floors	Daily
	• Dust all horizontal surfaces	Daily
	• Spot clean mirrors and glass surfaces	Daily
	• Clean mirrors thoroughly	Daily
	• Wet mop wood floors	Weekly
	• Wash and disinfect rubber floor surfaces	Daily
	• Clean HVAC ducts	Bi-monthly
	• Clean light fixtures	Bi-monthly
	• Clean the audio equipment	Bi-monthly
	• Wash the solid-surface walls	Quarterly to annually
	• Refinish wood-floor surfaces	Annually

Figure 21.3. Cleaning guidelines for fitness and group-exercise facilities

Facility Area	Cleaning Activity	Frequency
Gymnasium	• Remove trash • Dry mop and dust floors • Dust all horizontal surfaces • Spot clean all glass surfaces • Clean all glass surfaces thoroughly • Tack/wet mop the wood floors • Clean HVAC filters • Clean light fixtures • Refinish wood floors	Daily Daily Daily Daily Weekly Weekly Bi-monthly Bi-monthly Every two years
Racquet Courts	• Remove trash • Dry mop and dust floors • Dust horizontal surfaces • Spot clean walls and glass surfaces • Remove ball marks • Tack or damp mop the floors • Thoroughly clean glass surfaces • Clean HVAC vents • Clean light fixtures • Refinish floors (squash should be left unfinished, but sanded)	Daily Daily Daily Daily Daily Weekly Bi-monthly Bi-monthly Bi-monthly Annually
Tennis Courts	• Remove trash • Sweep/vacuum indoor hard courts • Blow outdoor courts to remove debris • Roll dry outdoor hard courts after rain • Sweep courts and brush lines for clay courts • Water clay courts • Scrape dead material on clay courts • Patch low spots on clay courts • Jet broom and sweep hard courts • Pressure wash hard courts • Recondition clay courts (add surface material) • Replace tape on clay courts • Resurface hard courts • Resurface clay courts	Daily Daily Daily Daily Daily Daily Weekly Weekly Weekly Bi-annually Semi-annually-to-annually Every two-to-three years Every three-to-four years Every three-to-four years

Figure 21.4. Cleaning guidelines for gymnasiums, racquet courts, and tennis courts

basis. Figures 21.3 to 21..5 provide an overview of the cleaning requirements for several of the key areas in a health/fitness club, including the fitness center, the group-exercise studio, gymnasium, racquet courts, tennis courts, offices, lobby and circulation areas, and massage rooms. (Note: cleaning guidelines for locker rooms and pools are not covered in these figures because they have been addressed in previous chapters.)

Facility Area	Cleaning Activity	Frequency
Lobby and Circulation Areas	• Remove trash	Daily
	• Vacuum carpets	Daily
	• Clean off walk and mats in lobby areas	Daily
	• Wet mop hard-surface floors (granite, tile, etc.)	Daily
	• Buff hard surfaces	Daily
	• Dust horizontal surfaces	Daily
	• Clean and polish furniture	Daily
	• Clean and polish mirrors, sconces, etc.	Bi-monthly
	• Clean light fixtures	Bi-monthly
	• Clean HVAC vents	Bi-monthly
	• Clean carpets	Quarterly-to-annually
	• Strip and refinish wood floors	Annually
Massage Rooms	• Remove trash	Daily
	• Vacuum carpeted floors	Daily
	• Dust horizontal surfaces	Daily
	• Remove all soiled linen	Daily
	• Clean and disinfect beds, tables, etc.	After each client
	• Clean and polish furniture	Daily
	• Wet mop the floors if wood or tile	Daily
	• Clean light fixtures	Bi-monthly
	• Clean HVAC vents	Bi-monthly
	• Clean carpets	Annually
Offices	• Remove trash	Daily
	• Vacuum carpeted areas	Daily
	• Dust horizontal surfaces	Daily
	• Clean and polish furniture	Daily
	• Wet mop the floors if wood or tile	Daily
	• Clean light fixtures	Bi-monthly
	• Clean HVAC vents	Bi-monthly
	• Clean carpets	Annually

Figure 21.5. Cleaning guidelines for the lobby, massage rooms, and offices

Accounting

Accounting operations are a sub-set of the financial management practices that were reviewed earlier in the book. As was noted, financial management encompasses a club's financial structuring and the types and kinds of reports the facility uses to monitor its overall financial performance. Accounting operations, on the other hand, are the processes, policies, and practices that the club employs to ensure that the money is handled in an appropriate manner, both on the revenue and the expense side. These processes, policies,

Accounting operations, on the other hand, are the processes, policies, and practices that the club employs to ensure that the money is handled in an appropriate manner, both on the revenue and the expense side.

Because accounts-payable practices focus on managing and making payments to the club's outside vendors, they are an integral element of controlling expenses.

and practices can normally be grouped into four distinct categories: accounts payable, accounts receivable, payroll functions, and financial reporting. Club operators have several resources available that can help them set up their accounting practices, including the GAAP (generally accepted accounting practices) principles, an accepted set of accounting principles, standards, and procedures that most (if not all) companies employ to compile their financial statements. In the United States, GAAP is administered by the Financial Standards Board that is headquartered in Norwich, Connecticut.

❑ *Accounts payable.* Accounts payable refers to the policies and practices that govern how the club/facility pays its vendors and employees for services. Because accounts-payable practices focus on managing and making payments to the club's outside vendors, they are an integral element of controlling expenses. Figure 21.6 lists several of the most relevant accounts-payable practices that clubs can adopt to assist them in managing their finances.

Accounting Operational Practice	Description/Purpose
Expense reports	The expense-report process requires employees to complete an expense report with accompanying receipts for all business-related expenses. The reports should be approved by a supervisor before payment.
Check requests	The check-request process requires department heads to complete a form requesting any check for payment of a service provided by a vendor. This form is usually approved by the manager before a check can be issued.
Purchase orders	A purchase-order system requires that before any items are ordered, the items desired be priced beforehand and put on a purchase order for approval. Once approved, the items can be purchased. The purchase order then serves as a check-and-balance mechanism against the packing slip and invoice from a supplier.
Par-stock inventory system	Every supply the club uses and every item/product sold should have a par-stock that is inventoried regularly. A point-of-sale software system typically does this for retail operations, but clubs need their own system for supplies.
Check and invoice approval and payment	To provide better control, each club should have a process that requires at least two signatures on a check request or invoice before a check is cut. Furthermore, every check should be reviewed against the invoices and signatures by someone other than the accountant or bookkeeper before it is released.

Figure 21.6. Accounts payable practices

Accounting Operational Practice	Description/Purpose
Monthly member billing	Creating the monthly member statements if the club bills its members directly
Daily charging activities	Applying all member charges to their member accounts in the event the club allows members to charge services on their membership account
Monthly EFT and charge handling	Most clubs use electronic funds transfer to bill and collect member payments. Accounting needs to correctly set-up each member's account for proper billing and collection
Bank reconciliation	This practice falls into both a payable and a receivable function, because it involves the daily undertaking of reconciling the books to make sure all deposits and debits are accounted for and that the bank account is liquid
Accounts receivable collection	Accounting has the responsibility of monitoring the club's accounts that are outstanding and making sure all past-due funds are collected. This involves 30-, 60-, and 90-day policies and practices that are focused on prompt collection of all past-due funds

Figure 21.7. Accounts receivable practices

❑ *Accounts receivable*. The accounts-receivable accounting operation involves the policies and practices that pertain to the billing and collection of funds from anyone (e.g., members) who uses the club's services. The primary focus of accounts-receivable accounting function is to ensure that the club receives all monies that are due for the services and benefits provided to anyone by the facility. Figure 21.7 illustrates several of the most relevant accounts receivable practices that clubs utilize to assist them in managing their finances.

❑ *Payroll functions*. Payroll functions refer to the policies and practices governing a club's handling of all compensation and benefits involving both employees and independent contractors. The main focus of payroll activities is to ensure that employees and contractors receive the proper compensation for the services they have rendered. Figure 21.8 details several of the most relevant payroll-related practices that clubs employ to assist them in managing their finances.

❑ *Financial reporting*. Financial reporting refers to the policies and practices that are involved in monitoring the club's overall financial performance. Financial reporting may also include activities that relate to the preparation of a club's budget and monitoring the facility's actual adherence to the budget (financial-wise). Figure 21.9 presents an overview of several of the most relevant financial-reporting practices that clubs can use to assist them in managing their finances.

The primary focus of accounts-receivable accounting function is to ensure that the club receives all monies that are due for the services and benefits provided to anyone by the facility.

Time sheets/time cards	Every club should have a system in place to set employee schedules, have the employees check-in, monitor the hours that employees work, provide reports on time worked, overtime hours, etc.
Preparing payroll and contractor checks	Involves preparing the payroll and contractor checks, and using the time-card and time-sheet information.
Monitoring overtime, vacation, and personal time	Most accounting departments are involved in monitoring overtime hours, vacation pay, and personal pay. In addition to monitoring, accounting handles all distributions of compensation related to those factors.
Employee benefits administration	Most accounting departments are responsible for the appropriate enrollment of employees in the club's benefit programs and handling the activities related to those benefits.

Figure 21.8. Payroll practices

Daily sales sheets	Daily sales sheets allow clubs to monitor the total sales each day. A daily sales sheet encompasses a tally of each sale that occurs that day. The daily sales sheet should reflect each sale, what it was for, the amount of the sale, the category of sale, whether it was cash or charge, etc.
Daily, weekly, and monthly financial reports	Clubs should have specific reports that can help them better understand their finances, including daily sales report, daily payroll report, weekly/monthly profit-and-loss statement, weekly/monthly balance-sheet report, weekly/monthly accounts-payable report, weekly/monthly accounts-receivable report, and monthly fixed-asset report.
Budget and forecast tools	Every club should have an annual budget for each department, as well as quarterly forecast reports for each department that reflect the expected revenue and expense outcomes of operations. Accounting is normally responsible for preparing and printing these reports, in conjunction with management.

Figure 21.9. Financial reporting practices

22

Club Spas

Chapter Objectives

According to *IHRSA's 2004 Profiles of Success*, day-spa services are offered in 11% of the clubs surveyed, while massage, considered a spa service, is offered in 59% of the facilities surveyed. According to research conducted by the International Spa Association, club spas have grown at an annual rate of 27% since the year 2000. Day spas have not always been such an important component of the club industry. As early as the mid-1990s, most club operators would have questioned the wisdom of devoting financial resources to build a day spa. Yet today, most club operators are aware of the value of a day spa in serving the needs of the marketplace and helping to grow the club's overall operating revenues.

This chapter presents an overview of the day-spa business as it applies to the successful operation of a health/fitness club. This overview addresses several factors attendant to a club spa, including:

- Defining the types of spas that exist, particularly those in the health/fitness club industry

- Describing the individuals who like to engage in the spa experience and how understanding these populations can assist in operating a spa for a particular type of club

- Detailing the basic facility and equipment needs of a successful club spa

- Identifying the basic program and service elements needed for a successful club spa

- Discussing the most effective approaches to marketing a club spa

- Reviewing several of the key issues involving spa staff

> Most club operators are aware of the value of a day spa in serving the needs of the marketplace and helping to grow the club's overall operating revenues.

Types of Spas

To many idividuals a spa is a retreat from the world; a place where they can escape from their normal daily regimen and pursue activities that they believe will help to enrich their lives. According to the International Spa Association (ISPA), spas have been in existence for a very, very long time. The original concept of a spa was derived from retreats that had hot springs and provided treatments that involved the use of these soothing hot-mineral springs. The original concept for spas emanated from baths filled with hot mineral waters that were believed to be beneficial for the body. Over the years, however, spas have evolved substantially, resulting in spas moving well beyond the original notion of hot-mineral baths.

In 2002, ISPA reported that approximately 9,600 spas existed in the United States and another 1,300 in Canada. Of that total, approximately 75% of those spas were day spas. According to research, in 2001, the spa industry generated a total of $10.7 billion in revenue (e.g., approximately 51% from treatment rooms), almost as much as the $12 billion that was generated by health/fitness clubs during that same year. Overall, spas experienced 156 million visits during 2001.

In 2002, ISPA reported that approximately 9,600 spas existed in the United States and another 1,300 in Canada.

Spas provide several services, including massages, facials, body wraps, manicures, pedicures, salon services, yoga, meditation, nutrition counseling, and exercise classes. The introduction of these multiple services into the spa environment has spawned numerous spa concepts. According to ISPA, several primary types of spas exist, including:

❑ *Medical Spas.* Medical spas are spa facilities that provide services that are medically focused. These services encompass therapeutic and rehabilitative treatments (e.g., therapeutic massage, exfoliation, detoxification, etc.) that are integrated with more conventional medical services. According to ISPA's 2002 survey, approximately 225 of the 9,632 (2.3%) spas in the United States are medical spas.

❑ *Resort/Hotel Spas.* Resort/hotel spas are spa facilities that are located in either a hotel or resort setting. The primary focus of these spas is to provide basic spa services (e.g., sauna, steam, whirlpool, massage) for hotel and resort guests. According to ISPA's 2002 survey, approximately 1,150 of the 9,632 (12%) spas in the United States are resort/hotel spas.

❑ *Destination Spas.* Destination spas are spa facilities that are located on resort properties that offer a complete destination experience. These spas fully engage the visitor in a spa experience that includes such endeavors as dining, exercise, and spa treatments (e.g., massage, body wraps, facials, pedicures, hot mineral baths, etc.), among others. These spas usually bundle their services into packages that involve designated time periods. According to ISPA's research, destination spas represent less than one percent of the total spas in the United States.

❑ *Mineral-Springs Spas.* Mineral-springs spas are spa facilities that offer spa services that incorporate the use of onsite sources, such as natural minerals, and naturally heated water and seawater, that are employed in hydrotherapy treatments. According to ISPA's 2002 survey, approximately three percent of the total number of spas that exist in the United States marketplace are mineral-spring spas.

❑ *Day Spas.* Day spas are spa facilities that focus on delivering easily completed spa services (e.g., hair, manicures, pedicures, facials, massage, etc.) that can be experienced in periods of 30 minutes to one day in length. Most day spas are located in affluent urban and suburban markets that serve individuals who want to have a spa experience without having to leave their community. Approximately 75% of the spas in the United States are classified as day spas, which generate nearly 80% of their traffic from women.

> **Research has identified three primary profiles for spa consumers: periphery spa consumers, mid-level spa consumers, and core spa consumers.**

❑ *Club Spas.* Club spas are day-spa facilities that are located within health/fitness clubs that focus on providing basic spa services, such as massage, facials, manicures, sauna, steam, etc., to club members and guests. According to ISPA's 2002 survey, approximately seven percent of the spas in the United States are club spas.

As the aforementioned review of the various types of spas indicates, the spa industry affords individuals multiple opportunities to engage in the pleasant environment afforded by spa treatments. One of the underlying themes among all of these spa offerings is the fundamental focus on providing an experience that can help enrich the individual's life.

Club Spa Consumers

In 2004, ISPA sponsored research that was designed to identify the characteristics of the individuals who use spas. This research identified three primary profiles for spa consumers: periphery spa consumers, mid-level spa consumers, and core spa consumers.

❑ *Periphery Spa Consumers.* Periphery spa consumers are individuals who tend to be impressed by well-operated spas and whose primary expectations concerning the spa involve indulging in cosmetic services that make them feel special and look beautiful. These consumers are price-

An analysis of the various categories of spa consumers indicates that approximately 70% of such users are female, who average 41 years old in age (42% are under the age of 35).

sensitive and tend to prefer the more superficial spa services (e.g., cosmetic or physical body). As a rule, they want to experience pleasurable and light spa services. These consumers are not into the wellness and spiritual aspects of spa services, rather they prefer massages, facials, and manicures. This consumer group is the predominant segment for which club-based spas should develop and target their facilities and services.

❏ *Mid-level Spa Consumers.* Mid-level spa consumers are people who tend to view going to spas as more of a wellness experience. These individuals want to achieve an emotional encounter, as well as experience the cosmetic and physical-body services that the periphery spa consumer typically pursues. These individuals prefer the isolation of a treatment room, seeking services such as massage, skin treatments, and body treatments. These consumers tend to be price-sensitive when the more esoteric services are involved. They are not as sensitive about price when it comes to less arcane services, such as massage, manicures, and facials. These consumers are interested in the therapist's credentials. In most instances, this group is a secondary market for club spas.

❏ *Core Spa Consumers.* Core spa consumers are individuals who have "adopted" the spa lifestyle. They tend to view the spa experience as being an essential part of their overall wellness routine. These consumers place a high level of importance on the entire spa experience, not just the actual treatment. They measure the spa experience, starting with their arrival, and continuing through the treatment that they receive and concluding when they depart. All factors considered, these individuals are the most demanding of the consumers who utilize the services of club spas. As a rule, they prefer not to interact with periphery and mid-level consumers. While this group will use a club spa, they also tend to expect to receive services and achieve experiences that are counter to the largest audience for the services offered by club spas.

An analysis of the various categories of spa consumers indicates that approximately 70% of such users are female, who average 41 years old in age (42% are under the age of 35). Over 50% of spa consumers have a college education. The average household income of a spa consumer is $72,000 annually (it should be noted that this is almost identical to the average household income of the average health/fitness club member). In essence, the demographic profile of a spa consumer closely parallels the demographics of health/fitness club members, with one notable exception—women are more likely to be spa consumers than club members.

Motivating Factors for Using Club Spas

Industry research shows that spa consumers at all levels indicate that they have three primary reasons for using a spa: indulgence, escape, and work.

❑ *Indulgence.* The most self-centered of the reasons for using a spa, indulgence is the primary driver for periphery consumers and a secondary driver for mid-level consumers. Accordingly, it is the factor that clubs should focus on when they design their spas. When consumers refer to indulgence, they often inject such talk by mentioning such factors as fun, playfulness, decadent, pampering, heavenly, joy, enjoyment, and personal time. As a rule, women, more than men, are willing to indulge themselves. Indulgence is highly dependent on household cash flow. In that regard, when the expendable income level of peripheral and mid-level consumers declines, they are less likely to engage in indulgent activities. The most common spa services that are categorized as indulgent are massages, facials, aromatherapy, body scrubs, and thermal treatments.

❑ *Escape.* Escape is the primary driver to use a spa for those consumers who are not engaging in spa services merely as a means to an end. In this instance, escape refers to achieving an experience that allows consumers to remove themselves from the everyday occurrences of life. This process entails a blend of mind and body factors. Escapist experiences involve spa treatments that create an environment that is characterized by a sense of calmness, respite, tranquility, seclusion, etc. This driver is likely to be one of the major reasons why mid-level or core consumers utilize a spa. The most common escapist spa experiences include body scrubs, body wraps, aromatherapy, and hydrotherapy.

❑ *Work.* Work is a driver for using a spa that is grounded in the desire of individuals to make improvements in themselves, whether it is to look better, feel better, or balance their life. Mid-level consumers and core consumers are more likely to be driven to utilize spas by work than either indulgence or escape, because they tend to see spas as being a more integral element in their overall lifestyle.

With regard to spas, the club industry has the greatest opportunity to be successful when they provide spa experiences that appeal primarily to periphery spa consumers and to mid-level consumers to a lesser degree. As such, the group of core spa users is relatively small. In reality, if that group is targeted, it will often drive away the other two consumer audiences.

Industry research shows that spa consumers at all levels indicate that they have three primary reasons for using a spa: indulgence, escape, and work.

Club Spa Facilities and Features

The typical club spa can encompass one or more types of treatment spaces, including massage rooms, facial rooms, multipurpose-treatment rooms, wet-treatment rooms, manicure and pedicure spaces, relaxation space, and reception area/retail space. It should also be noted that one of the most recent trends in spa facilities is the inclusion of rooms where couples can receive massages, facials, and wet treatments. Each of the various types of treatment spaces in spa facilities has its own unique features.

> All factors considered, multipurpose treatment rooms are the most important spaces in the club spa, because they are in area in which peripheral spa consumers are most likely to engage in spa services.

❑ *Multipurpose-Treatment Rooms.* In the spa industry, the average multi-purpose treatment area includes five massage rooms (48% of room space) and three facial rooms (33% of room space). Primarily utilized for performing massage services and facials, these rooms typically range in size from 100-to-120 square feet. Couples rooms are usually larger—150-to-200 square feet. As a rule, multi-purpose treatment rooms include:

- Indirect lighting that is controlled through dimmer switches

- Floor surfaces that are easily washable and provide cushioning for the therapists. The best surfaces are soft vinyl floors or treated wood floors. Some surfaces, such as tile, are relatively easy to clean, but are not good for the therapists. On the other hand, carpeting can be difficult to keep clean.

- Built-in sound systems that can be controlled by the therapists

- Built-in millwork that includes a hard counter surface, sink, storage spaces, and retail-display cabinetry

- Wall surfaces that can easily be cleaned, as well as being able to help provide a soothing environment

- Individual room thermostats that can help maintain the proper air temperature

- Added sound attenuation construction to reduce transmission of sound

All factors considered, multipurpose treatment rooms are the most important spaces in the club spa, because they are in areas in which peripheral spa consumers are most likely to engage in spa services.

❑ *Wet-Treatment Rooms.* In the spa industry, the average wet-treatment area consists of two rooms (18% of the total treatment space). Wet-treatment rooms are utilized primarily for spa treatments that involve the use of water. Among the treatments that are performed in these rooms are body wraps, body scrubs, and hydrotherapy treatments, which involve such implements as hydrotherapy tubs, Vichy showers, Scottish hose, etc. These rooms typically range in size from 120-to-150 square feet, while rooms for couples are closer to 200 square feet. As a rule, these rooms include:

- Indirect and direct lighting, both on dimmer switches
- Floor and wall surface that is water resistant and easy to clean. The most suitable surface for the floors and walls is tile (e.g., ceramic or porcelain). At the least, the walls in these areas need to have a four-foot wainscot of tile. Custom vinyl surfaces can also be used, in lieu of tile.
- Built-in shower and additional water faucet fixtures. The additional fixtures can be used for hydrotherapy tubs or Vichy showers.
- Floor drains
- Built-in sound systems that can be controlled by the therapists
- Built-in millwork that includes a hard counter surface, sink, storage spaces, and retail-display cabinetry
- Added sound attenuation construction to reduce the transmission of sound

Because wet-treatment rooms mostly appeal to mid-level and core consumers, they are not essential to the successful operation of a club spa.

❑ *Manicure and Pedicure Spaces.* The manicure and pedicure spaces require a more social and open atmosphere than do the multipurpose and wet-treatment rooms. These spaces not only are designed to provide manicures and pedicures, but also to facilitate social interaction between the therapists and customers. These spaces typically include the following features:

Pedicure space (in spa industry, the average pedicure space has three stations):

- Approximately 50-to-60 square feet per pedicure station (chair, foot bath, and therapist chair)
- Floor and wall surfaces that are water resistant and easy to clean. The most suitable surface for the floors and walls is tile (e.g., ceramic or porcelain). At the least, the walls in this area should have a four-foot wainscot of tile. Custom vinyl surfaces can also be used in lieu of tile.
- Floor drains
- Soft, yet bright, lighting
- Built-in sound systems that can be controlled by the therapists
- Negative exhaust system to help pull fumes out of the space

Manicure space (in the spa industry, the average manicure space has four stations):

- Approximately 40-to-60 square feet per manicure station (table and two chairs)

The manicure and pedicure spaces require a more social and open atmosphere than do the multipurpose and wet- treatment rooms.

- Floor surfaces that are either carpet or a solid material (e.g., vinyl, wood, or tile)
- Lighting that is soft, yet bright
- Built-in sound systems that can be controlled by the therapists
- Negative exhaust system to help pull fumes out of the space

Individuals consider manicure and pedicure services as both an indulgence and work. Accordingly, the services offered in these spaces tend to appeal equally to core spa consumers and peripheral spa consumers. Club-based spas should view these spaces as being somewhat less essential than multipurpose treatment rooms.

❑ *Relaxation Space.* A relaxation space is most commonly found in club spas that have more than six treatment rooms. The relaxation room serves as a transition space between the treatment rooms and the rest of the club, an area in which the client is allowed to relax prior to entering a treatment room, or wind down after a treatment, before returning to the locker room or leaving the spa. Some of the larger club spas have both a men's and a women's relaxation area. As a rule, these rooms typically range in size from 100-to-200 square feet and include the following features:

- Soft floor surfaces (e.g., carpet or wood with throw carpets)
- Indirect soft lighting
- Sound attenuation construction that facilitates a quiet environment
- Millwork with display cabinets, hard-surface countertops, and built-in refrigerators
- Built-in sound system

Relaxation rooms appeal mostly to core spa consumers and, as a result, are not an essential element when developing club spas. On the other hand, if the club wants to appeal to core consumers, then relaxation rooms are a must.

The relaxation room serves as a transition space between the treatment rooms and the rest of the club, an area in which the client is allowed to relax prior to entering a treatment room, or wind down after a treatment, before returning to the locker room or leaving the spa.

❑ *Reception Area/Retail Space.* A reception area/retail space is not normally incorporated into the design of most club-based spas. These spaces, which provide a separate entry and retail space specifically for the spa, are normally not required, unless the club spa is designed to drive a large non-member level of business. This space normally consists of a reception desk, retail displays (e.g., wall-mounted cabinets, floor displays, etc.), and a soft-seating area. This space typically features:

- Wood, granite, or similar hard surface flooring
- Extensive millwork with retail displays
- Indirect soft lighting

- Custom wall treatments and furniture
- Sound system

In addition, if the club spa has more than four treatment rooms, then a separate storage and employee room should be provided. Such an area can be used for several purposes, including storing the various treatment supplies, preparing the treatment materials, and serving as a location for therapists to relax.

Club Spa Space Requirements

A club spa can be simply as small as a single multipurpose treatment room or as large as a 20-room, full-service facility. The typical fitness club has between one and four treatment rooms, with two treatment rooms being the norm. A few club companies, such as Lifetime Fitness, Sports Club/LA, and Western Athletic Clubs, offer club spas that encompass from six-to-12 treatment rooms, while other club operations have spas that consist of over 20 rooms. According to ISPA's research, the median size of a club spa is approximately 10,000 square feet.

When developing a club spa, facilities should evaluate several factors, including the following:

❑ *Internal Market Demand*. How many current club members would be interested in using spa services? Typically, a club that serves either a family market or a predominately female market will have greater demand for spa services.

❑ *External Market Demand*. How large is the non-member market, and what type of traffic can be generated?

❑ *Target Audience*. Which spa consumer group will be the club's desired audience?

❑ *Available Space in the Facility*. What space is available for renovation or conversion to spa-related services?

❑ *Costs of Development*. What will it cost to develop a spa, and what will be the expected return on the investment?

While no actual club-industry averages exist for how many rooms should be incorporated into a club spa, a list of the general guidelines on how to proceed in this regard includes the following:

The typical fitness club has between one and four treatment rooms, with two treatment rooms being the norm.

- Provide a minimum of one treatment room/station per 1,000 memberships and a maximum of two treatment rooms/stations per 1,000 memberships. For example, if the club has 3,000 memberships, it should have a minimum of three treatment rooms and a maximum of six treatment rooms.

- For club spas that have no more than four treatment rooms, all of them should be designed as multipurpose treatment areas. If a facility has more than four treatment rooms, it should consider providing one wet-treatment room (only if its intent is to appeal to mid-level and core consumers). In most instances, a club spa will never need more than one wet-treatment room.

- The club spa should include relaxation space if the facility has at least six treatment rooms and the decision has been made that the spa is going to target core spa consumers. If the spa facility wants to attract a relatively large number of women, the club should consider having both a women's and a men's relaxation room.

- As a rule, manicure and pedicure areas normally never have to exceed two stations each, unless the club is offering a full-service spa that attempts to appeal to all levels of spa consumers. In the event that the club has a full-service spa, the number of spaces for pedicures and manicures depends upon the assumed traffic level.

- Depending on the number of specialized rooms (e.g., treatment areas, manicure/pedicure spaces, and relaxation rooms) that are included in the club spa, the typical club spa facility ranges in size from 600-to-2,000 square feet. It should also be noted that the median free-standing (spas that are not located in a club) spa in the United States is 3,200 square feet, according to statistics provided by IPSA.

> The variety and quantity of equipment in a club spa is dependent upon the services provided by the spa and the facility spaces that exist.

Club Spa Equipment

The variety and quantity of equipment in a club spa is dependent upon the services provided by the spa and the facility spaces that exist. Figure 22.1 presents a list of the basic equipment requirements in the various types of club-spa areas.

Club Spa Service Offerings

The three leading service offerings in the spa industry are massages, facials, and wet treatments. According to industry research, 48% of treatment-room space is used for massages, 33% for facials, and 18% for body/wet treatments. From a revenue perspective, massage drives approximately 49% of spa revenue, while facials account for approximately 34% of revenue.

Multipurpose Treatment Room	Wet Treatment Room	Manicure/Pedicure Space	Relaxation Room
• Massage/facial table (adjustable) • Therapists stool • Bolster pads • Stone heater and stones • Warmers for oils and lotions • Hydro collator • Paraffin heater/ bath • Facial system (rotary brush, vapo-steamer, vacuum/spray, high-frequency galvanic stimulator, and magnifying lamp) • Towel-heater cabinet • Sterilizer/autoclave • Mixing bowls • Blankets and sheets	• Wet/dry table • Vichy shower unit • Hydrotherapy tub (optional) • Heat lamp • Hydro collator • Mixing bowls • Paraffin heater/bath • Shower • Step stool • Therapist stool	• Manicure table • Task chairs • Pedicure chair with footbath • Nail-drying station • Foot spa • Pedicure stool • Paraffin heater/bath • Storage cart	• Soft seating (sofas and chairs) • Coffee table • Magazine racks • Refrigerator • Cabinets for retail displays and storage • Dispenser system for drinks

Figure 22.1. Equipment options for a club spa

The services that a club spa provides depend upon several factors, including the market it intends to serve (periphery, mid-level, or core), the space it has available, and its overall revenue and profitability goals. Industry research indicates that club spas should focus most on those consumers who are seeking indulgences (first) and escapes (second). As a result, providing massage and facial services should be a top priority for clubs with a spa, while offering pedicures and manicures should be a secondary priority for facilities, with wet treatments a distant third.

❑ *Massage Services.* Massage encompasses a vast array of treatments, ranging from soothing massage modalities to therapeutic modalities. The most frequently offered massage services include:

• *Swedish massage.* A gentle relaxing massage modality that focuses on enhancing circulation and relaxing the musculature.

• *Sports massage.* A more therapeutic massage modality that centers on addressing specific sport/activity-related issues. This type of massage tends to involve deeper massage, designed to release deep tension and break up scar tissue.

• *Trigger-point massage.* A modality based on Asian massage techniques that focus on applying pressure to specific trigger points to release tension. While this type of massage can be painful at first, it is excellent as a therapeutic modality.

The services that a club spa provides depend upon several factors, including the market it intends to serve (periphery, mid-level, or core), the space it has available, and its overall revenue and profitability goals.

- *Hot-stone massage.* A modality that employs pre-heated stones, placed along the musculature, to help release tension. The stones are moved periodically to other areas of the body's surface.

- *Aromatherapy massage.* A modality that involves the use of aromatic oils, in combination with Swedish massage techniques. Some individuals consider this type of massage to be both relaxing and therapeutic.

In addition to the aforementioned massage techniques, a host of more esoteric techniques exist that vary in popularity, depending upon the facility's geographic location. These activities include such techniques as Thai massage, reflexology, and shiatsu. Most massage treatments involve time periods ranging from 25-to-90 minutes.

The most common type of club-spa facials encompass the use of special lotions to exfoliate the skin, followed by gentle massage, and finally, the application of lotions to hydrate the skin.

❏ *Facial Services.* Facials involve a combination of treatment applications, including exfoliation, detoxification, hydrating, and massage. The most common type of club-spa facials encompass the use of special lotions to exfoliate the skin, followed by gentle massage, and finally, the application of lotions to hydrate the skin. Recently, day and club spas have begun to utilize microderm abrasion to provide a more thorough exfoliation of the skin surface. It is common for spas to provide special names for their various facial treatments, based on the lotions and techniques used, for example, executive facials, spa facials, European facials, eye-contour treatments, acne treatments, back facials, facial peels, fruit-based facials, facial masks, make-up applications, etc.

❏ *Body Treatments and Wet Treatments.* Body treatments and wet-treatments are services that the majority of club spas provide in their wet treatment rooms. The body treatments normally involve some use of water, while wet treatments (as the term implies) directly incorporate the use of water. The most frequently offered body and wet treatments include the following:

- *Body scrubs.* Body scrubs are treatments that involve the use of brushes, sponges, and/or lotions to exfoliate the targeted skin surface. Some of the most common types of body-scrub treatments are deep-sea salt scrubs, body polish, essential oil scrubs, Turkish body scrubs, and fruit-based body scrubs.

- *Body wraps.* Body wraps are treatments that involve wrapping the entire body or a segment of the body with special products, such as seaweed or mud. These treatments focus on both detoxification and exfoliation. Examples include herbal wrap, mud wrap, essential oil wrap, spirulina wrap, silk wraps, etc.

- *Hydrotherapy tub treatments.* These are treatments that are conducted in a hydrotherapy tub and involve the use of water jets to stimulate and massage the body.

- *Vichy shower and Scottish hose treatments.* The Vichy shower involves the use of multiple water jets to massage the body. In most cases, the client is prone on a wet table while the Vichy treatment is conducted. A Scottish hose is a more intense water treatment that involves the use of a powerful water jet that is sprayed on the body to create intense stimulation of the skin and underlying body tissues.

❑ *Other Services That Club Spas Can Offer.* In addition to certain basic services, such as massage, facials, and body treatments, club spas should also consider providing the following services, based on the audience to which they are attempting to appeal:

- Manicures

- Pedicures

- Waxing (a fast-growing service-treatment segment)

- Paraffin treatments for the hands and feet

- Cosmetic application (assisting clients in the proper use and application of cosmetics)

Clubs should always conduct the proper market research before establishing the spa services that they will offer and the prices that they will charge for those services.

Club Spa Financial Parameters

The price that club spas place on their services depends upon many factors, including the geographic region in which the spa is located, the club's initial investment in the spa facility, the target audience, the surrounding demographics, and the role the spa plays in the club's overall business strategy. Clubs should always conduct the proper market research before establishing the services that they will offer and the prices that they will charge for those services. Club-based spas, on average, offer their services at a lower price point than day spas, resort/hotel spas, and destination spas. If the club is trying to grow the business and appeal to periphery spa consumers, the price points for its services must be carefully considered, since this group of consumers is extremely price sensitive. Figure 22.2 illustrates the general ranges for several of the most common club-spa service price points.

According to ISPA research, the average freestanding day spa generates approximately $221 per square foot of treatment space. The ISPA data also indicated a mean revenue of $40,000 per treatment room for day spas.

As such, the average club spa can expect to generate between $3,000 and $6,000 a month per treatment room and, $1,000-to-$3,000 a month per manicure/pedicure station. The net income generated by a club spa should be

Club Spa Service	Price Range
Swedish and sports massage (one hour)	$50 - $90
Aromatherapy/ Stone Massage (one hour)	$60 - $100
Facial (50 minutes to an hour)	$60 - $100
Manicure	$20 - $35
Pedicure	$25 - $45
Body wrap (one hour)	$60 – $90
Body Scrub (one hour)	$50 - $80
Paraffin treatment (30 minutes)	$25 - $40

Figure 22.2. Price-point ranges for club-spa services

Ideally, a club spa should pull 50% of its clients from the club's existing membership base and 50% from non-members who either reside or work within the locale of the club's primary market.

approximately equal to 20%-to-35% of the gross revenues of the spa. For example, a club spa with six treatment rooms, two manicure stations, and one pedicure station could expect to generate revenues of $27,000-to-$45,000 a month, with a net profit of $5,500-to-$13,500 a month.

Marketing the Club Spa

The marketing efforts of a club spa depend, in large part, on the audience that the club is attempting to attract. Ideally, a club spa should pull 50% of its clients from the club's existing membership base and 50% from non-members who either reside or work within the locale of the club's primary market. This duality of markets requires a club to pursue two distinct approaches to marketing. First, it must establish a marketing approach that effectively draws members from its target market. Second, it must develop a marketing strategy that attracts non-members to the spa without impacting any sense of overall exclusivity of the club that the facility might be attempting to establish. Club operators who view the spa as a prospecting source for membership often incorporate efforts to promote the spa to non-members as part of their overall membership marketing campaign. Several successful strategies can be employed to help market club-spa services, including:

❑ *Strategies Used to Market the Spa to Members:*
  • *New-member coupons.* When individuals first become a member, many clubs provide them with a coupon for either a complimentary spa service or a spa service at a discounted rate. Clubs that offer a discount rate should quote the discount in absolute dollars, rather than percentages.

- *Club displays.* Some of the best efforts to market the spa involve internal spa displays that touch the various senses, by incorporating visual, auditory, touch, and smell elements.

- *Spa demonstrations.* Clubs can program monthly or even weekly demonstrations that offer members the opportunity to experience the club's spa services on a complimentary basis. For example, the club's complimentary spa offerings could include five-minute chair massages, one nail manicure, aromatherapy, etc.

- *Special classes.* Many clubs have found that offering special classes, such as massage classes for couples or classes in skin care, can help introduce members to the club's spa services.

- *Posters/flyers.* The use of custom-designed posters and flyers that are displayed in appropriate areas of the club can also help bring attention to the club's spa services.

- *Member spa-appreciation days.* Once a quarter, clubs can schedule special spa-appreciation days that offer members special prices on the various spa services.

- *Special-event invitations.* Special days and holidays, such as Valentine's day, mother's day, birthdays, etc., represent great opportunities for attracting members to the club's spa services. Clubs can send special invitations and gift certificates to their members during these time periods to help attract them to the spa.

- *Spa brochures.* Producing an attractive spa brochure that can be displayed in the club, as well as distributed to the membership, can be another excellent marketing tool.

- *Member-referral program.* One proven strategy to market a club's spa services is to reward members who invite other members to experience the facility's spa services.

- *Spa website.* Developing a website for the spa that is directly linked to the club's spa website can be helpful by providing a source of updated information on the spa's services (e.g., spa menu) and even allowing on-line scheduling of appointments for the spa.

❑ *Strategies Used to Market to Non-Members:*

- *Spa brochures.* Producing an attractive spa brochure that can be distributed to the market via direct mail and retail displays can be an excellent marketing tool.

- *Direct-mail invitations/certificates.* Targeted direct-mail invitations and gift certificates can be employed to attract non-members to the club spa.

- *Spa fairs.* Special massage events involving local corporations or local community groups can be conducted that can provide targeted consumers with a sampling experience of the club's spa services.

Special days and holidays, such as Valentine's day, mother's day, birthdays, etc., represent great opportunities for attracting members to the club's spa services.

Clubs can develop a sponsorship program that rewards members for inviting non-members to the club to engage in spa services.

- *Special-event invitations.* Special days and holidays, such as Valentine's day, mother's day, father's day, Christmas, birthdays, etc., represent great opportunities for attracting non-members to the club's spa services. Clubs can send special invitations and gift certificates to targeted non-member audiences during these time periods that are designed to help draw them into the spa.

- *Member-sponsor program.* Clubs can develop a sponsorship program that rewards members for inviting non-members to the club to engage in spa services. For example, each time a member brings in a non-member, the member could be given a special discount or a credit for fees due.

- *Club website.* Clubs can create a spa website that is linked to the club's primary website. This spa site can provide updated information on services and allow online appointment scheduling of the spa's services for non-members. If feasible, the website could also be linked to search engines for spas.

In addition to the aforementioned strategies concerning the most effective approaches for promoting a facility's spa services, clubs can also employ less-targeted marketing approaches, such as newspaper ads, magazine ads, and radio spots, to make non-members in the marketplace aware of their spa-related offerings.

Club Spa Staff

Club operators have two basic options concerning the most effective approach for staffing their spa. They can either hire or retain employees to operate the spa or recruit independent contractors to do the job. The benefits and limitations of these two options are reflected in Figure 22.3.

Employees		Independent Contractors	
Benefit	Downside	Benefit	Downside
• The club has control of schedules, hours, pricing, and services. • Employees will blend with the overall club culture. • Employees will likely take more ownership in connecting the spa with the rest of the club. • Performance- based compensation can be established that supports spa and club goals.	• Added costs related to benefits • Possibly not as recognized in the community	• No payroll or payroll costs involved • Ability to use well-known business operator from the community • Costs are more directly tied to revenues generated; no downtime costs. • Potentially lower operating costs	• Less likely to have an integration of the spa with the club • The club has limited control of services and pricing. • The club has potentially less opportunity to generate revenues.

Figure 22.3. Benefits and downsides of hiring employees vs. using independent contractors in a club spa

Position	Compensation	Competency	Role
Spa director (normally in club spas with greater than four treatment rooms)	Base salary range of $18,000-to-$40,000, plus commission on retail sales (two-to-five percent) and commission on total spa gross revenues or net revenues. Therapists are paid a commission on any treatment sessions they perform.	College degree or spa experience; either licensed massage therapist or licensed esthetician preferred.	Supervises the spa and is responsible for all aspects of the spa's operation. In smaller spas, this individual also performs treatments.
Massage therapist	Commission for services ranges from 35%-to-60% of revenue generated. Range of 40%-to-50% is most common. Base wage of six-to-eight dollars an hour during administrative times.	Licensed registered or certified by the state in massage therapy (varies by state); previous work experience	Performs all massage treatments and also can do other body treatments, such as body scrubs, body wraps, etc., if they have undergone the appropriate training
Spa therapist	Commission for services ranges from 35%-to-60% of revenue generated. Range of 40%-to-50% is most common. Base wage of six-to-eight dollars an hour during administrative times.	Licensed as a massage therapist or esthetician preferred. No licensing is required in most states for those individuals who conduct body wraps, scrubs, etc., if they have undergone the appropriate training.	Performs the body treatments and wet treatments, except does not do any massage or facial work; appropriate training in modalities required
Esthetician	Commission for services ranges from 35%-to-60% of revenue generated. Range of 40%-to-50% is most common. Base wage of six-to-eight dollars an hour during administrative times.	Licensed by the state as an esthetician; previous work experience	Performs all manicures, pedicures, and facials; can also conduct body-treatment sessions if they have undergone the appropriate training.

Figure 22.4. Club spa staff positions, compensation, and credentials (based on research conducted by ISPA)

Once the decision has been made to utilize either employees or independent contractors, the next decision that has to be made involves the make-up of the staff and the compensation that should be accorded to each of the designated positions. The most common job roles in a club spa, the accompanying compensation ranges, and the job skill requirements for those positions are shown in Figure 22.4.

Some of the larger club spas also have receptionists. For most club spas, the receptionist's responsibilities can easily be filled by other staff members during times when they are not performing treatment sessions.

Key Points to Consider

Club spas are among the fastest growing amenities in the club business, expanding by 27% on an annual basis since the year 2000. As the population continues to age (e.g., baby boomers) and the demands on an individual's time increases, a club spa that provides a refuge for personal indulgences and escapes will remain as both a valuable revenue source and an effective tool to enhance membership retention for health/fitness clubs.

International Health/Fitness Club Industry

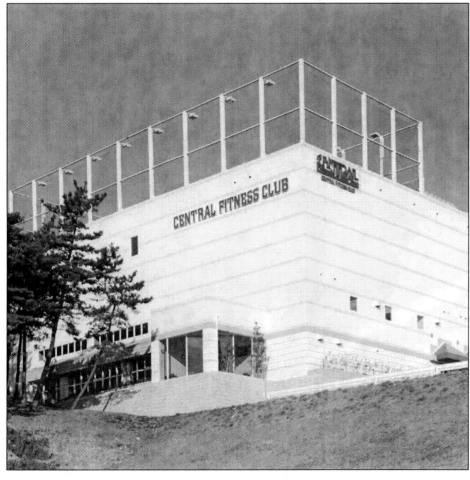

- Chapter 23: International Health/Fitness Club Market

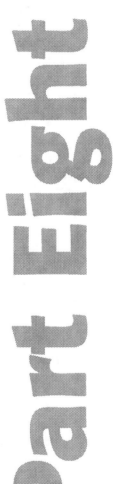

23

International Health/Fitness Club Market

Chapter Objectives

Understanding the dynamics of the international market can help facilitate a greater understanding of the competencies involved in managing and leading a successful health/fitness club business. With regard to the world market for health/fitness clubs, six countries account for approximately 80% of the total—the United States, Canada, the United Kingdom, Germany, Japan, and Brazil. This chapter presents a basic overview of the international health/fitness club market that includes not only a brief history of the international health/fitness club industry, but also a discussion of the current dynamics of the market. The review addresses critical factors and issues attendant to each of the major continents, in particular the European and Asian markets.

Historical Perspective

❑ *The Early Years*. Similar to the domestic U.S. market, private clubs (particularly athletic-oriented clubs) evolved in the international arena in the 1800s. The earliest private clubs were established in the United Kingdom, with Germany and France entering the market shortly thereafter. The first health/fitness clubs in Europe featured gymnastics and related sports, such as boxing, wrestling, weightlifting, and running. In 1812, Fredrick Jahn became the first individual to formally put together a gymnastic organization, which he called Turnvereins. In the mid-1840s, Hippolyte Triat opened Gymnase Triat in Paris, France—one of the inaugural efforts in the international health/fitness club market. Triat's gym and others that followed during that time period primarily focused on athletic-related program offerings, such as gymnastic activities, boxing, and wrestling.

The first health/fitness clubs in Europe featured gymnastics and related sports, such as boxing, wrestling, weightlifting, and running.

One important delineating factor of the modern era was the formation of companies dedicated to operating multiple clubs to serve the fitness and sports needs of the marketplace.

The earliest United Kingdom clubs were organized around social relationships and athletic endeavors, such as court tennis, cricket, squash, snooker, and lawn tennis. One of the first facilities in this regard was the All-England Lawn Tennis and Croquet Club, which was founded in 1868 and began operations in 1877, just outside London. The Fitzwilliam Lawn Tennis Club in Dublin, Ireland, which was founded in 1877, lays claim to actually operating as a club before the aforementioned All-England Club. These facilities were representative of the earliest form of recreational sports-driven clubs that subsequently were developed in the United Kingdom. With a strong social component, these facilities provided men with the opportunity to engage in physical activity. The programming focus in these clubs tended to involve either physical-culture activities (e.g., physique improvement, combat sports, and acrobatics) or court sports (e.g., court tennis, squash, tennis, etc.). As such, these early European efforts led to the development of America's first social/athletic clubs, such as the New York Athletic Club. Subsequently, the concept of a social/athletic facility was also exported to Asia by expatriates, thus creating this type of club in Hong Kong and other major Asian markets.

❑ *The Modern Era.* The birth of the modern era of the international health/fitness club industry occurred in Europe about the same time it did in the United States—the 1960s and early 1970s. (Note: The modern era is defined as the period during which health/fitness clubs became part of the culture and opened their doors to the general public to provide a means of improving physical health.) One important delineating factor of the modern era was the formation of companies dedicated to operating multiple clubs to serve the fitness and sports needs of the marketplace. About this same time period, health/fitness clubs also began to take root in Japan and somewhat later in other Asian countries. In fact, several organized health/fitness club operations were established throughout Asia, such as Central Sports, which opened in 1969 and The People Company, which started in 1973. However, it wasn't until the late 1970s and early 1980s that health/fitness clubs became a significant business venture in the international arena. It is interesting to note that this scenario coincided closely with the consequential changes that were occurring in the United States marketplace.

In the early 1980s, club groups such as Archer Leisure, Vardon Leisure, David Lloyd Leisure in the United Kingdom, and DIC in Japan entered the market, followed a few years later by health/fitness industry groups, such as G&P Gockel in Germany, Health and Racquet in South Africa, Living Well in the United Kingdom, and Clark Hatch in Asia. During the same period, the health/fitness club industry also began to take off in a number of other segments of the international market, including Spain, Sweden, Norway, Italy, and the Netherlands. The 1980s also ushered in the beginning of large-scale operators, which in turn drove the international industry. Figure 23.1 presents an overview of the growth of the industry leaders in the international market during the period 1995-2004.

The real renaissance of the health/fitness club industry internationally occurred in the 1990s. The international health/fitness club market exploded during this decade, with England, Germany, France, South Africa, and Japan experiencing the most significant growth. Figure 23.2 illustrates the enormous growth that has occurred in market penetration in the various international markets through 2004.

In the 1990s, the United Kingdom was the center of attention in the international health/fitness club market because of the explosion of quality facility operations in England, such as David Lloyd Leisure, Esporta, Holmes Place, Cannons, Dragons, and LA Fitness. These various operations featured business models that took British consumers by veritable storm and created an incredible buzz in the financial markets. David Lloyd Leisure was sold to Whitbread for approximately $350 million dollars, which, at the time, involved a high multiple of earnings and became the benchmark that the financial markets in England employed to judge the other up-and-coming health/fitness club operations. Besides David Lloyd, companies such as Cannons, Holmes Place, Esporta, and Fitness First also went public in the mid-to-late 1990s and were very well received by Britain's financial markets.

During the later half of the 1990,s several of these businesses traded at 30-to-40 times earnings, far in excess of the four-to-eight times earnings multiples that were the norm in the United States. One of the most unique factors about the British market, other than the incredible multiples on earnings, was the fact they did not experience the price wars and discounting practices that had plagued the United States. The market in the United Kingdom focused on establishing quality benchmarks and avoiding the price markdowns and strong sales tactics that the U.S. industry experienced during its early years. In addition, British clubs were able to work closely with England's national health insurance group to create several important synergies for the market.

During this period, British clubs could be grouped into three basic categories, based on price and amenities. Clubs, such as Fitness First and LA Fitness, were what would be termed in the U.S. domestic market as affordable and convenient fitness-only facilities. Focused primarily on fitness-related activities, this group of facilities operated smaller, well-outfitted ventures that were both convenient and affordable to the masses, particularly to single individuals. In contrast, a number of British health/fitness operations, such as Esporta, were structured on a larger fitness-club model, one that targeted families, and provided slightly more amenities and services at a higher price. In the United States, such a facility would be called a mid-price level, family-fitness club. The third type of facility focused on the high end of the market. This group featured full-

The real renaissance of the health/fitness club industry internationally occurred in the 1990s.

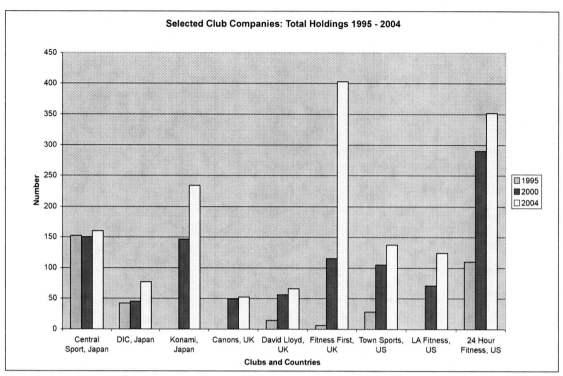

Figure 23.1a. Selected club companies: total holdings 1995-2004

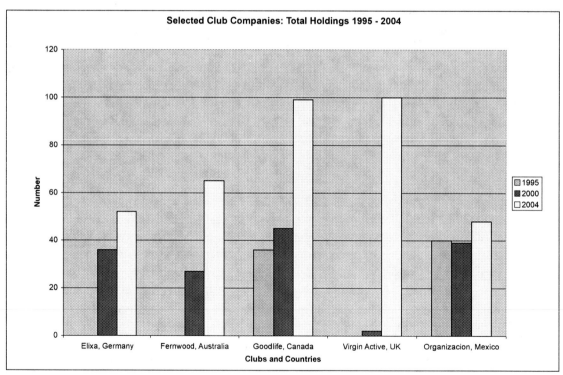

Figure 23.1b. Selected club companies: total holdings 1995-2004

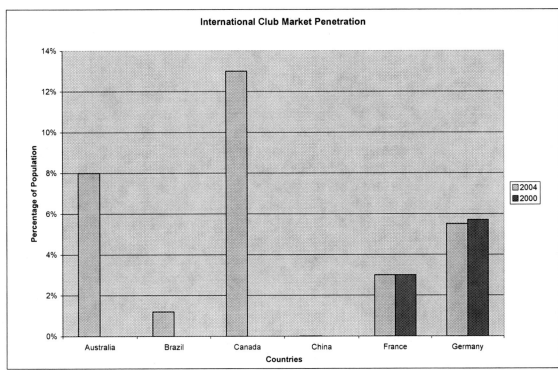

Figure 23.2a. International club market penetration

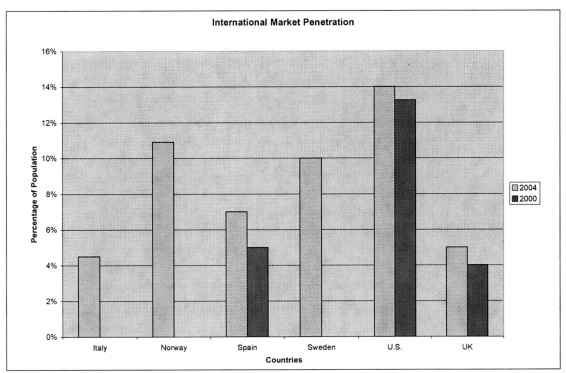

Figure 23.2b. International club market penetration

service, multipurpose clubs that offered both great programming and exceptional service. These high-end operations emphasized an appropriate blend of fitness, recreation, and social interaction (e.g., David Lloyd Leisure, Cannons, Holmes Place).

During the 1990s, the health/fitness club industry also began to thrive in other European countries, such as Germany, Italy, Belgium, France, Sweden, and South Africa. For example, a French company, Compagnie Gymnase, grew to 116 clubs by the mid-to-late 1990s. A significant portion of Compagnie Gymnase's clubs were subsequently sold to Club Med, which, in turn, branded them as Club Med Gyms. A chain in South Africa, Health and Racquet, reached over 60 clubs by the mid-to-late 1990s. Eventually, this chain expanded into both Europe and Australia (under the brand name Healthlands). However, because of legal and financial problems, it had to divest of its holdings. At the present time, the former Health and Racquet clubs in South Africa and Europe are operated by Virgin Active, which had created its own unique brand of health/fitness clubs during this same period.

Since the 1990s, Japan has strengthened its dominant position as a commanding factor in the international health/fitness club industry.

In markets such as Germany, Italy, Spain, and Sweden, several smaller multiple-club companies opened their doors and brought a number of innovative (for their respective areas) programming emphases to their respective markets. For example, Kieser opened a number of small clubs in Germany that focused entirely on delivering a resistance-training environment. 24 Hour Fitness made its presence in the international market by purchasing several facilities in the Scandinavian region (e.g., Denmark, Norway, and Sweden). At one point, 24 Hour Fitness had approximately 70 clubs in the Scandinavian region. Subsequently, these clubs were sold to Nordic Capital and are currently part of the SATS club group.

During the late 1990s, Fitness First, based in London, seized a dominant position in the Australian market, by purchasing the clubs that were formerly operated by Health and Racquet of South Africa (e.g., Heathlands). Starting with approximately 15 clubs, Fitness First grew its Australian club's holdings to over 40 strong. Before Fitness First entered the Australian market, most of the health/fitness clubs down under were either small independent operators with less than 10 clubs or community swimming centers that were operated by the local government bodies. In an attempt to emulate Fitness First's success in Australia, a second major player in the industry, Fernwood, emerged in Australia. In fact, in 2004, a third major player, Zest Health Club, entered the fray.

Since the 1990s, Japan has strengthened its dominant position as a commanding factor in the international health/fitness club industry. At the present time, three companies—DIC, Central Sports, and Konami (formerly, the clubs operated by the People Company)—operate close to 25% of the health/fitness facilities in the Japanese marketplace and generate close to

40% of the total revenue produced by clubs in the market. These Japanese operations feature facilities that provide exceptional fitness, group-exercise, and swimming programming. Swimming is an extremely popular activity in Japanese clubs, as is group exercise.

During the 1990s, the Asian market (exclusive of Japan) was primarily driven by small fitness centers that were located in hotels and residential developments. One of the first individuals to recognize the opportunities that existed in Asia was Clark Hatch, who has since opened over 60 clubs in markets such as Singapore, Hong Kong, Malaysia, Thailand, and the Philippines, most of which, if not all, are associated with hotel properties. During the later half of the 1990s, some U.S. entrepreneurs also decided to enter the larger Asian markets. For example, California Fitness, founded by Ray Wilson, became one of the first health/fitness club chains to enter Hong Kong. In fact, its first facility reached over 12,000 members in its initial year of operation. Another organization that established a presence in Asia was 24 Hour Fitness, which created a subsidiary that now operates those aforementioned California Fitness clubs. In addition to 24 Hour Fitness, Fitness First, based in London, and Gold's Gym and Bally's from the U.S. have made significant inroads into the emerging Asian market. Currently, the prevailing approach to the Asian market seems to be licensing or franchising. In that regard, Gold's and Bally's have aggressively attempted to franchise facilities in China.

Similar to Europe and Asia, South America also witnessed substantial growth in the demand for health/fitness clubs in the 1990s. This demand was particularly strong in Brazil and Argentina. At the present time, these markets remain fertile grounds for a growing industry. Since 2001, IHRSA has conducted a Brazilian conference for health/fitness club owners—a true sign that the South American market has achieved noteworthy status.

In 2004, the international markets represented just over 52% of the total membership base and over 60% of the gross revenues in the global health/fitness club industry (refer to Figure 23.3). The average monthly dues in the international health/fitness market (in euros) is shown in Figure 23.4. In other words, what was once considered primarily a North American industry, has developed into an international industry, one in which North America—particularly the United States—is just another player in a global marketplace. Figure 23.3 presents a quantitative overview of the international health/fitness industry.

The Future

In the late 1990s, IHRSA reported that, with regard to the global marketplace, one of the goals of the health/fitness club industry was to reach 100 million club members by the year 2010, with 50 million in the United States and 50 million in the various international markets. Less than a decade later,

During the 1990s, the Asian market (exclusive of Japan) was primarily driven by small fitness centers that were located in hotels and residential developments.

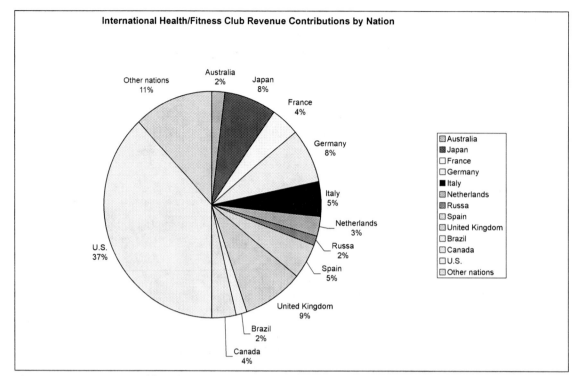

Figure 23.3. International health/fitness club revenue contributions by nation

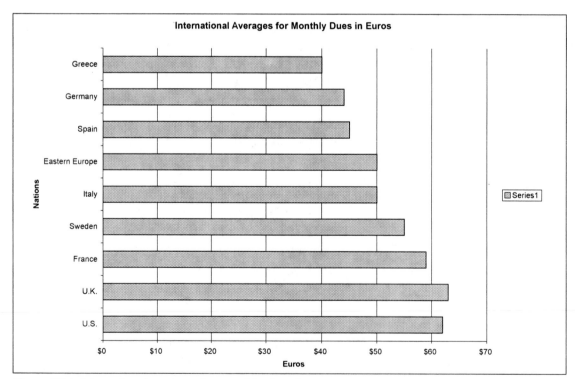

Figure 23.4. International averages for monthly dues in euros

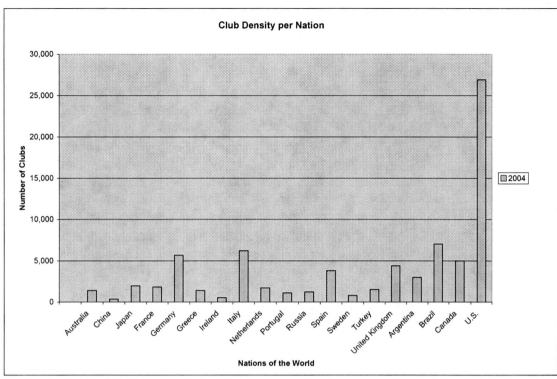

Figure 23.5. Club denisty by nation

substantial progress had been made toward achieving that goal. As of 2004, clubs worldwide had an estimated 84 million members, with 41 million in the United States and 43 million internationally. What once seemed a lofty goal for the global health/fitness club industry currently seems very likely. In fact, that objective will likely be achieved well in advance of the year 2010 (the actual number could easily reach 110 million).

The future of the international health/fitness club industry appears to be as promising as its past. In that regard, the following trends may continue to have a substantial impact on the international marketplace:

❑ *Domestic Growth.* The health/fitness club industry in the United Kingdom and mainland Europe will continue to evolve, with companies focusing their developmental efforts within their respective countries. The rapid expansion in the industry that occurred in an earlier part of this century caused many clubs to be unable to adapt their business models to the markets in their non-native countries. As a result, a renewed interest in refining and growing their domestic businesses emerged in a number of health/fitness organizations. Hopefully, this renewed focus on addressing the needs and interests of individuals within their respective countries will produce a significant increase in their ability to penetrate the market. The move from a publicly traded industry to more of a private-equity industry may also help fuel this movement. The exceptions to this rule may be

David Lloyd and Virgin Active, who have recently (as of 2001) made acquisitions in mainland Europe (Italy, Portugal, and Spain).

> **At the present time, the international market, as a whole, only penetrates approximately three-to-four percent of the eligible population.**

❑ *Market Penetration.* At the present time, the international market, as a whole, only penetrates approximately three-to-four percent of the eligible population. While the level of penetration in Europe is higher at 5.5%, it is still well below the 14% level that exists in the United States and the 10% rate of market penetration that is achieved in countries such as Norway and Sweden. These statistics reflect the fact that a huge opportunity exists to provide a product that can tap into these relatively overlooked markets. One of the challenges will be creating a workable model that fits within the cultural and financial conditions attendant to each specific country. For example, in the United States, the average annual club dues—as a percentage of per capital income—are 1.9% and .85-to-one percent of household income for those individuals who are club members. In contrast, in Europe, the average annual dues are just over two percent of the per capita income. In order to make fitness more accessible, clubs will have to price their offerings at a level that is appropriate to the income levels that exist within each nation.

❑ *Tackling a Growing Problem.* With regard to obesity, the global marketplace is confronted with similar challenges. In the last decade, the level of obesity has increased in every country, in both genders, and across all age groups, races, and types of backgrounds to a point where it is currently a worldwide epidemic. In fact, obesity represents the single largest global opportunity for the health/fitness club industry to have a meaningful impact on the health of the planet.

❑ *Favorable Circumstances.* The emerging markets of China and southeast Asia offer a significant growth opportunity for the health/fitness industry. In reality, the success of these markets will depend on several factors, including the continued growth of a capitalistic economy, the sustained emergence of an evolving middle class, and the introduction of professionally conducted fitness operations in these countries. Another fertile international area for the health/fitness club industry will be the Eastern European block of nations, who are just now beginning to enter the marketplace.

❑ *A Changing of the Guard.* The major health/fitness-club operations in the United States will lose their place as the top performers in the industry. Substantial potential exists that relatively large health/fitness-club organizations in the United Kingdom, Europe, and possibly even Asia may become the leading club operations in the latter part of the early 21st century. As of September 2005, Fitness First, based in the United Kingdom, has become the largest operator of clubs worldwide (based on the number of clubs).

❑ *An Appropriate Blend.* Fitness will continue to evolve into a format that can be best termed as "fusion fitness," in which the interests and practices of various international cultures are "blended" into unique modalities. Companies that are able to integrate the diversity of the various cultures into their branding and operating practices will become international leaders in this area.

❑ *Growing Older.* Statistics indicate that the population of the world is aging. In fact, the over-50 population is projected to be the largest segment of the world's population over the next 10-to-15 years. The efforts that international clubs undertake to target this market will, in large part, determine their financial success in the coming decade.

❑ *Growing Up.* The under-25 population may represent the biggest challenge for the health/fitness club industry. Possibly the most globally influenced group of individuals in the history of mankind because of the world to which they have been subjected, this relatively young population has been raised on fast foods, video games, sedentary living, and quickly evolving technology. The challenge is to find a fitness model that appeals to this young audience and engages them in physical activity. It is a challenge that will benefit from the combined wisdom and innovation of the industry's international partners.

❑ *A United Front.* The major segments of the international health/fitness industry must communicate with each other to help create a united front that can work with the global community in order to heighten the public's awareness of the industry's role in enhancing the health and well-being of every person on the planet. In this regard, the major international health/fitness club operations, including those in the United States, must find a way to establish non-profit fitness opportunities for those nations and populations that cannot afford to pay for fitness memberships. Unfortunately, the health/fitness club industry (home and abroad) has slowly morphed into a marketplace where the available fitness opportunities are limited to those individuals who have the financial resources to take advantage of the existing circumstances. However, the

The major segments of the international health/fitness industry must communicate with each other to help create a united front that can work with the global community in order to heighten the public's awareness of the industry's role in enhancing the health and well-being of every person on the planet.

The international markets, with the exception of the United Kingdom, have not differentiated themselves as significantly as have the U.S. and Canadian markets.

real potential for having a meaningful impact on the global marketplace lies in reaching those who currently cannot afford the services provided by the industry.

❑ *Setting Themselves Apart.* The international markets, with the exception of the United Kingdom, have not differentiated themselves as significantly as have the U.S. and Canadian markets. Over the next few years, these international players can be expected to create greater brand differentiation in their efforts to reach the smaller niche markets in their countries.

(Note: Additional information on the global health/fitness club marketplace can be obtained by contacting IHRSA.)

THE FUTURE OF THE HEALTH/FITNESS CLUB INDUSTRY

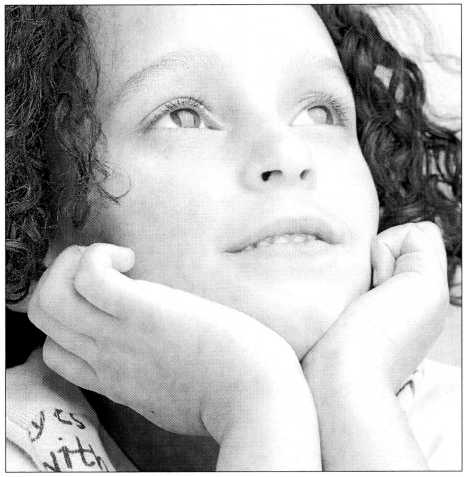

- Chapter 24: The Future of the Health/Fitness Club Market

Part Nine

24

The Future of the Health/Fitness Club Market

Chapter Objectives

The health/fitness club industry is an evolving entity, both domestically and internationally. While it is more of an accepted part of the American culture and lifestyle than it was 25 years ago, the industry remains somewhat susceptible to the whims of changing demographics and trendy popular culture. Several factors involving these demographics and the popular culture may have a significant impact on the club industry over the next several years. The more clubs are aware of these factors and respond accordingly, the more the industry will be able to sustain continued growth and profitability. This chapter details several of the factors that can have a meaningful bearing on the future of the health/fitness market.

Demographic and Psychographic Factors

❏ *Demographic and Psychographic Factors That May Impact the Industry from 2006 to 2015*:

- *Aging of the baby boomers*. Over the next 10 years, 78 million baby boomers will either reach age 50 or will have passed it already.

- *The echo boomers*. The under age-18 population, involving approximately 77 million individuals, will be entering the traditionally "clubbable market" of 18-to-34.

- *Melting together*. The fusion of America will result in a greater mix of ethnic diversity, with no distinct majority or minority. America will truly be a melting pot of cultures, each with a differing set of expectations for physical activity, based on their cultural background.

While it is more of an accepted part of the American culture and lifestyle than it was 25 years ago, the health/fitness industry remains somewhat susceptible to the whims of changing demographics and trendy popular culture.

- *Growing problem.* The number of overweight and obese individuals in America will continue to increase. In fact, these individuals will become more the norm than the exception, as the number of factors that have contributed significantly to the epidemic of sedentary lifestyles and obesity (e.g., technology, television, the elimination of the physical education requirement in schools, the protracted growth of the fast-food industry, etc.) carries on unabated.

- *Expanding boundaries.* Cities and suburbs will continue to push ever outward, creating a loosely centered culture.

- *Living together.* Two-family households will continue to impact the industry.

- *Refurbishing the cities.* Urban revitalization will continue to influence the domestic and international markets, bringing work and home close to each other.

- *Unfolding developments.* Former third-world countries will continue to evolve into significant and influential markets.

- *Recognizing opportunities.* The financial markets will continue to look at the health/fitness club industry as a viable investment opportunity.

Projected Expectations

❑ *Projected Expectations for and from the Industry by 2015:*

By 2015, over 66% of the individuals who join health/fitness clubs will be older than 40 and will have at least one health-related risk factor.

- The average age of the prospective health/fitness club member will continue to increase. By 2015, over 66% of the individuals who join health/fitness clubs will be older than 40 and will have at least one health-related risk factor. As a result, clubs must be even more aware of the safety factors involved in working with an older adult population that has one or more serious health risks and must establish appropriate operational guidelines and practices.

- Health promotion and risk prevention will become a universal theme as a result of the increasing number of health risks that exist within the population (e.g., obesity. diabetes, arthritis, heart disease, etc.). Because fitness clubs will be perceived as a viable form of alternative medicine, many clubs will focus their marketing efforts on the fact that regular exercise helps keep people healthy (i.e., prevent illness) as a means of attracting new members.

- The cultural blend that is occurring in America will put greater emphasis on the need for clubs to develop more diverse program offerings. As such, culturally related factors may result in the segmentation of clubs, depending on the culture that is found in a particular geographic region or area. It is possible that new niche markets will open up to serve specific cultural segments that exist in the United States, as well as in international markets.

- Clubs will need to focus even more on their community "roots" in the market in which they are located in order to maintain their identity and avoid the commoditization that can result when differentiation is reduced to pricing and facility factors.

- Franchised fitness operations will continue to grow, as club owners enter a period of niche offerings. In particular, small franchise opportunities with specialty themes (e.g., Curves, Cuts, Golf Fitness Centers, Heart Care Centers, etc.) will become an integral part of the industry's landscape.

- Functional fitness and core fitness, as well as rehabilitative fitness, will receive even more attention in the industry.

- The demand for soft-style Eastern martial arts (e.g., tai chi) and soft-style Western movement programming activities (e.g., pilates) will increase.

- Equipment manufacturers will continue to push the envelope on issues and factors involving entertainment and connectivity. Some equipment will incorporate features that are more like home furnishings.

- Consolidation of the industry will continue, with the realistic possibility that more than 50% of the industry will eventually be controlled by a few large companies.

- Many of the larger privately held club companies will go public or evolve into more extensive well-financed operations that expand into international markets.

- Fitness professionals will be seen in the same light as other healthcare professionals, resulting in the need for them to be either registered or licensed.

- Clubs will face the challenge of offering entertaining experiences to the new echo-boomer market. Brought up on video games, echo boomers will demand constant stimulation in their club experience. As a result, program offerings in clubs must include an entertainment dimension in order to attract and retain these individuals as members.

- Suburban clubs will be confronted with the expectation that they serve as one-stop lifestyle malls.

- Supply and demand will result in some shrinkage in the number of local clubs that, financially, are performing at a marginal level. This scenario will have an ever greater impact in those club chains that tend to all look the same.

- Capital will continue to flow into the industry. At the same time, the club industry will begin to look more like McDonald's and Walmart. As part of this change, local facility operators will capitalize on their ability to provide personalized club experiences.

Consolidation of the industry will continue, with the realistic possibility that more than 50% of the industry will eventually be controlled by a few large companies.

No one can accurately predict the future of the health/fitness industry. The real key to success for club owners over the next decade will be to understand the rich culture of the industry, protect it, and then evolve their facility's offerings, based on societal influences, without changing the base culture of the industry.

The real key to success for club owners over the next decade will be to understand the rich culture of the industry, protect it, and then evolve their facility's offerings, based on societal influences, without changing the base culture of the industry.

CASE STUDIES IN THE HEALTH/FITNESS CLUB INDUSTRY

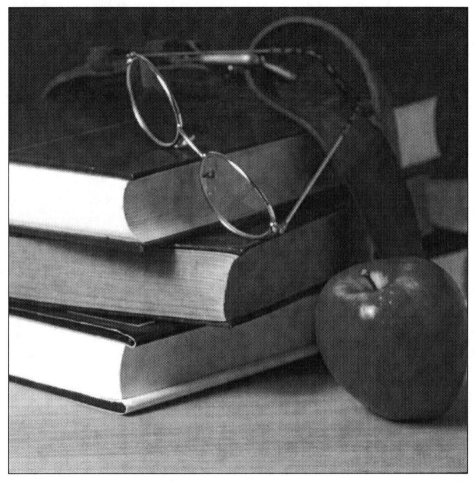

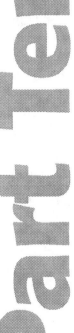

- Chapter 25: Customer and Member Chronicles
- Chapter 26: Employee Chronicles
- Chapter 27: Big Business Chronicles

My first manager called it, "baptism by fire." He was referring to the leadership and management scenarios that occur in the health/fitness club industry that are not taught in textbooks. Later in my career, I decided that his primary point was that the only way to really learn management and leadership is by dealing with the unique and unexpected situations that often transpire when working with members and employees. Most first-time managers and leaders enter their new roles armed with a rudimentary understanding of the basic principles of financial management, leadership, programming, sales and marketing, member/customer relations, and employee relations. In reality, such basic competencies will only carry a person so far in business. Individuals who want to operate a great club—one that is known for its outstanding member/customer service—must be prepared to lead and manage during challenging and unexpected circumstances. Addressing these events in an appropriate manner is an ever-evolving process that can benefit from continual nurturing. Among the steps that can be undertaken in this regard is to study and learn from the problem-solving efforts of others in particular situations.

The only way to really learn management and leadership is by dealing with the unique and unexpected situations that often transpire when working with members and employees.

This part of the book presents a recap of several of the most demanding and challenging situations that actually occurred in the club business and how seasoned and not-so-seasoned leaders and managers dealt with them. Information about these scenarios has been provided by some of the industry's most seasoned professionals. Collectively, the individuals who shared their experiences and the actions they took to address them have over 300 years experience in the health/fitness club industry. It is important to note that each of the scenarios recounted in chapters 25-to-27 represents events that actually occurred. The individuals involved are actual people, either club members or employees (although for privacy reasons, no names are used in the chronicles, and the locale of each story has been changed). The chronicles presented in this part are grouped into three basic scenarios. Chapter 25 addresses scenarios that involved customers and members of clubs. Chapter 26 deals with employee scenarios, while chapter 27 features a series of synopses involving business scenarios.

Each management scenario is defined in three parts. The first part describes the event or scenario; the second summarizes the solution or response of management; and the third discusses the event and solution.

The primary objective of Part X is to provide an opportunity to consider and examine selected leadership/managerial-related scenarios that typically are not addressed in either formal schooling programs or company-sponsored managerial training efforts. Equally important is seeing and reflecting on how experienced professionals dealt with each set of circumstances. All factors considered, studying these unique business scenarios can help individuals to be better prepared to lead through the most challenging of situations.

25

Customer and Member Chronicles

Chapter Objectives

The situations recounted in this chapter focus on events and experiences involving the customers and members of health/fitness clubs. Each of these stories represents a unique situation that required extraordinary leadership and management.

Sun Wars

❑ *Scenario.* In the mid-80s, a high-end club located in the northeast had just completed an extensive renovation. Serving approximately 2,000 memberships with an average household income in excess of $200,000 annually, the club had a fitness center, group-exercise studios, locker rooms, dining area, pool, and sun deck.

The new fitness director had just been hired. One of the first stories he heard from his colleagues concerned the "sun wars" that were occurring on the club's sun deck, which was located eight stories above street level. He was told that over the past few summers, members had hit each other, stole others items from the sun deck, and thrown lifeguards in the pool—all in an effort to get one of the 30 lounge chairs that were located on the sun deck. Rather than take these stories at face value, the new fitness director decided to observe the actions of the club's members and staff. Since the sun deck did not officially open until Memorial Day, the fitness director felt that by observing events in the spring, he might be able to gain a better idea of what was really happening. After a couple of sunny weekends, the fitness director observed a litany of troubling events, including one of the facility's lifeguards being hit and thrown into the pool, member's clothes that were hanging on lounge chairs being thrown off the deck, members pulling each other's hair as they pulled each other off

> Rather than take these stories at face value, the new fitness director decided to observe the actions of the club's members and staff.

lounge chairs, members yelling at each other when they thought it was time for them to have a lounge chair, and verbal and physical threats beingmade against staff by members.

❑ *The Solution.* The fitness director met with his senior-level department heads and a few members to try to identify a possible solution that would eliminate the dangerous situation and, hopefully, produce a mutually satisfactory outcome for all involved. After considerable discussion, a solution was proposed that included the following elements:

- A reservation system for lounge chairs was developed that would allow members to reserve a specific chair up to seven days in advance.

- Each lounge chair would be marked with a number and a corresponding reservation card, and a chair-reservation book would be prepared for the summer and kept at the front desk.

- A sun deck map was devised that showed the location of the lounge chairs.

- A ten-dollar charge to reserve a chair for a two-hour time period would be implemented.

- A cancellation and no-show policy would be instituted. If someone failed to cancel their chair reservation at least 24-hours in advance or if they did not show to claim their reservation, they would be charged the full amount for their lounge chair.

- The reservation, which had to be made in person or over the phone, could be made no earlier than seven days in advance.

- A concierge would be provided for the deck and would circulate every couple of hours with the reservation sheet to verify reservations and to pass out complimentary beverages.

- Details about the chair-reservation program would be communicated to the members, approximately two months before it was set to begin. Such efforts would include such steps as sending a personal letter to each member, placing posters up in conspicuous locations in the facility, putting notices in the club's member newsletter, and having the staff speak to the members they know.

> The fitness director met with his senior-level department heads and a few members to try to identify a possible solution that would eliminate the dangerous situation and, hopefully, produce a mutually satisfactory outcome for all involved.

When the chair-reservation program was first introduced to the members, the club received considerable feedback from the membership, most of which was not very flattering. And yet, one week before Memorial Day, all of the lounge chairs had been reserved, and a waiting list had been created. Over the course of the first summer, the chairs were 100% booked each weekend in two-hour time slots, with a waiting list of at least 10 people each weekend. By the July 4th weekend, the club had introduced food-and-drink service. During the first summer of the program, only one argument ensued. As a result, the club's members and staff did not have to deal with all of the fights and disorder that had previously existed. Another positive by-product of the new policy was the fact that the club generated approximately $1,000-to-$1,500 in revenue each weekend.

❑ *Discussion*. The aforementioned scenario is an example of a club not listening to its membership and understanding that a membership need existed that was not being addressed with an appropriate service-delivery process. The members wanted to see and feel the sun, a goal that was not so easily attained in this northeastern market. The members also needed to know that once they had a spot on the sun deck, that someone could not just walk up and take it. In essence, it was a basic supply-and-demand situation that had evolved into a member/customer relations headache for the club and, in the end, had led to a considerable degree of member/customer outrage. The proposed solution worked for the following reasons:

- The staff took the time to talk with members and staff, as well as observe the situation before attempting to identify a solution. Because the club got everyone involved in the situation in its efforts to understand the attendant circumstances, those individuals took ownership of the subsequent solution.

- The solution leveraged the supply-and-demand issue and provided the facility's customers and members with the opportunity to get what they wanted on a relatively exclusive basis.

- Value was created where it did not exist before. By putting a time limit on the use of a chair, setting a price for the service, and requiring reservations, the club had established a value for the sun deck.

- The club communicated its intentions sufficiently in advance so that it could address any concerns that might arise well before the program went into place.

- The club took a dynamic approach to the solution by continually offering new services to the members.

In reality, other possible solutions to the situation existed, including closing the deck, incorporating a reservation system but not charging for it, selling the chairs for the season, etc. Ultimately, the solution that was implemented achieved its desired goal of preventing more fights. It also resulted in an unexpected benefit—additional revenue and cash for the club.

The solution leveraged the supply-and-demand issue and provided the facility's customers and members with the opportunity to get what they wanted on a relatively exclusive basis.

Odor Eaters

❑ *Scenario*. This situation occurred in the mid-90s and involved a high-end club that was located on the west coast. The club had 2,500 memberships and provided full-service amenities. One of the unique services of this club was that all of the members rented lockers ($25 a month), which included access to such amenities as laundry service and shoeshines. Each individual paid an initiation fee of $1,000 to join this facility and $100 monthly dues to maintain their individual membership.

The fitness director, who had responsibility for the locker rooms and the fitness areas of the club, was approached by several members complaining about one of the club's most prominent constituents. Their grievance involved the fact that this particular individual had a very distinct aroma about him, both when he exercised and in the locker room. In fact, several of the complaining members stated that they would resign their membership if the offensive odor problem was not resolved. These members made it clear who the offending member was and that they did not want it to be known that they had complained. His pungent aroma made it difficult not only for other people to be on the exercise floor at the same time with him, but also (and possibly worse) to be in the locker room area around his locker.

The member and fitness director agreed to take several steps, including the club would provide the member with free laundry service for his clothes and provide him with his own soap solution that he could keep in his locker.

❑ *The Solution.* Understandably, the fitness director was very concerned. He was fully aware of the fact that the offending individual was an important member who spent a considerable amount of money in the club. He also knew that the club could not afford to lose the other members. The effort to identify a possible solution to this problem involved the following steps:

- He talked privately with the members who had complained in an attempt to get a better handle on the issues. He also told them that he would be taking action on their concerns.

- He spoke with his staff to get additional information on the situation. In addition, he checked out the offending member's locker during after-hours.

- He subsequently contacted the offending member by phone and asked if there was a time that they could meet. A meeting was set up in one of the private offices of the club. During the meeting, the fitness director told the individual about the other club members' concerns. The fitness director then asked the individual to express his feelings about the issue. The member was upset and wanted to know who was complaining. The fitness director replied that he understood the member's hurt feelings and that he would like to work with him to resolve the issue.

- The member and fitness director agreed to take several steps, including the club would provide the member with free laundry service for his clothes and provide him with his own soap solution that he could keep in his locker. Furthermore, the club agreed that they would always check to make sure that the member's laundry was done, even if he did not leave it out for laundering.

- The fitness director got in contact with the members who had complained and informed them that he had talked with the member who had the odor problem and that a solution had been reached. He told them that he appreciated their bringing this matter to his attention and asked that they let him know if the proposed solution did not work to their satisfaction.

❑ *Discussion*. This scenario is one that will likely occur at some point in every health/fitness club, especially if the facility provides rental lockers. When a facility has a diverse membership that extensively utilizes the club's services during the hours that it is open, it can expect situations such as this to occur. While no "perfect" solution to this kind of situation and problem exists, the club in this scenario handled the circumstances in a professional manner. The aforementioned solution worked for several reasons, including:

It is always difficult to share unfavorable news with members, especially when it is unflattering.

- The manager took the time to gather information about the situation by talking to members and staff and by personally observing what was occurring.

- The manager made sure to let the members who were complaining know that he would address the situation and get back to them.

- The manager set up a private appointment with the offending member. During that meeting, as professionally as he could, he discussed the situation that had been brought to his attention. Furthermore, he asked the member how he felt about the issue and made sure that the member had the opportunity to express his feelings about the situation.

- The manager worked with the offending member to identify a solution that would be appropriate for everyone involved.

- The manager made sure to follow-up with those individuals who had complained to thank them and let them know what actions had been taken. He also asked these members to feel free to contact him if the proposed solution did not seem to be working.

It is always difficult to share unfavorable news with members, especially when it is unflattering. Whether it is odor or any other difficult issue, it is important to remember that the privacy and feelings of everyone involved should always be accorded an appropriate degree of attention and respect. When dealing with such a situation, the manager should communicate openly, but with a sense of empathy. Managers who are open-minded, are good listeners, and demonstrate that they can be trusted, will likely elicit favorable responses from the members.

Naked Man on the Loose

❑ *Scenario*. This scenario took place in an urban fitness club that was located along the northeast corridor. Open for just over 10 years, the club served a rather upscale market of business professionals who lived in the area.

The club had just hired a new operations manager, who was experiencing his first week on the job. At the time, he was going through his initial training with the club's staff. On this particular day, he was training with one of the facility's sales directors. This particular sales director was giving a tour to a couple in their 40s. The operations director was tagging along to learn more about how to conduct a tour of the club.

As the tour proceeded towards the locker-room areas (the men's and women's locker rooms were located across the hall from each other), a man suddenly ran out of the locker room completely naked and confronted the sales director. The member jumped up and down in front of the sales person, prospects, and operations manager, shouting that someone was in the locker room rifling through lockers. He demanded that the situation be taken care of immediately, thinking nothing of the fact he was standing naked in front of a group of people—several of whom were complete strangers to him.

❑ *The Solution*. Within seconds of the man appearing naked and screaming at the sales director, the following actions took place:

- The first step that the sales director took was to tell the member that the club's operations manager would be right in to address the situation.

- The sales director then turned to the prospects and apologized to them for the member's behavior. She attempted to diffuse the awkwardness of the moment by casually mentioning that in this city anything was possible. The sales director affirmed that having a member of the club stroll the hallways in the nude was not a normal part of the sales tour. She added that the operations manager would address the member's issues and invited everyone to proceed with the tour.

- The operations manager immediately escorted the member into the locker room, and then contacted security to let them know that a stranger was in the club who was stealing from member's lockers.

- After making the call to security, the operations manager continued through the locker room and found the culprit. He tried to retain him, but he escaped to the freight elevator.

- Subsequently, security personnel captured the would-be thief as he left the freight elevator and contacted the operations manager to give him an update about the situation.

> He demanded that the situation be taken care of immediately, thinking nothing of the fact he was standing naked in front of a group of people—several of whom were complete strangers to him.

- The operations manager then met with the member who had originally seen the thief and let him know how the situation had turned out. Furthermore, he informed him that, in the future, it would be more appropriate if he would at least wrap a towel around himself before leaving the confines of the locker room.

- The operations manager then let the sales director know what had occurred so that she could communicate it to the prospects.

❑ *Discussion.* While having a naked member run out in front of everyone when a tour is being conducted is not likely to happen often, it does represent a situation that can be embarrassing for everyone involved. As such, it requires quick thinking on the manager's part. The staff involved in this situation handled it professionally. Their response and solution were effective because of several factors, including:

Paying attention (listening), apologizing, taking action, and finally, following-up are all critical steps in dealing with any member or customer issue that arises in the club.

- The sales director maintained her calm and responded to the member's concerns at once by indicating that immediate action to address the situation would be taken.

- Exhibiting a professional presence, the sales director immediately apologized to the prospects. Her efforts to apologize also included a touch of humor that helped diffuse any tension that was present.

- The operations manager escorted the member back into the locker room and then immediately contacted security.

- The operations manager, after contacting security, searched for the thief and attempted to retain him until security personnel arrived.

- After the thief was apprehended, the operations manager contacted the sales director and gave her an update on the actions that had been taken. He also made sure to inform the member who had originally brought the matter to the club's attention.

Paying attention (listening), apologizing, taking action, and finally, following-up are all critical steps in dealing with any member or customer issue that arises in the club. Furthermore, by maintaining a calm, professional presence, the team was able to put the member and prospects at greater ease.

Peace and Harmony During the Holiday Season

❑ *Scenario.* This scenario occurred in a small suburban fitness club in the southwest. The club was a fitness-only facility that served a corporate market. The club had been in business for several years at the time of the event.

It was the holiday season, and the club was brightly decorated. The club, as was its usual practice each holiday season, was filled with the sounds of joyful holiday music. While most of the club's members enjoyed the holiday music, one particular member felt that it was inappropriate music to listen to while working out. All of a sudden, one member of the club started arguing with another member over the music that was being played. The manager noticed that these two individuals were arguing over the music and asked them to separate. The two members then retreated to the men's locker room. Subsequently, the manager heard from yet a third member of the club that the two men were now in a fistfight.

In almost every situation when a fight breaks out between members, the manager's best course of action is to break it up, ask the members to leave the facility, and schedule time to talk with each of the members at a later date about their behavior.

❑ *The Solution.* The manager immediately got hold of one of the male personal trainers and had him go into the locker room. The personal trainer separated the men and broke up the fight. The manager told the trainer to communicate to both of the individuals that the manager would like to meet with them. Subsequently, one of the combatants met with the manager, who explained to him that his behavior was completely unacceptable. Indignant, the member offered a series of excuses. Eventually, he was asked to leave the club by the manager and did. The other member was so angered that he just left the club without talking to the manager. Later on, the manager met with him the next time he was in the club.

❑ *Discussion.* In reality, disputes over music are not that rare. It is relatively amazing how something as simple as the choice of music can cause grown men to get into a fistfight. In this particular scenario, the manager handled the situation very well by taking the following steps:

- Terminating the argument on the exercise floor, and when it continued in another area of the club, having a personal trainer of the same gender enter the locker room and break it up.

- Talking with both of the combatants to let them know that their behavior was unacceptable.

- Requesting that the one recalcitrant member immediately leave the club.

In almost every situation when a fight breaks out between members, the manager's best course of action is to break it up, ask the members to leave the facility, and schedule time to talk with each of the members at a later date about their behavior. In some instances, suspending a member from the club might be necessary.

With regard to music selection—a factor that causes problems more frequently than most would like to believe—clubs should establish a music policy that is made known to the members. By having a clearly communicated music policy, members are aware of what they can expect and are less likely to behave in an antisocial manner.

Beware of the Nose

❑ *Scenario*. This scenario took place in a fitness club that was located in an urban market in the deep south. The facility served a reasonably high-end corporate membership. At the time of the incident, the club had been in business for over 20 years.

> The situation involved a member of the club who ran on a treadmill a few times each week. Several of the club's members and employees complained about the member's behavior while he was using the treadmill. Their complaint involved the fact that every time the member ran on the treadmill, he would perform a "farmer's blow" (i.e., blowing his nose into his hands) and then would touch the treadmill. The fitness director was informed by both the staff and several members that they found the exerciser's disgusting behavior repulsive, to a point where no one wanted to work out in the same area of the club when this member was on the treadmill.

When an individual does something that results in unhygienic conditions and impacts the ability of other members to enjoy the club, it is the responsibility of management to address the issue with that member.

❑ *The Solution*. The fitness director decided to contact the member in question by letter. He felt that if he initially met with the member in person, he might embarrass that individual if the conversation was overheard by others. He sent the letter to the member's home. The letter detailed the member's unacceptable conduct and emphasized how important it was to keep the club clean and hygienic for all of the members. The letter indicated that his actions were insulting to other members and impacted the club's overall cleanliness. The member responded to the letter by contacting the fitness director personally and thanking him for sharing what he did and doing so in a confidential manner. Going forward, the member did not exhibit the offensive behavior any more.

❑ *Discussion*. It is not uncommon for some members to be disrespectful of the club and other members when it comes to hygiene. In this particular scenario, the fitness director handled the circumstances appropriately. As a result, the behavior came to a halt. Among the steps that enabled this situation to be dealt with successfully were:

- The fitness director contacted the member confidentially, thus helping to limit any possible embarrassment.

- The fitness director focused his efforts on addressing the offending behavior, not the member. He ensured that the member knew that his behavior was causing a problem for other members of the club. In essence, he "de-personalized" the issue.

When an individual does something that results in unhygienic conditions and impacts the ability of other members to enjoy the club, it is the responsibility of management to address the issue with that member. To the

Management decided that because they were asking the young woman to seek medical clearance, the club had to be prepared to provide emotional and financial assistance if it was determined to be warranted.

extent possible, this effort should always be kept private to help prevent any embarrassment for the member. Furthermore, the endeavor should focus on the behavior of the offending individual and its impact on other members and staff, rather than making it a personal issue.

Clubs can help head off situations similar to these by having house rules that clarify how members should respect the club, other members, and employees and what behaviors are unacceptable. These rules can be very simple and shared with each individual through a member's handbook, a notice on the website, or other appropriate forms of media (e.g., signage, mailings, etc.).

To the Rescue

❑ *Scenario.* This scenario occurred in the mid-Atlantic region of the U.S. in a facility that was a well-operated multipurpose club serving a family market. In this particular set of circumstances, club management had become aware of a young woman who they believed had an eating and exercise disorder. Management had noticed that this individual, who was in the club almost every day, had become ever-increasingly emaciated over the last several weeks. Management believed that it had an obligation to become involved in the situation, but was not sure how to do so without overstepping its expertise or abusing the privacy and feelings of the member involved.

❑ *The Solution.* After considerable discussion among the senior leaders of the club, an intervention was identified that everyone agreed upon. As such, management decided to take the following actions:

- They identified the club's resident registered nurse as the most appropriate staff person to open a dialogue with the young woman.

- Management asked the nurse to open a dialogue with the young woman and request that she obtain a medical clearance from her physician before continuing with her use of the club.

- Management decided that because they were asking the young woman to seek medical clearance, the club had to be prepared to provide emotional and financial assistance if it was determined to be warranted.

- The nurse set up a private meeting with the member involved in the situation and informed her that the club would require her to obtain medical clearance before she would be allowed to continue using the club's facilities. At first, the young woman was defensive, but then became offended by the club's request.

- After informing the young woman of the club's position, the nurse told her that the club was willing to lend her assistance, both financially and emotionally. Upon hearing this, the young woman's attitude changed dramatically, and she expressed her thanks. Subsequently, the young woman indicated that she was aware that she had a problem and had been struggling to identify a clinic or program that could meet her needs (note: her parents had previously washed their hands of the situation).

- Upon hearing the young woman's comments, the staff nurse researched the clinical options until she found a facility that seemed to offer what the young woman needed. Once the clinic was identified, the nurse and staff worked with the young woman to help her get accepted into the clinic's eating disorder program. Subsequently, after the young woman had been admitted to the program, she reported that she had a fear of travel since losing one of her favorite travel companions a few years earlier (e.g., a stuffed animal).

- The nurse proceeded to purchase a special travel companion for the young woman, which she presented to her prior to her departure to the clinic for the first time.

- The young woman made a commitment to the club to successfully complete her treatment program and to come back healthy.

❑ *Discussion*. This set of circumstances is one of the most challenging situations that management can face. The dilemma facing management involved several interrelated factors: the privacy of a member, the medical diagnosis (which is not the club's role), the endangerment of the member's health, and the self-esteem of the member. By any reasonable standard, determining an appropriate solution to this particular situation could have been very difficult. In this situation, however, management took several steps that led to a successful resolution of the problem, including:

> **The dilemma facing management involved several interrelated factors: the privacy of a member, the medical diagnosis (which is not the club's role), the endangerment of the member's health, and the self-esteem of the member.**

- The staff met as a team and identified the steps that would be taken. Subsequently, the measures were perceived as a team solution, which is the best basis for attempting to resolve any situation.

- The staff person most qualified to deal with this particular issue (e.g., a registered nurse) was identified.

- The nurse spoke privately with the young woman and asked her to obtain medical clearance.

- The club expressed its willingness to provide assistance—both financially and emotionally—to the young woman.

- The club followed through on its commitment.

Collectively, the net effect of management's actions was a young woman who opened up about her problems and was able to make a commitment to pursue much-needed therapy.

Clubs are not (and should not be) in the business of making medical diagnoses and must not assume that a member has a particular health problem unless the individual informs them or provides them with a note from a physician that informs them of that fact.

Several points should be emphasized to anyone in a leadership position in a club who may be confronted by a situation like this in the future. First, clubs are not (and should not be) in the business of making medical diagnoses and must not assume that a member has a particular health problem unless the individual informs them or provides them with a note from a physician that informs them of that fact. Second, a club is obligated to seek medical clearance from any member or prospective member who has known risk factors that would increase that person's likelihood of experiencing a health or medical problem as a result of exercising. The key for a club, in this regard, is to make sure that it is consistent in how it applies the use of medical clearance to all of its members. Third, all factors considered, the facility should seek advice from its legal council before proceeding in situations like this. Fourth, when the club initiates dialogue with the member, it is best if it involves someone who already has a positive, trusting relationship with the member. Finally, the club should be prepared for the likely responses in such circumstances (e.g., denial of any problem, an expression of anger and hurt, and a refusal to obtain medial clearance).

I had two experiences with a member whom we believed had anorexia. In both instances, steps similar to the ones undertaken by the club in this scenario were initiated, with the exception that we talked with our attorney, and we had a physician (rather than a registered nurse) from our medical-advisory committee talk with the member. In both cases, the member was hurt and angered, and we ended up having to remove their membership.

The solution developed and successfully implemented by the club in this scenario is an excellent example of a management team that, through empathy and a commitment to its members, was able to turn a potentially perilous situation into a life-changing one for the member involved.

Cell-Phone Enforcer

❑ *Scenario.* This scenario took place in a mid-western multipurpose club that served a relatively affluent membership base of approximately 4,000 individuals. This particular club had a policy that disallowed camera phones in the locker rooms. One member of this facility was convinced that any individual using a cell phone in the locker room was actually taking pictures of him. Over a period of time, this particular member had become obsessed about cell-phone usage in the locker room and had decided to take it upon himself to be the club's enforcer with regard to camera phones and cell phones. The club's policy concerning this issue was clear. If a member notices that a camera phone is in use in the locker room, that person should contact management and allow staff to deal with the situation. Disregarding the club's policy, this member had begun accosting other members and verbally abusing any individual he saw with a cell phone in the locker room. When this member was approached by the manager on duty about his behavior, the abusive member verbally assaulted him.

❑ *The Solution.* The club management took the following steps to resolve the situation to the satisfaction of everyone involved:

  • The operations manager contacted the member by phone to rationally discuss the concerns of other members and of club management in an attempt to reach a reasonable solution to the problem. The member responded by saying that the club should ban all cell phones from the club and that furthermore, he would physically accost any individuals whom he found with a cell phone.

  • The executive director of the club then contacted the member and explained to him that his behavior was unacceptable. The executive director also informed the member that the club could not ban all cell phones (even if it wanted to), because several of the members were physicians who might need to be reached. On the other hand, he indicated to the member that the club's policy did ban the use of camera phones and that if he noticed another member with one, he should please contact a member of the staff, and management would address the situation.

  • Finally, the executive director informed the member that if he continued his verbal attacks on members that he would face expulsion from the club and possible criminal action.

❑ *Discussion.* Cell phones (camera phones in particular) have become a big issue in the club industry. Most clubs have instituted policies that ban the use of camera phones in their facilities. This particular situation arose possibly out of a member's safety concerns and his inability to clearly understand the club's policies. The member's subsequent actions were totally inexcusable and caused serious problems with the other members. The response of management in this situation was effective because of several reasons, including:

  • The club had a senior manager talk directly with the member in a manner that did not embarrass him.

  • When the member did not respond appropriately to the club's initial efforts to resolve the situation, a senior-level manager spoke with him in a private setting.

  • That manager reinforced the club's policies concerning the use of both cell and camera phones and detailed the member's options involving situations that warranted attention. The senior-level manager also

Cell phones (camera phones in particular) have become a big issue in the club industry.

communicated his displeasure with the member's actions and informed him that if he continued, that the club would consider banishing him from the club.

When dealing with situations similar to this one, the club should do the following:

While prohibiting camera phones in the locker room is a good rule, this policy should apply throughout the club.

- Develop house rules and policies that address such issues and take steps to ensure that each member is aware of these rules and policies. Not only should these policies address the use of cell phones, they should also deal with other issues that are important to maintaining the club's atmosphere and sense of privacy. These rules should also detail guidelines concerning what actions management can take in the event that the policies are violated. For example, the club should have a policy that states that management maintains the right to expel any member of the facility if that individual blatantly ignores the policies and rules of the club.

- Consider having the most noteworthy policies, such as camera-phone rules, posted in the locker rooms and even inside the lockers. Ensuring that the members are fully aware of all key policies and rules of the club is important.

- Establish a hierarchy of management for responding to these types of situations.

- Ensure that all conversations with members concerning the possible violation of the club's rules and policies are conducted in private.

- Document the member's activities and the resulting actions of management concerning those activities and place the report in the member's file.

While prohibiting camera phones in the locker room is a good rule, this policy should apply throughout the club. Prohibiting the use of these phones in only one area of the facility can cause problems. All factors considered, it is better to preclude their use anywhere in the club. It should be emphasized that it is always advisable for a club to get its legal council's advice before establishing any policy concerning the use of camera phones in the facility.

26

Employee Chronicles

Chapter Objectives

The scenarios related in this chapter involve situations that entail employee experiences in health/fitness clubs. Resolving them required both insight and thoughtful managerial acumen.

Health Hearsay

❑ *Scenario*. This scenario took place in a large upscale club during the mid-to-late 1980s, which was located in an affluent residential neighborhood on the east coast. At the time, the club had approximately 3,000 memberships, for which it charged approximately $120 a month for dues for a single membership. The club offered approximately 150-to-200 personal training sessions a week at an average cost of $40 each. These workouts were supervised by a group of eight personal trainers, two of whom conducted about 35-to-40 sessions each week.

One of the most popular trainers was a gentleman who had been in the personal training business for a considerable time period and had a reputation as being one of the best in his field. Subsequently, several female members approached the fitness director with their concerns about the trainer. They indicated that they thought the trainer had AIDs (because of a quite noticeable skin condition) and that he should not be allowed in the club. Within days, over 40 members had come to the fitness director and indicated that they had heard this particular employee had AIDs and asked what the club was going to do about it. Eventually, a number of the club's employees went to the fitness director and reported that they believed that this personal trainer had AIDs and should be dismissed from the club. In only a few short days, over 100 complaints about this individual had been received, all based on a similar rumor.

In only a few short days, over 100 complaints about this individual had been received, all based on a similar rumor.

❑ *The Solution*. The fitness director decided to investigate the situation. His first step was to speak with the other employees and members, each in private. During his talks with these individuals, he informed them that he wanted to initially determine whether a problem existed. If and when he discovered an issue that needed attention, he would address it as appropriately as possible. Subsequently, he took the following steps:

- He met with the manager of the facility to share with him what was occurring and asking for his guidance. The manager replied that he would talk with the club's legal counsel.

- The fitness director then had a private meeting with the personal trainer in question and informed him that some of the club's employees and members had expressed their concern that he might have a contagious virus. Although he was slightly offended, he assured the fitness director that he was fine and that he had a minor illness that was being treated, which posed no problem to others.

- The fitness director, taking the trainer at his word, went back to the manager and detailed their conversation. In addition, the fitness director met privately with the members and staff who had expressed their concern and told them that he had met with the personal trainer, that they had discussed the person's health, and that the rumor was false.

- Subsequently, the manager informed the fitness director that he wanted the trainer to see a physician and be screened for AIDS. The fitness director replied that although he personally felt that such a request was inappropriate, he would reluctantly ask the trainer to do as the manager wanted and get a note saying that he was healthy and not contagious. The manager then announced that the fitness director had no choice; either get the individual screened for AIDs or else.

- Consequently, the fitness director met privately with the physical trainer and told him that the club was willing to pay for him to visit a local physician, undergo a physical, and get a clearance note. Furthermore, he informed the trainer that this step would put the concerns of the members and management to rest. No mention was made of AIDS testing. The personal trainer consented and a physician's appointment was made for him.

- On the day of the appointment, the trainer was accompanied to the doctor's office by his direct supervisor at the club. When the trainer got to the physician's office, he received a physical, but was then asked to sign a sheet regarding undergoing a blood test for AIDS, a request that angered him a lot. He took the blood test, but immediately returned to the club.

- The fitness director then met with the personal trainer and his supervisor and discussed the events that had occurred. The fitness

The fitness director then had a private meeting with the personal trainer in question and informed him that some of the club's employees and members had expressed their concern that he might have a contagious virus.

director apologized to the trainer for not telling him about the AIDS test beforehand. In reality, he said that he was very uncomfortable about the situation and wanted to avoid that issue if he could, but felt that there was no other way for him to handle it.

- After considerable discussion, the personal trainer and fitness director came to a mutually agreed upon resolution. The trainer would not come to work for a few days, so he could gather himself. Subsequently, however, the trainer would return for full duty.

- The blood tests indicated no evidence of AIDS, but did show a treatable virus that was affecting his skin. Medicine was provided to him, and his virus was successfully treated.

- The fitness director met with both the members and the employees who had lodged a complaint about the trainer's perceived medical condition. He informed them that the issue had been addressed and that the rumors were blatantly untrue.

❑ *Discussion.* This situation involved a very challenging employee issue that required total privacy. Unfortunately, the situation was not handled as well as it should have been. As a result, the trust of an employee was lost, and the integrity of a leader was negatively impacted. While eventually the matter was addressed to the satisfaction of those who were concerned with the medical condition of the personal trainer, it was not handled in an appropriate manner from the employee's perspective. In fact, the staff's actions could have exposed the club and fitness director to a lawsuit. Several key observations could be made regarding the situation and how it was handled, including:

- The fitness director responded appropriately at first by talking with his manager and collecting information from the concerned members and staff.

- The fitness director also acted in a responsible manner by speaking with the personal trainer in question and soliciting feedback from him.

- On the other hand, the fitness director should never have sent the employee to see a physician under false pretenses, no matter how much pressure was applied by senior management. Because his integrity and character were at stake, the fitness director should have taken a firmer position with senior management.

- Failing that, the fitness director should have been up-front (honest) with the trainer and should have asked him to please bring in a note from his physician that confirmed that he was not contagious. The fitness director should not have recommended a physician, unless asked to do so by the trainer. The choice of which physician to utilize should have been left to the trainer.

The fitness director should never have sent the employee to see a physician under false pretenses, no matter how much pressure was applied by senior management.

> It cannot be overemphasized how important it is for managers to respect their employees and be truthful with them at all times, no matter how challenging or difficult the situation.

- Much earlier in the sequence of events, the fitness director should have informed the members that he had addressed the situation with the personal trainer and that it had been safely resolved. Furthermore, the matter (including the members' concerns, complaints, and accusations) should have been dropped at that point.

It cannot be overemphasized how important it is for managers to respect their employees and be truthful with them at all times, no matter how challenging or difficult the situation. Furthermore, managers must always respect the privacy of both employees and members and never do anything that might compromise their privacy. In addition, managers should address issues truthfully. Parsing the facts or their words is never the right approach for dealing with any situation. Managers should also remember that making the right decision is the proper course of action, even when doing so might cause them to lose their job. Finally, when dealing with members, managers should inform them that they have addressed the issue in a manner that they feel is appropriate. If the members don't feel comfortable with that, it is their problem. Managers should let the members deal with it, rather then try to go too far in appeasing them. A fine line always exists that managers should not cross when attempting to address issues that arise between members and employees.

A Lover's Quarrel

❑ *Scenario.* This scenario occurred in an urban racquet club that was located along the northeast corridor during the early part of the 1990s. Serving an upscale membership base, this facility provided fitness and racquet-sport services for its members.

The situation involved a female assistant general manager with four years experience who was on duty at the time of the incident. This employee started her career at the front desk and, through hard work and stellar performance, had been promoted to her current position. Also on duty during the same shift was the front-desk concierge, who had been with the club for six months and had been, to that point, an exemplary employee. As happens with matters of the heart, both employees had recently begun seeing each other on a personal level.

About 5:00 p.m. that day, during the club's prime time, the front desk was very busy. The desk was manned by the assistant general manager, the front-desk concierge, and two other staff personnel. In addition, at least ten members where checking in at the desk at the time. All of a sudden, without any warning, the assistant general manager and the front-desk concierge began screaming at each other, a situation which quickly escalated into a full-scale battle. Subsequently, the front-desk concierge slapped the assistant general manager, who then punched the front-desk concierge in the head. The fight continued to escalate, with swearing, hissing, and the further threat of physical violence.

❏ *The Solution*. The manager and owner of the club almost immediately became aware of the situation and responded as follows:

- The manager immediately separated the two employees and brought them into his office. He then scheduled meetings with each of them for the next day and sent both home for the rest of the day.

- The manager first met with the assistant general manager and informed her of his dissatisfaction with the behavior that had occurred the prior evening and reiterated with her the type of behavior that was expected. He then suspended her for two weeks without pay.

- The manager next met with the front-desk employee and conveyed his displeasure with the actions that had occurred the prior evening and shared with that individual the type of behavior that was expected of all club employees. The manager then told the front-desk employee what action had been taken against the assistant manager. The front desk employee got angry, indicated that this was not the end of the situation, and then proceeded to quit.

❏ *Discussion*. Situations such as this one can happen in any business, including the club industry. When employees work together for extended periods of time, the possibility of romantic relationships occurring will increase. While most clubs have policies against employees having relationships with each other, it is still difficult, if not almost impossible, to prevent personal relationships from transpiring. In this particular set of circumstances, the manager handled the situation well by doing the following:

- Immediately separating the two employees and getting them into his office. The manager also did the right thing in sending both employees home separately, but only after scheduling meetings with each of them for the next day. It is important that after such an emotional event, both parties involved be given a cool-down period before meeting with each of them privately.

- Holding private meetings or counseling sessions with each employee was an appropriate next step. In the case of the assistant general manager, the two-week suspension provided a clear message as to the serious nature of the violation. On the other hand, it let the employee know that the manager valued her (she could have also been fired). The other employee quit before further disciplinary action could be taken.

To prevent instances such as this one from occurring, clubs should establish policies and practices that clearly communicate the expectations of the facility with regard to personal relationships between employees. Once instituted, those policies and practices should be enforced on a consistent

To prevent instances such as this one from occurring, clubs should establish policies and practices that clearly communicate the expectations of the facility with regard to personal relationships between employees.

basis. When it involves personal relationships between supervisors and employees, those policies and practices must be particularly explicit and straightforward. It is never a good idea for supervisors to have a romantic relationship with an employee who reports to them. If and when management becomes aware of a personal relationship between employees, especially those between a supervisor and employee, they should reiterate and reinforce the club's policy concerning such associations with each participant in the relationship. In most instances, when a relationship between a supervisor and an employee happens and management counsels these individuals, one of the following actions should occur:

- The supervisor and subordinate must agree not to see each other any more.

- One of the two employees should be asked to leave; in most cases it will be the employee with less tenure and perceived value to the club.

By undertaking the necessary steps, a situation such as the one detailed in this scenario can be prevented. However, in the event it does, the actions taken by this manager provide an excellent template to follow.

Anyone Up for a Dip?

❑ *Scenario*. This scenario took place in a high-end club that was located in the southwest part of the country. The club offered a variety of sports and recreation-related programs. One of the club's most valued features was its outdoor swimming pool. During the outdoor season, the outdoor pool had a staff of six lifeguards, all between the ages of 18-and-20, and one head lifeguard, who was female. The manager of this operation had had great success with this team for the entire outdoor season. The pool closed each evening around 9:00 p.m.

Near the end of the outdoor season, the manager was returning from a dinner meeting with one of the members, at approximately 10:30 p.m. The manager was walking to his car in the lot when he heard some strange noises coming from the pool. Since the pool supposedly closed over an hour earlier, the manager decided to take a look. As he approached the pool, he heard laughing and loud noises, including some emanating from the club's head lifeguard. When he got up to the edge of the pool, his head lifeguard had swum up to the edge to greet him. There was a moment of silence, until the manager explained to her that everyone must get out of the pool. The head lifeguard did not move. Puzzled, the manager again asked the lifeguards to get out of the pool. All the lifeguards, with the exception of the head lifeguard, proceeded to get out at the other end of the pool. It was then that the manager noticed that his entire staff had been "skinny dipping." Dismayed, he turned away so the head lifeguard could leave the pool.

If and when management becomes aware of a personal relationship between employees, especially those between a supervisor and employee, they should reiterate and reinforce the club's policy concerning such associations with each participant in the relationship.

❑ *Solution.* Once the pool had emptied and the lifeguards had gotten dressed, the manager had them depart, but only after scheduling meetings with each of them for the next day. He then proceeded to clean up and close the pool area.

The next day, he met with each of the lifeguards. He explained to them how disappointed he was with them and how inappropriate their behavior was. Because the club still had to serve the members, the option of dismissing the entire staff was not one that could be taken. Instead, after meeting with each individual, he wrote each one up for behavior unbecoming of staff. In addition, he spent extra time in counseling the head lifeguard. Finally, he spent the remainder of the outdoor pool season working evenings to make sure no further problems occurred.

❑ *Discussion.* It is not uncommon when dealing with a young staff (a common circumstance in the fitness industry), especially when the supervisors are young themselves, for foolish and inappropriate behavior to occur. In this situation, the staff demonstrated a lack of maturity, disregard for leadership, and disrespect to the membership. The manager dealt with the situation in a professional and satisfactory manner by performing the following steps:

- Clearing the pool upon noticing what was occurring

- Respecting the employees by not making a spectacle of them at that time

- Scheduling time to meet the next day with each individual and counseling them on their behavior

- Providing the employees with written warnings concerning their behavior that would go on their employee records

- Monitoring the actions of the staff after the event to ensure that such behavior did not occur in the future

Had a need not existed to have the lifeguards on duty for the remainder of the outdoor pool season, the manager indicated that he would most likely have dismissed all of the employees. From a professional perspective, it would have been wise to suspend the head lifeguard immediately. This step would have sent a relatively strong message to the other lifeguards. While it would have undoubtedly subjected the manager to a heavier workload, the end result of suspending the head lifeguard would have sent the message that the other lifeguards needed to hear.

As individuals in a position of leadership, managers sometimes need to make a strong statement about values, respect, and trust. Suspending or dismissing a supervisor who has demonstrated behavior that is totally inappropriate can be a necessary step in order to maintain long-term stability and respect among the rest of the team.

As individuals in a position of leadership, managers sometimes need to make a strong statement about values, respect, and trust.

A Little Affair

❑ *Scenario.* This scenario took place in a suburban club that was located in the southwest. Designed to serve an affluent family market, the club provided a host of networking and social activities for the members. The facility's membership roster was small, and most of the members knew each other.

Late in the evening one day, the club was nearing the end of another successful member social event. Many of the members and employees in attendance decided to continue the party at a local pub. The manager decided to attend the after-hours event to make sure that nothing inappropriate occurred. The manager noticed that a senior member of the staff was receiving some flirtatious looks from one of the club's female members. The manager thought about the situation for a moment, but figured this employee was a top supervisor and the member was a married woman with children. He felt that he could go home and nothing would happen.

The manager decided that it was in the best interest of everyone involved to keep this situation under wraps.

The manager arrived home around midnight and was immediately told by his wife that the security company had called and that an alarm had gone off at the club. The manager immediately returned to the club. When he arrived, he noticed two cars in the lot, one of which was the supervisor's car. The manager then went into the club and kept calling out to see if anyone was there. Hearing no response, he searched the entire club and found nothing. Just before departing, he decided to go to his office. Upon opening the door, he found his employee and the member in a very compromising position, both with blank stares on their face.

❑ *The Solution.* Once the manager had entered the room, the member pleaded with him not to tell anyone. The manager asked the member to leave and told her that he would meet with her the next day. The manager then had the employee get dressed, after which he read the employee the riot act. He told the employee he would meet with him the next morning.

The manager met with the member first. The member told her side of the story and pleaded for confidentiality. She promised not to place the club or the manager in that situation again. She did not want this to get out and end her marriage. The manager decided that it was in the best interest of everyone involved to keep this situation under wraps. The manager then met with the employee and explained to him that this event was to remain confidential and that he would not be dismissed because it would bring unwanted attention to the situation. On the other hand, the manager did share with him that if word did leak out, he would be immediately terminated. The manager took the time to explain the member's request for confidentiality to the employee. The employee apologized to the member and the manager.

While the manager indicated that he was not sure he did the right thing, he did feel, at the time, that it was important to protect the member. As a result, he did not punish the employee to the degree he might otherwise have.

❑ *Discussion.* As hard as it may be for some individuals to believe, employees and members occasionally enter into inappropriate relationships. When employees work closely with members and begin seeing each other in a social context, situations such as this scenario can arise. In this particular instance, the employee and the member both showed poor judgment—not just by having an affair, but consummating it on club property. The manager, in this instance, handled the situation as best he felt he could, given the fact that he faced a dual dilemma of having to discipline an employee and maintain the privacy of the member, both of which were critical factors. The manager's response dealt satisfactorily with the situation, particularly from the member's perspective, because he undertook the following steps:

- Once he came upon the employee and member together, he separated them and sent the member home.

- He immediately talked with the offending employee to make sure that he knew the gravity of the situation.

- He met privately with the member and kept the situation in total confidence. He maintained the level of trust that is essential in a situation of this magnitude.

- He met privately the next day with the employee and recounted the details of the meeting with the member. He further counseled the employee and gave him a warning that any leak of the information involving the situation would result in his immediate termination.

While the situation seemed to end reasonably well, the manager should have written the employee up and suspended him. While cause certainly existed to dismiss the employee, which would have been a perfectly appropriate response, a suspension would have worked just as well. With regard to the member, he could have suspended her from the club and asked her not to return. Since this member was married and had a family, the manager decided to focus his efforts to resolve the situation on the member's circumstances, rather than doing something that might cause further damage to her. Considering the social nature of the club and the family situation, this was a good decision. Had the member been single, the more appropriate option might have been to suspend her from the club.

Club managers should be aware of the fact that member-and-employee relationships can and will occur. Accordingly, it is important for clubs to have policies in place that make it clear that such behavior is unacceptable and

In this particular instance, the employee and the member both showed poor judgment—not just by having an affair, but consummating it on club property.

Club managers should be aware of the fact that member-and-employee relationships can and will occur. Accordingly, it is important for clubs to have policies in place that make it clear that such behavior is unacceptable and inappropriate for employees.

inappropriate for employees. A club should also have house rules that address this type of situation from a member's perspective as well. Such policies should be reinforced regularly. If and when these policies are violated, the proper discipline should be administered.

27

Business Chronicles

Chapter Objectives

The situations detailed in this chapter encompass stories involving business-related circumstances. Resolving them required sound leadership and managerial skills.

Closing a Club and Gaining Fans

❑ *Scenario*. This scenario took place in a large multipurpose club that was located in the south. Approaching its 10th anniversary, the facility was recognized as the number one adult club in the marketplace and served a membership base of over 2,000 individuals. The building in which the club was located had been sold to new owners in the past year. The new owner had a reputation for demanding premium leases.

The club, which was part of a chain, had not funded all of the necessary capital improvements that it needed over the past several years. As a result, during its 10th anniversary year, the indoor pool experienced problems, causing it to empty into the tenant's space below it. In order to get the pool up and running, the club manager and regional manager sought a capital infusion of a couple of hundred thousand dollars to repair the pool. Concurrently, the new building owner was seeking to ignore the club's request for a lease extension and increase the club's base rent by 200%.

The manager and regional manager went before senior management asking for capital to repair the pool and for help with negotiating with the new landlord. While the club had contributed significant cash flow to the company in the past, the prospect of investing a couple of hundred thousand dollars and having the cost of the lease at least double caused senior management to make the difficult decision to close the club. Senior

> While the club had contributed significant cash flow to the company in the past, the prospect of investing a couple of hundred thousand dollars and having the cost of the lease at least double caused senior management to make the difficult decision to close the club.

management informed the regional manager and manager that they had decided to close the club. Unable to change the minds of senior management, the regional manager and manager received permission to have a 90-day window in which to close the facility.

❑ *The Solution.* Once the decision to close the club had been communicated to the regional manager and club manager, they went into action. Among the steps that they took to address the club's closing were the following:

- The regional manager and manager initially decided that the best course of action was to develop a strategy for closing the club that they would review with the senior staff before settling on a final plan.

- The regional manager and manager met with the senior staff in a private setting and informed them that senior management had decided that the best course of action for the club was to close its doors. In this meeting, the regional manager and manager encouraged the senior staff to share their feelings concerning the situation. As a team, they then identified the best strategy for going forward.

- Before communicating further with either the staff or members, the manager and regional manager determined the steps that would be undertaken to help ensure that both the members and employees ended up in the best possible situation, including:

  ✓ The manager and regional manager would get each employee a severance package that paid that individual all accrued vacation and sick time, as well as one week's pay for every year worked for hourly employees and two week's pay for every year worked for salaried employees.

  ✓ The regional manager would arrange job opportunities with other clubs within the company for the supervisory staff.

  ✓ The manager would contact other local clubs to make special membership arrangements that would allow the club's members to transfer to these other clubs with full privileges and not have to pay for them for a specified period of time (the club would pay the dues for those members for that time period).

  ✓ The manager and regional manager would arrange to sell the equipment in the club to help offset the costs of closing the facility.

  ✓ The senior staff would take responsibility for developing a closing party and would designate a charity that would be the recipient of any funds that would be raised at the party.

- Next, the regional manager and manager met with the entire staff. At this meeting, the regional manager shared the news about senior management's decision and stated the reason for closing the facility. At

> Once the decision to close the club had been communicated to the regional manager and club manager, they went into action.

the meeting, all of the arrangements regarding compensation payments, new jobs, etc. were discussed. In addition, the plans for handling the membership were reviewed. Employees were given the opportunity to go to their new jobs immediately or remain with the club until it closed. Everyone chose to stay and get new jobs after the closing.

- The regional manager and manager then met with a group of vocal and influential members of the club to share the news and seek their ideas on how best to communicate the closing to the entire membership. At that time, management told the group about plans for a closing party and the arrangements made with the other local clubs.

- Management then informed the entire membership about the closing and what was going to occur. Initially, this communication was accomplished through personal letters that were sent to each member and signed by the manager. Once the letters went out, special message boards were put up around the club for member viewing. In addition, the manager and the facility's senior staff met personally with each of the members that they knew. Their dialogue with these individuals included the following information:

  ✓ That there would be a special closing party on the final day. That they could bring a guest, and that all entry fees ($20 a person) would go to a local charity.

  ✓ That the party would include a cash bar and a live band.

  ✓ That the club had made arrangements with other local clubs, and that representatives of those clubs would be available for the members to meet with and sign them up for memberships in those clubs.

  ✓ That the staff would do whatever they could to help members with the transition.

- Management, including the regional manager, kept their doors opened over the next 60 days for anyone who wanted help with a closing-related issue, assisting members with the transition, supporting employees with any problem that they might have, and preparing for the final closing.

- On the final day, the closing party was the highlight event. The staff worked the party so that members and guests could enjoy the party. A total of 2,000 individuals attended the party. In the process, over $10,000 was raised for charity. The party lasted for over five hours, and closed with a special funeral procession.

- The event featured celebrations and storytelling. A local TV station covered the event and collected stories from members. The next day, the by-line of the local station's nightly newscast was "local landmark closes."

The regional manager and manager then met with a group of vocal and influential members of the club to share the news and seek their ideas on how best to communicate the closing to the entire membership.

Closing a club is one of the most challenging tasks that leadership will ever face.

- After the party, members called and stopped by to say how much they appreciated how the closing was handled and that they hoped that someday the club would return.

❏ *Discussion.* Closing a club is one of the most challenging tasks that leadership will ever face. Members and employees who have been involved with a facility for any period of time take a sense of ownership in the club. As a result, they often feel an incredible loss when a club closes. Accordingly, club owners and operators need to realize that closing a facility can be traumatic for both members and employees. How the club closes not only impacts the facility's relationship with its members and employees, but also the community. In this particular instance, the facility had been a great club for almost 10 years. The closing, although lamentable, was handled in such a way that the employees, members, and community all retained their sense of pride about the club. Among the keys to this particular closing's success were the following:

- Management took the time to initially communicate and discuss the event with the facility's senior staff. Concurrently, they solicited feedback from the staff regarding what would be the right way to close the club.

- Management informed members at various levels about the closing and made the process as personal as possible.

- Before meeting with the club's employees and members, management made sure that they would be able to answer any important questions that might come up during the meeting.

- Management made the closing a celebration and made it an event that demonstrated that the club was still an important part of the community by contributing proceeds from the closing party to a local charity.

- Management made arrangements for members and employees before the meeting in an effort to help lessen the shock of the closing.

- Management, staff, and members worked together until the end, instead of becoming adversaries.

- Until the very last moment, management's approach was to be upbeat and positive, to view the process of closing the club as a change, instead of an end point.

- If staff or members wanted to talk about the closing on a personal level, the manager and regional manager made themselves available, rather than hiding behind their doors.

While closing a club is not a frequent experience for managers, nonetheless, it is an experience that many managers will have. The ability to close a club, while maintaining the relationships and integrity of the club in the eyes of employees, members, and community, is a sign of exceptional leadership. One key lesson that can be learned from this particular scenario is that managers should never burn a bridge; instead, they should continue to build, since they never know when they might return.

Drive-In Fitness Anyone?

❑ *Scenario.* This scenario occurred in a suburban fitness club in the southwest. Located along a major thoroughfare, the club leased space in a corporate business park. The facility served a corporate market and had approximately 800 memberships. The club opened at 5:30 a.m. and closed at 9:00 p.m. on weekdays.

One night at approximately 1:00 a.m., the manager received a phone call from the building's landlord who informed him that a car had just driven through the exterior window of the club and was lodged in the fitness center. The manager immediately came to the club to find a car situated inside the club, with shattered glass everywhere. Not only had the car broken a significant portion of the exterior window, it had destroyed two offices and part of the fitness floor. Glass was strewn throughout the entire fitness area. Subsequently, the police arrived and had the vehicle towed out of the club.

❑ *The Solution.* Upon surveying the situation, the manager proceeded to take the following actions:

- The manager immediately contacted the staff who were scheduled to open the club the next morning at 5:30 a.m. to let them know what happened and discuss a plan of action.

- The manager showed up at the club prior to 5:30 a.m. the next day and met with the staff. The staff then made signs that explained what happened and what actions would take place.

- Subsequently, the manager and employees greeted the club's members as they arrived at the facility and directed them over to another club for their morning workouts (the manager contacted that club upon arriving to make arrangements for his club's members to use that facility at no cost to them).

- During the course of the day, members were greeted by the facility's staff and manager who informed them of the club's closing and let them know that they would have access to and privileges at another club during the clean-up period.

- The manager brought the entire staff into the club later in the morning, and everyone worked all day cleaning up the space. The building landlord also sent staff down to help clean up.

> Managers should never burn a bridge; instead, they should continue to build, since they never know when they might return.

- The manager also contacted the club's insurance agent to get that process activated.

- The club was cleaned and open to members the next afternoon.

- For a couple of weeks, the club operated with plywood on several of its windows. Within 30-days, however, the window, carpet, and broken equipment were replaced.

- No members left the club as a result of the incident.

❏ *Discussion.* A car driving through the club is not a normal event. Obviously, had it occurred during the club's normal operating hours, serious harm could have resulted. The real challenges in this particular scenario were having to address the members' needs the next morning, get the club repaired, and make sure that staff was completely informed about the situation. Furthermore, an event such as this could have resulted in the loss of members. The club manager did an excellent job on short notice of ensuring that the members were taken care of in an appropriate manner. Among the key actions that helped resolve this situation were:

- The manager visited the site right away and surveyed the situation.

- The manager immediately contacted the club's opening staff to inform them of what happened and made sure that they had a plan upon arriving in the morning.

- The manager and staff got to the club early and greeted the members as they arrived, explained the situation to them, and got them access to another club.

- The manager made arrangements for the members to use another club at no cost to them.

- The staff, with assistance from the landlord, was able to get the club cleaned up and open within one day.

- The manager made sure that the club maintained communication with the members throughout the period of the incident.

Situations such as the one recounted in this particular scenario cannot be predicted. If they arise, however, the critical factor is the ability of management to communicate with the members to lessen the shock and confusion that can accompany such an event and provide every possible opportunity for the members to pursue their fitness activities, with as minimal a level of disturbance as possible.

The real challenges in this particular scenario were having to address the members' needs the next morning, get the club repaired, and make sure that staff was completely informed about the situation.

Now, Where Did You Say the Fitness Area Was?

❏ *Scenario.* The club involved in this scenario was located along the northeast corridor in a dense urban market. The club had been open for several years and had a membership of approximately 1,600. Recently, the club had decided to go through a three-million dollar renovation that would take approximately 12 months to complete. During the renovation, the facility's goal was to grow membership by at least 500. The club had also decided that during the course of the 12-month renovation, it would remain open for the members and keep its dues pricing unchanged.

❑ *The Solution*. Once the decision to renovate the facility and remain open during the renovation was made, the club's leadership team developed a game plan to tackle the process. In that regard, some of the most important actions that took place included:

- The club had models and color floor plans of the renovation produced that could be used to share information with the members about the renovation process.

- The club created a renovation calendar that provided approximate timelines for each phase of the renovation, including what areas of the club would be under construction, when these spaces would be worked on, and what changes in the facilities would occur during each stage.

- The renovation calendar and pictures were included with a letter that was forwarded to each member. In addition, a notice on the club's plans for renovation was put in the newsletter. These communication efforts occurred approximately 90 days in advance of the start of the project and again at 60 days and 30 days prior to work beginning.

- The club set up a renovation hub in the club that members could refer to every day regarding the status of the project. This hub had a model of the new club, pictures of the new equipment, copies of the renovation calendar, and a daily update poster that showed what was happening each day.

- The staff had daily meetings and updates so they could communicate effectively with the club's members.

- The locker rooms had to be switched on four occasions, with the women utilizing the men's lockers on one occasion, and during another period, the men and women using the locker rooms on alternate days. A special area for lockers was set up so that even during the time that radical changes were occurring in the location of locker rooms, the members always had a locker in which to store their items.

- The club provided special treats and drinks each day to help ease any pain caused by the renovation efforts.

- When the exercise studios were closed, the club provided members with hard hats and held classes in the construction areas after hours.

The club created a renovation calendar that provided approximate timelines for each phase of the renovation, including what areas of the club would be under construction, when these spaces would be worked on, and what changes in the facilities would occur during each stage.

One of the most challenging experiences that managers will encounter in the club business is operating a facility and serving the members during a period of major renovation.

This step was facilitated by using special flooring that the staff could roll out on the concrete floors after the construction workers had left for the day.

- Special classes and programs were offered that provided members with the opportunity to exercise at times they might not otherwise have worked out.

- The manager and department heads made themselves available to the members in 12-hour shifts to address the members' complaints and deal with any other issues that they might have.

- Each time a phase of work was completed, the club held a relatively small celebration party.

- Each of these parties provided an opportunity for special instructors and celebrities to visit the club during those days on which the festivities were held in order to further enhance the experience.

After 12 months of renovation, the club's membership had increased from approximately 1,600, when construction began, to 2,400 at the time of completion. Furthermore, the member retention rate remained at the same level as it was prior to the renovation work.

❑ *Discussion.* One of the most challenging experiences that managers will encounter in the club business is operating a facility and serving the members during a period of major renovation. Clubs cannot afford to just close their doors during renovation, or they would lose their revenue stream from dues. Clubs have to find ways to continue operating at full bore and provide the same (or better) service during periods of renovation. Because the health/fitness club industry changes frequently, clubs will be challenged at one time or another with having to make a facelift—sometimes a major facelift. The key to successfully meeting such a challenge is whether the club can continue to operate and drive revenues during a period when members will be inconvenienced.

Club owners and operators who are involved with facilities that will be undergoing renovation must find a way to succeed at delivering their club experience under times of high duress. Without question, members will complain during renovation. At the beginning of the renovation efforts, most members will be excited about the changes that are occurring and tolerate the inconveniences that are being caused by the construction. As the construction wears on, however, usually at about six months, members will begin to complain and will become less accepting of any inconveniences that might arise. Concurrently, the staff will be challenged to have to provide satisfactory service under the most trying of circumstances. As members begin to complain more, the employees will be subjected to additional stress.

The aforementioned circumstances require extraordinary leadership if the club's renovation efforts are to proceed smoothly, with minimal disruption to the membership. In this particular scenario, club management did an outstanding job of turning a long renovation into a successful operation. Among the most critical steps that allowed management to be successful in this situation were the following:

- Management created an entire game plan around the renovation that addressed the concerns of both members and staff.

- Management informed the membership well in advance what was going to occur and repeated efforts to communicate with the members throughout the process.

- Management created a communication center that provided daily updates concerning the renovation efforts.

- Management developed a series of newly created experiences that were designed to help take the members' and employees' minds off the actual renovation process.

- Management and staff undertook several activities (e.g., parties, social events, and special classes) that helped lend a measure of excitement to the renovation process.

- The employees pulled together under a common cause to help make the situation better for the members.

- Management provided additional support to the employees so that they, in turn, could take better care of the members during the renovation process.

- A club can do a number of things to help make a renovation, such as this one, relatively palatable to everyone involved. The key point that should be emphasized is that if the management and employees are able and willing to plan and act in an appropriate manner, the entire renovation experience can be somewhat rewarding for members and employees alike, rather than an unnerving, strife-filled struggle.

The key point that should be emphasized is that if the management and employees are able and willing to plan and act in an appropriate manner, the entire renovation experience can be somewhat rewarding for members and employees alike, rather than an unnerving, strife-filled struggle.

A. Leading Health/Fitness Industry Associations and Organizations
B. Leading Health/Fitness Industry Trade Publications
C. Profiles of Leading Health/Fitness Club Companies
D. Brand Logos for Selected Health/Fitness Club Companies
E. Profiles of Leading Health/Fitness Club Equipment Manufacturers
F. Sample Job Descriptions
G. Sample Compensation Agreements
H. Sample Structured Interview Questioning Format for a Fitness Director Applicant
I. Sample Strategic Planning Forms
J. Selected Front-of-the-House Operational Forms
K. Selected Heart-of-the-House Operational Forms
L. Sample Design and Construction Checklist
M. Sample Construction Project Budget
N. Sample Member Satisfaction Survey
O. Sample Corporate Sales Checklist
P. Selected Health/Fitness Industry Programming Practices
Q. Selected Risk Management Forms
R. Suggested References

Appendices

Appendix A: Leading Health/Fitness Industry Associations and Organizations

American College of Sports Medicine 401 West Michigan Indianapolis, Indiana 46202 317-637-9200 www.acsm.org	Research, education and certification for fitness professionals, physicians, and individuals in related sports medicine fields.
American Council on Exercise 4851 Paramount Drive San Diego, California 92123 800-825-3636 www.acefitness.org	Education and certification for fitness professionals.
Aerobic and Fitness Association of America 15250 Vetura Blvd. Suite 200 Sherman Oaks, California 91403 877-968-7263 www.afaa.com	Education and certification for fitness professionals.
IDEA Health and Fitness Association 10455 Pacific Center Court San Diego, California 92121-4339 800-999-4332 www.ideafit.com	Education for fitness professionals.
International Health, Racquet and Sportclub Association 263 Summer Street Boston, Massachusetts 02210 800-228-4772 www.ihrsa.org	Trade association for the health, fitness, racquet and sports club industry. Public policy and education
International Spa Association 2365 Harrodsburg Road, Suite A325 Lexington, Kentucky 40504 888-651-4772 www.experienceispa.com	Trade association for the spa industry. Education for the spa industry.
National Academy of Sports Medicine 123 Hodencamp Road, Suite 204 Thousand Oaks, California 91360 866-292-6276 www.nasm.org	Education and certification for fitness professionals.
National Strength and Conditioning Association 1885 Bob Johnson Drive Colorado Springs, Colorado 80906 800-815-6826 www.nsca-lift.org	Education and certification for fitness professionals.
National Wellness Association 1300 College Ct., P.O. Box 827 Stevens Point, Wisconsin 54481-0827 800-244-8922 www.nationalwellness.org	Association involved in education and communication for professionals with an interest in wellness and health promotion.

Appendix B: Leading Health/Fitness Industry Trade Publications

ACSM's Health and Fitness Journal Published by Lipponcott, Williams and Wilkens 16522 Hunters Green Parkway Hagerstown, Maryland 21740 800-638-3030	Publication for fitness professionals. Can be obtained by non-ACSM members. Published six times a year.
ACE Certified News 4851 Paramount Drive San Diego, CA 92123 800-825-3636	Publication of ACE. Published six times a year for certified members of ACE. Covers a wide array of health and fitness-related topics.
ACE Fitness Matters 4851 Paramount Drive San Diego, CA 92123 800-825-3636	Bimonthly publication that is geared to the consumer. Provides information on health, wellness, and exercise.
Aquatics International A Hanley Woods publication 6222 Wilshire Boulevard, Suite 600 Los Angeles, California 90048 323-801-4900	Monthly publication for aquatic professionals serving in all market segments.
Athletic Business 4130 Lien Road Madison, Wisconsin 53704 800-722-8764	Monthly publication for athletic, fitness and recreational professionals. Focuses on issues concerning recreation centers, universities, military, and commercial health/fitness clubs.
Club Business International Magazine of IHRSA 263 Summer Street Boston, Massachusetts 02210 800-228-4772	Monthly publication for members of IHRSA. Focus is on the commercial club industry.
Club Business Entrepreneur Magazine of IHRSA 263 Summer Street Boston, Massachusetts 02210 800-228-4772	Quarterly publication targeted at owners and managers of independent health/fitness clubs.
Club Industry Primedia Publications 9800 Metcalf Avenue Overland Park, Kansas 66212 913-341-1300	Monthly publication for the commercial health/fitness club industry
Club Insider News Box 681241 Marietta, Georgia 30068 770-850-8506	Monthly publication for anyone involved in the health/fitness club industry. Offers inside news typically not provided by other publications.
Exercise Standards and Malpractice Reporter PRC Publishing 3976 Fulton Drive, N.W. Canton, Ohio 44718 330-492-6063	Monthly publication targeted at professionals in the fitness industry. Focus is on legal and risk-management issues.

Fitness Management Leisure Publications 4160 Wilshire Boulevard Los Angeles, California 90010 323-964-4800	Monthly publication targeted at fitness professionals involved in supervisory roles within the industry.
IDEA Fitness Journal 10455 Pacific Center Court San Diego, California 92121 800-999-IDEA	Monthly publication targeted at personal trainers and group-exercise instructors.
Pulse A publication of ISPA 2365 Harrodsburg Road, Suite A325 Lexington, Kentucky 40504 859-226-4429	Monthly publication targeted at professionals who own and operate spas.
Recreation Management CAB Communications 50 North Brockway Street, Suite 4-11 Palatine, Illinois 60067 847-963-8740	Monthly publication targeted at recreation professionals. Addresses an array of industry-related issues.
Strength and Conditioning Journal Professional Journal of NSCA 1885 Bob Johnson Drive Colorado Springs, Colorado 80906 800-815-6826	Bimonthly publication targeted at NSCA members.

Appendix C: Profiles of Leading Health/Fitness Club Companies

24 Hour Fitness

Year Founded	1983	Company Overview
Number of clubs	350 plus	Primary markets served are 18 to 24 and 25 to 34 year olds and HH incomes between $25 k and $50 k. Brand based on 24 hour convenience, lots of equipment, convenience, nationwide access and affordable pricing. Focused on multiple sites within a geographic region. Offers fitness only and also sports and super sports clubs with gyms and courts. Also has celebrity clubs supported and promoted by such celebrities as Andre Agassi, Lance Armstrong, Magic Johnson and Jackie Chan. Company has a high volume membership sales focus and strong focus on personal training sales and supplement sales. Drives sales through national, regional and local advertising. Preference is membership contracts, but month by month offered. Group exercise programming reasonably good. Fitness clubs range in size from 15,000 to 30,000 s.f. with sport clubs as large as 50,000 s.f. The company was purchased in 2005 for approximately $1.5 billion by Fortsmann Little and Company.
Number of members	3 million	
Revenues (2004)	$1.1 billion	
Markets served	USA and Asia	
Principals	Mark Mastrov, CEO Fortsmann Little and Company	
Individual Dues Pricing	$29 to $49 a month	

Bally's Total Fitness

Year Founded	1962	Company Overview
Number of clubs	400 plus	Primary markets are 18 to 24 and 25 to 34 year olds and HH incomes between $25 k and $50 k. Brand built on trendy, hard bodies, glitz, convenience, nationwide presence and affordable pricing. Focuses on multiple sites within a geographic region. High volume membership sales with focus on membership contracts. Limited service focus. Drive sales through national and regional advertising. Strong focus on personal training and supplement sales. Group exercise programming is strong. Most clubs range in size from 15,000 to 30,000 s.f. The company is publicly traded.
Number of members	4 million	
Revenues (2004)	$1 billion	
Markets served	USA, Canada, Asia	
Principals	Paul Toback, President	
Individual Dues Pricing	$9 to $49 a month	

Club One

Year Founded	1991	Company Overview
Number of clubs	104	Primary market is young professionals (25 to 50) in dense corporate markets, with some suburban clubs serving a stronger family market. Targets HH incomes between $75 k and $100 k. Brand built around the corporate market, convenience, service and education. Commercial clubs mostly on the West Coast, with corporate centers throughout the USA. Clubs range from under 10,000 s.f. to 50,000 s.f., though a few clubs approach 100,000 square feet in size. Balanced focus on sales and service, with strong programming.
Number of members	100,000	
Revenues (2004)	$70 million	
Markets served	USA	
Principals	John and Jill Kinney, Founders Jim Mizes, CEO	
Individual Dues Pricing	$49 to $100	

Gold's Gym International

Year Founded	1965	Company Overview
Number of clubs	620 plus	Majority of clubs are franchised operations, with 38 clubs owned. The initial market was young bodybuilders and hard bodies, but in many markets the franchisees target the family market. Primary market is 18 to 24 and 25 to 34 with HH incomes of $25 k to $50 k. The market can vary depending on franchisee. Brand based on the Gold's logo that speaks to serious workouts, plenty of equipment, and the home of champions. Clubs range in size from under 10,000 s.f. to 50,000 s.f. Focus is on membership contracts in most clubs and sales focus and service focus can vary by market. High volume logo merchandise sales.
Number of members	2.5 million	
Revenues (2002)	NA	
Markets served	International	
Principals	TRT Holdings, LLC, Gene Lamott, CEO	
Individual Dues Pricing	$29 to $49 a month	

L.A. Fitness International

Year Founded	1984	Company Overview
Number of clubs	124 plus	Primary market is 18 to 24 and 25 to 35 with HH incomes between $25 k and $50 k. Brand built on very affordable, convenience, lots of equipment and expansive facilities. Offers limited amenities in its clubs. Most clubs are 30,000 to 50,000 s.f. High volume membership sales with minimal attention to service. Membership contracts are the primary form of membership. Drive sales through regional and local advertising. Limited programming and service. Privately held. Since 2002, one of the fastest growing club companies in the US.
Number of members	500,000 plus	
Revenues (2004)	NA	
Markets served	USA	
Principals	Chin Yi, Chairman	
Individual Dues Pricing	$19 to $49 a month	

Life Time Fitness

Year Founded	1990	Company Overview
Number of clubs	44 plus	Primary market is young and upcoming families with HH incomes between $50 k and $100 k with adults between 25 and 40. Strong focus on attracting the entire family. Brand built on its grand facilities with every imaginable facility amenity with high visibility for its kid's areas and water entertainment areas. 24 hour accessibility another key aspect of their brand. Most facilities are between 90,000 and 120,000 s.f. Most clubs target at least 10,000 memberships. High volume membership sales. Limited focus on service and programming, but do provide every imaginable fitness and recreational opportunity. Company went public in 2004 and has been well accepted by the public market. Stock was trading at 30x earnings in July 2005. One of the fastest growing club companies in the USA.
Number of members	300,000 plus	
Revenues (2004)	$312 million plus	
Markets served	USA	
Principals	Bahram Akradi, CEO	
Individual Dues Pricing	$39 to $69 a month	

Spectrum Clubs

Year Founded	1999	Company Overview
Number of clubs	20 plus	Primary markets are 25 – 34 and 35 to 44, with household incomes between $50 k and $100 k. In Texas serves more of a family market, while in CA serves more of an individual market. Brand is different in CA and TX, with CA being built on programs, facility offerings and facility appeal. In TX, the brand is known more for community involvement, affordable cost and convenience. Most facilities range from 30,000 to 50,000 s.f., with some clubs significantly larger. Strong sales focus with good volume, but balanced on the service end. Use local and regional advertising. Offer considerable program diversity.
Number of members	100,000 plus	
Revenues (2004)	$86 million plus	
Markets served	CA and Texas	
Principals	Brentwood & Associates. Matthew Stevens, President	
Individual Dues Pricing	$49 to $99	

Sport & Health

Year Founded	1973	Company Overview
Number of clubs	28	Clubs have several distinct markets, ranging from clubs that serve the 25 to 34 market with HH incomes between $25 k and $50 k and clubs that serve families with HH incomes over $100 k. Brand is not consistent across all clubs, but known for facility convenience, its programming and member service. Clubs range from 20,000 s.f. to over 120,000 s.f. Strong membership sales focus, but balanced by almost equal focus on member service. Advertises in local media, but also member referral is an important part of the sales process.
Number of members	NA	
Revenues (2004)	$80 million plus	
Markets served	Washington DC area	
Principals	Purchased in late 2005 from previous owners	
Individual Dues Pricing	$49 to $100 plus a month.	

Tennis Corporation of America

Year Founded	1969	Company Overview
Number of clubs	41 plus	Primary market is 35 to 54, individuals and families with HH incomes over $75 k and in many markets over $100 k. A few clubs serve younger and less affluent markets. Brand originally built on great tennis, but since expanded to be built on great tennis and great service. Clubs range from 20,000 s.f. to close to 200,000 s.f. Exceptional reputation in the tennis industry. Membership sales are based more on referral and community involvement. Strong focus on member service and active programming. Tenured leadership team.
Number of members	90,000 plus	
Revenues (2004)	$80 million plus	
Markets served	USA and Canada	
Principals	Alan Schwartz, Chairman Steven Schwartz, CEO	
Individual Dues Pricing	$60 to $150 a month	

Town Sports International

Year Founded	1974	Company Overview
Number of clubs	137 plus	Two primary markets are individuals between 25 and 34 in an urban setting and families in the 30 to 50 range in a more suburban setting. The HH income range is diverse, but would be $50 k plus in the urban markets and above $75 k in the suburban markets. Strong brand in its markets. Brand built on convenience, accessibility and affordability. Clubs in urban markets range from 10,000 to 25,000 s.f. and suburban clubs range from 40,000 to over 100,000 s.f. High volume membership sales supported by strong and creative advertising in major media. Group exercise is strong in urban markets and strong kids programs in suburban markets. Tenured leadership team.
Number of members	380,000 plus	
Revenues (2004)	$350 million	
Markets served	NE Corridor of USA	
Principals	Mark Smith, Chairman and Bob Giardina, CEO	
Individual Dues Pricing	$60 to $90 a month	

The Wellbridge Company

Year Founded	1983	Company Overview
Number of clubs	43 plus	Company has three distinctly different club types. In the upper Midwest, clubs are family oriented with a primary market of 25 to 44 and household incomes in the $50 k to $100 k range. In the southwest the clubs are family oriented and serve a similar age demographic, but slightly lower HH income. Finally there are the higher end clubs spread in multiple markets that serve a 35 to 54 market, individual and couple and HH income in excess of $100 k. Brand is based on wellness and health, customer service and educated staff. Facilities range from 20,000 s.f. to well over 100,000 s.f. Strong sales focus, but not high volume. Known for wellness focus, educated fitness staff and programming.
Number of members	100,000 plus	
Revenues (2004)	$179 million	
Markets served	USA	
Principals	Starwood Capital and Chilmark Partners. Ed Williams, CEO	
Individual Dues Pricing	$60 to $100 a month	

Western Athletic Clubs

Year Founded	1977	Company Overview
Number of clubs	11	Clubs have two primary markets based on urban or suburban location. In all cases it is individuals or families, 35 to 54 and HH income in excess of $100,000 annually. Brand is based on a sport resort that pampers the member with great facilities, high service levels and great programming. Facilities range from 40,000 to over 100,000 s.f. Excellent sales focus, with emphasis on community involvement. Rely on member referral and have high retention percentage. Clubs known for service and programming, as well as educated fitness staff. Tenured leadership team.
Number of members	42,000 plus	
Revenues (2004)	$90 million plus	
Markets served	West Coast	
Principals	James Gerber, president	
Individual Dues Pricing	$70 to $150 a month	

In addition to the aforementioned nationally based companies, the following club companies are leaders in their respective regional communities:

Regional & Local Leaders

❏ **DMB Sports Clubs, Scottsdale, Arizona**. DMB is a chain of four clubs based out of Scottsdale, Arizona. Clubs are high end sport resort type clubs serving an affluent family market. Clubs are multipurpose and range from 50,000 to over 100,000 S.F. Brand build on resort feel family offerings and service level. Most clubs have between 2,000 and 3,000 memberships. Pricing varies, but individual dues may range between $75 and $100 a month. Known for their family programs and customer service. Company had total sales of approximately $17 million in 2004.

❏ **Equinox Clubs, New York, New York**. Equinox is primarily a New York based chain, but in the last several of years has spread to Chicago, San Francisco and other major metropolitan markets. The clubs serve an affluent, middle age urban market. The Equinox brand is built on trendy facilities, trendy programs and services and association with the "star wannabes" in their respective communities. The clubs range in size, but most are in the neighborhood of 25,000 to 40,000 S.F. The clubs have between 4,000 and 6,000 memberships per club. Pricing varies, but in all cases is in excess of $100 a month for an individual membership. Equinox is known for their personal training and great group exercise classes. Strong advertising in the local media.

❏ **Fitcorp Fitness Centers, Boston, Massachusetts**. Fitcorp is a regionally based company that has built is reputation in the corporate market. Fitcorp operates and manages both corporate fitness centers and commercial clubs (e.g. total of 32 properties) serving a strong corporate market. Brand built on great service, well trained staff and wellness programming for the corporate market. Has one of the best corporate sales strategies in the industry. Clubs range from 10,000 to 30,000 s.f. pricing varies, but in most cases individual dues are between $75 and $100 a month. The company had sales of approximately $14 million in 2004.

❏ **Fitness Formula, Chigaco, Illinois**. Fitness formula owns and operates nine clubs in the Chicago market with approximately 26,000 memberships. The clubs are primarily urban, though they do have a couple of suburban clubs. Market is middle income to affluent individuals (families in suburbs). Brand built on programming, facilities and people. A multiple club membership is offered. Clubs range from 30,000 s.f. to 100,000 s.f. Pricing ranges from $70 to $100 a month for an individual. Clubs do market in the local media. In 2004 the company had sales approximating $28 million.

❏ **Healthworks, Boston, Massachusetts**. Healthworks is a women's only group of clubs in the Boston area that has distinguished itself as one of the best in the business. Healthworks serves both an urban residential and corporate market, as well as a suburban market of women. Target market is middle income to affluent women. The company has established a separate foundation that serves the less advantaged women and families in the Boston area and provides membership opportunities to those who could not normally afford membership. Brand built on the "women's only" environment and community involvement, but known for great group exercise, Pilates programs and customized wellness programs for women. Pricing differs in clubs, but in most cases an individual membership is over $70 a month.

❑ **Leisure Sports, Pleasanton, California**. Leisure Sports operates six high end multipurpose clubs in California, Oregon and Nevada. Leisure Sports focuses on an affluent (over $100,000 HH income) family market by offering a full service multipurpose facility. Brand is distinguished by the connection of a high end sports club with a high end hotel. The position is a sports club and resort. Facilities range from 70,000 to over 100,000 s.f., with a few thousand memberships per club. Monthly dues vary, but in most cases individual dues will fall between $90 and $120 a month. Focus is on service and programming.

❑ **Lifestyle Family Fitness Centers (LFFC), St. Petersburg, Florida**. LFFC operates twenty seven clubs in the central Florida market. Originally serving the Tampa and the St. Petersburg markets, LFFC has expanded into other major central Florida markets such as Orlando and Jacksonville. The owners have indicated that they will eventually reach a total of fifty clubs. LFFC clubs serve both the individual and family market and target those with HH incomes between $25 k and $75 k annually. Brand build on being affordable and convenient and having great facilities and group exercise programs. Clubs normally under 30,000 s.f. Monthly dues for an individual are under $50. Clubs do considerable advertising in the local media and have a strong leadership team.

❑ **Wisconsin Athletic Clubs (WAC), Milwaukee, Wisconsin**. WAC clubs own and operate over a half dozen clubs in the Milwaukee, Wisconsin market. WAC clubs serve primarily a family market, targeting homes with HH incomes between $50 k and $75 k. Clubs vary in size, but most are under 40,000 s.f. Company's first clubs were racquetball clubs. Brand is based on accessibility in the local market, convenience, good facilities, service focus and programming. Monthly dues for an individual would be $55 to $75 a month. Clubs do advertising in the local media.

The statistical and numerical data provided in this section is based on information in the *2005 Global Report on the State of the Industry* produced by IHRSA. The company overview was generated from observations made through first hand knowledge of each company.

Appendix D: Brand Logos for Selected Health/Fitness Club Companies

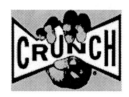

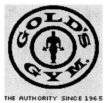

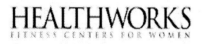

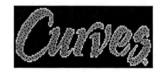

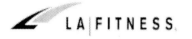

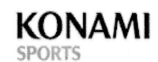

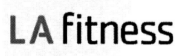

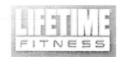

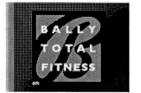

Appendix E: Profiles of Leading Health/Fitness Club Equipment Manufacturers

This appendix provides an overview of seven leading manufacturers of equipment in the health/fitness industry.

❑ *Cybex International; Medway, Massachusetts*

Cybex is a full-service equipment manufacturer that offers a full array of cardiovascular and resistance training equipment. Cybex originally was a manufacturer of medically based isokinetic equipment used in rehabilitative medicine. In the 1980s, Cybex purchased Eagle Resistance Equipment, which moved the company into a new arena focused on variable-resistance equipment and free-weight equipment. During its first several years of business, Eagle made significant inroads into the resistance-training equipment market that was dominated at the time by Nautilus. During the early 1990s, Cybex became the biggest player in the resistance training arena. Cybex also created a line of isokinetic cardiovascular equipment targeted specifically for the fitness and health club industry. The Cybex Upper-Body Ergometer was considered one of the best, if not the best, of its type in the industry. During the early 1990s, Cybex was known for its quality, service and its isokinetic cardiovascular equipment. Cybex was bought by Trotter in the 1990s to form the new company, called Cybex International. The new company, Cybex International, inherited the treadmills and other cardiovascular equipment that Trotter had developed over the years. At the present time, Cybex sells over $100 million in equipment annually, and its line of equipment offerings includes variable-resistance equipment, free-weight benches, plate-loaded equipment, treadmills, bicycles, and its newest creation, the ARC Trainer. Much of Cybex's popularity in the industry is a result of the variety of its equipment offerings (e.g. it can outfit an entire club); the quality of its resistance-equipment lines and its ability to provide financing to clubs for the purchase of its equipment.

❑ *Life Fitness; Franklin Park, Illinois*

Life Fitness was founded by Augie Neito in the early 1970s, when he first started marketing the Lifecycle. At the time, the Lifecycle became the "Band-Aid" brand for the fitness industry. Life Fitness was the first manufacturer to establish a leadership position in the cardiovascular equipment arena. The Lifecycle, lead to the development of the Lifestep and subsequently to the manufacture of a full line of cardiovascular equipment, including treadmills, recumbent bikes, and elliptical trainers. Life Fitness cardiovascular equipment was branded by its unique control panel and special programming features that included the hill and random programs. Life Fitness became (and to this day remains) the largest manufacturer of cardiovascular equipment in the industry. In the early 1990s, Life Fitness bought High Tech, a company that manufactured resistance-training equipment, and created the Life Fitness strength line. In the later half of the 1990s, they bought Hammer Strength. The merger of the cardiovascular, variable resistance and Hammer products created the largest equipment company in the industry. At the present time, Life Fitness has over $500 million in sales annually. Life Fitness is regarded as a leader in each product category, with the Hammer line being tops in the plate-loaded category, its bikes being the top in their class, and its treadmills among the top three in their category. Life Fitness's strength is based on its ability to completely outfit a club (e.g. treadmills, bikes, stairclimbers, ellipticals, resistance machines, and free weights), the quality of its products from a technical and customer perspective, the innovative nature of its products, the tenure of its personnel, and its inclusive marketing and sales efforts.

❏ *Nautilus Group; Vancouver, Washington*

Nautilus was founded in the 1970s by Arthur Jones in Deland, Florida. Its first product offering was the highly popular (and widely innovative at the time) Nautilus variable-resistance equipment. During its first ten to fifteen years of its existence, Nautilus was the most recognized brand in the industry and the top producer of resistance-training equipment. In the early 1990s, Nautilus lost considerable market share. While its brand remained highly visible, its sales slumped, causing it to experience some difficult financial times. In the early part of the 21st century, Nautilus was bought by Direct Focus, based in the state of Washington (a publicly traded company that is known for its popular home product, the Bowflex). Subsequently, Direct Focus also acquired StairMaster, Quinton Treadmills, and Schwinn. The new combined company changed its name to the Nautilus Group and instantly became one of the top five manufacturers and sellers of commercial fitness equipment in the industry. The company product mix includes Nautilus variable-resistance and plate-loaded equipment, free weight benches, StairMaster-branded bikes, elliptical machines, Stairmaster branded treadmills (these are the original Quinton treadmills), stairclimbers, and Schwinn-branded group-exercise bicycles. Nautilus's total commercial sales are well in excess of $100 million annually. Nautilus's strengths lie in the diversity of its products (e.g. it can outfit an entire club), the brand recognition of its products (Nautilus, Schwinn and StairMaster), the quality of its products, and its marketing reach.

❏ *Precor, Inc.; Woodinville, Washington*

Precor got its start by making cardiovascular equipment for the home market. In arena, it became the first leader in home sales of equipment such as bikes and treadmills. Precor entered the commercial club market in the late 1980s with treadmills, bikes and stairclimbers. The Precor treadmill established a unique niche in the market because of its ability to adjust to both positive and negative grades. Precor became a big market player when it introduced the EFX Elliptical Trainer in the mid 1990s. The EFX became a landmark phenomenon in the equipment industry – one that changed the landscape of the club industry. By the late 1990s and early 21st century, Precor had become one of the top three players in the cardiovascular arena in the industry, lead by the EFX and its treadmills. During this period, Precor also introduced its Stretch Trainer. As a result, Precor became highly regarded for innovation in equipment design, equipment esthetics and a desire to introduce new concepts to the market. In 2004, Precor purchased Icarian, a leading manufacturer of variable-resistance equipment and free-weight benches. Precor also bought Cardio Theater in 2004. At the present time, Precor offers a complete line of equipment (e.g. treadmills, elliptical trainers, bikes, stair-climbers and resistance equipment), as well as cardio entertainment. It is the third largest player in the industry, with approximately $200 million in annual sales. Precor's primary strength lies in its approach to innovation, its ability to offer a complete package of equipment, the aesthetics of its product offering, and its marketing and sales efforts.

❑ *Star Trac; Irvine, California*

Star Trac got its start in the early 1980s as Unisen. As Unisen, it produced the electronics for Life Fitness equipment during the early years of Life Fitness. Around 1990, Star Trac entered the market as Star Trac by Unisen and positioned itself as a leading producer of commercial treadmills. Star Trac introduced one of the first commercial treadmills that was customer-friendly, technically sound, and reasonably affordable. Since its inception, Star Trac has expanded its line of commercial treadmills and has added stationary cycles, stairclimbers, elliptical machines, and group-exercise bikes. Star Trac established it self as a leader in the area of cardiovascular equipment by offering quality equipment with innovations that served the needs of the end user. Star Trac's treadmills are the only machines of its kind with built-in fans and its bikes and recumbent bikes are the only ones with an innovative design that includes fans and comfort seating. Recently, Star Trac obtained rights to the "Johnny G" line of group-exercise bikes. In 2005, Star Trac expanded its offerings into cardio entertainment and concurrently the resistance equipment area with the purchase of Flex. Star Trac sales currently are in the neighborhood of $75 million to $80 million annually. Star Trac's strengths lie in the innovation of its products; its focus on producing user-friendly products, its level of exceptional customer service, and its relationships with its customers.

❑ *Technogym USA; Seattle, Washington*

Technogym is second only to Life Fitness in total global sales, with over $250 million in total annual sales worldwide. Technogym burst on the domestic scene in the United States in the early 1990s, after establishing itself as the leading manufacturer of commercial cardiovascular and resistance equipment in the European market. Technogym set itself apart when entering the domestic U.S. market on two fronts. First, it branded itself as the "wellness" company and provided educational support to the industry. Second, it introduced the technology platform that tied its equipment together through a "key" that contained all of a user's workout information. The "key" remains a benchmark feature for Technogym, since it still offers this particular upgrade. Technogym also introduced the flare of contemporary European design to resistance machines and free-weight benches. Its efforts in this regard have helped change the way other manufacturers design their resistance training equipment. Technogym's product offerings includes treadmills, bikes, stairclimbers, elliptical machines, resistance equipment, and free-weight equipment. Technogym's strengths lie in the technical quality of its equipment, the innovative design of its equipment, its focus on wellness, and its ability to outfit an entire club.

❑ *York Barbell Company; York, Pennsylvania*

The York Barbell Company, founded in 1938 by Bob Hoffman, is one of the oldest and most established manufacturers of free weights (e.g., barbells and dumbbells), free-weight accessories (e.g., bars, handles, etc.), and free-weight benches (e.g., flat benches, incline benches, squat racks, etc.) in the industry. Renowned at the time for the phrase, "The Strongest Name in Fitness," which it employed to help promote its products and image, York's claim to fame was driven by the vision and passion of its leader, Bob Hoffman, who established York, Pennsylvania as the home of weightlifting – a location that was often referred to as Muscletown USA. The resulting success of the York Barbell Company was, in large part, driven by the close association between the company and the numerous national, world, and Olympic weightlifting champions (e.g., 105 national champions, 28 world champions and 13 Olympic gold medalists) and the many world-famous bodybuilders (e.g., John Grimek) who attributed their success, in all or part, to Bob Hoffman and the York Barbell Company.

From its inception in 1938 and through the early 1970s, York Barbell was the premier manufacturer of free-weight equipment in the world. In the mid -1970s, York's position of dominance began to decline somewhat when other manufacturers of free-weight equipment appeared on the scene. In the 1990s, York underwent several internal changes that enabled it to again establish a position as one of the preeminent manufacturers of free-weight equipment in the industry.

Appendix F: Sample Job Descriptions

This appendix contains sample job descriptions for various generic positions in the fitness and health club industry.

❏ **Fitness Director**

Position Title: Fitness Director
Position Description Summary:

The position of fitness director is responsible for the overall operations and programming of the fitness facility, with primary oversight of the operating standards, systems and practices as they directly impact the overall operating excellence of the department.

Essential Accountabilities & Functions:

1. To oversee all financial aspects of the fitness department operations, including working with other department heads and supervisors as needed to insure that the financial performance of the fitness department meets budget.

2. To select, hire, coach, mentor and educate fitness department employees in a manner that reinforces the club's values and philosophies and insures the operation of the department meets company standards and provides an environment that promotes membership retention.

3. To oversee all operating practices, policies and systems that are necessary for achieving the department's and club's strategic and business plan goals.

4. To oversee all fitness programming and marketing practices, policies and systems that are necessary for achieving the department's and club's strategic and business plan goals.

Specific Job Accountabilities

1. To select, hire, educate and lead department employees in all work areas, including locker rooms, front desk, childcare, fitness floor, group exercise, massage, racquet sports, etc. This includes managing all aspects of the selection, hiring and education process and providing the leadership for the team on a daily basis.

2. To conduct regular meetings and education sessions for employees, including monthly department meetings and daily line-ups.

3. To oversee the financial success of the fitness department through: correct pricing of services, monitoring and management of employee payroll and lesson payments, daily and monthly audits of sales, forecasting department performance on a monthly basis and whatever other actions must occur for the department to meet its budget and forecast goals.

4. To handle the daily, weekly and period payroll functions for the department, including, but not limited to, collecting and auditing employee commission sheets, doing all payroll activities, managing payroll and commission expense to plan, etc.

5. To create, implement resource and/or execute the necessary actions steps required to successfully meet the fitness operating standards of the club.

6. To create, coordinate, resource, implement, market and sell fitness programs and services. In doing so, to insure proper systems are implemented so as to insure that the club program's meet the needs of membership and drive member participation in such a manner as to create and enhance Member retention.

7. To utilize the available resources of the club in executing the responsibilities of fitness director. This includes incorporating any standards and systems the club has established for operations and programming.

8. To assist in the delivery of department services as required, including providing specific services as qualified to do so by training (examples are working the floor, performing personal training, instructing a class, handling front desk duties, cleaning, etc.)

9. To meet regularly with the manager and other department heads/supervisors to make sure there is complete cooperation between departments in the club and to insure that there is regular communication to other employees in the club regarding the department's services and operation.

10. To assist with any required job activity of the department, as may be needed, so as to insure members are always served in accordance with the club's overall service philosophy.

11. To conduct oneself at all times in a manner of professionalism that aligns with the values, philosophies and standards of the club.

Reporting Relationships:

Reports to:	Club Manager
Directly Supervises:	Front desk staff, locker room staff, childcare staff, fitness floor staff, group exercise staff, massage staff, and racquet sport staff.
Indirectly Supervises:	

Work Experience:

1. Minimum of one year's experience in a supervisory or similar department head role.
2. Minimum of five years experience in the club and/or fitness industry.

Education:

1. College Degree in health, fitness or recreation related field.
2. Master's Degree in related field preferred, but not required.

Certification/License

1. Certification in CPR.
2. Certification from national organization such as ACSM, ACE, NSCA, etc. required..

Working Conditions/Environment

(describe the club's specific facilities and general environment)

Specific Working Conditions

Squatting	Bending	Kneeling
Reaching	Twisting	Crawling
Ladder Climbing	Stair Climbing	Other Climbing
Walking on Rough Ground	Exposure to Temperature Change	Exposure to Dust, Fumes & Gas
Near Moving Machinery	Working from Heights	Cleaning/Scrubbing
Dialing	Collating	Filing
Opening/Closing	Sorting	Stamping
Stapling	Folding/Unfolding	Inserting/Removing

Max. Weight Lifted Occasional	State Weight Lifted if Above 100 lbs.
Max. Weight Lifted Frequently	State Weight Lifted if Above 100 lbs.
Max. Weight Carried Occasionally	State Weight Carried if Above 100 lbs.
Max. Weight Carried Frequently	State Weight Carried if Above 100 lbs.
Max. Weight Pushed Occasionally	State Weight Pushed if Above 100 lbs.
Max. Weight Pushed Frequently	State Weight Pushed if Above 100 lbs.
Max. Weight Pulled Occasionally	State Weight Pulled if Above 100 lbs.
Max Weight Pulled Frequently	State Weight Pulled if Above 100 lbs.
Sit: Hr. Day	Sit: Frequency
Stand: Hr. Day	Stand: Frequency
Walk: Hr. Day	Walk: Frequency
Drive: Hr. Day	Drive: Frequency

❑ Fitness Instructor

Position Title: Fitness Instructor/Personal Trainer
Position Description Summary:

The position of fitness instructor/personal trainer is responsible for providing a safe and effective exercise environment for club Members through supervision of Member exercise programs, education of the Members in exercise and a focus on establishing a personalized program of exercise for each Member.

Essential Accountabilities & Functions:

1. To provide supervision of the exercise and fitness areas of the club, including assisting Members with their exercise and fitness program.

2. To evaluate Member fitness needs and provide the appropriate exercise program for meeting those Members needs, including providing personal instruction if necessary.

3. To connect Members to other Members through ongoing contact with the Members and promotion of club activities.

Specific Job Accountabilities

1. Conduct new Member fitness orientations in accordance with club standards.

2. To provide exercise floor supervision, including greeting each Member and servicing their fitness needs..

3. To create personalized exercise/fitness programs for Members, including providing personal coaching and education of the Member in the program.

4. To insure that all exercise areas and equipment are in safe and effective working condition, including cleanliness being maintained to club standards.

5. To assist with any required job activity of the department, as may be needed, so as to insure Members are always served in accordance with the club's overall service philosophy.

6. To conduct oneself at all times in a manner of professionalism that aligns with the values, philosophies and standards of the club. This includes being in club-approved uniform and nametag.

7. To attend all scheduled employee meetings.

Reporting Relationships:

Reports to: Fitness Director
Directly Supervises:
Indirectly Supervises:

Work Experience:

1. Minimum of one year's experience in the fitness or exercise industry.

Education:
1. College Degree in health, fitness or recreation related field.

Certification/License

1. Certification in CPR.
2. Certification from national organization such as ACSM, ACE, NASM, etc. preferred.

Working Conditions/Environment

(describe the club's specific facilities and general environment)

Specific Working Conditions

Squatting	Bending	Kneeling
Reaching	Twisting	Crawling
Ladder Climbing	Stair Climbing	Other Climbing
Walking on Rough Ground	Exposure to Temperature Change	Exposure to Dust, Fumes & Gas
Near Moving Machinery	Working from Heights	Cleaning/Scrubbing
Dialing	Collating	Filing
Opening/Closing	Sorting	Stamping
Stapling	Folding/Unfolding	Inserting/Removing

Max. Weight Lifted Occasional	State Weight Lifted if Above 100 lbs.
Max. Weight Lifted Frequently	State Weight Lifted if Above 100 lbs.
Max. Weight Carried Occasionally	State Weight Carried if Above 100 lbs.
Max. Weight Carried Frequently	State Weight Carried if Above 100 lbs.
Max. Weight Pushed Occasionally	State Weight Pushed if Above 100 lbs.
Max. Weight Pushed Frequently	State Weight Pushed if Above 100 lbs.
Max. Weight Pulled Occasionally	State Weight Pulled if Above 100 lbs.
Max Weight Pulled Frequently	State Weight Pulled if Above 100 lbs.
Sit: Hr. Day	Sit: Frequency
Stand: Hr. Day	Stand: Frequency
Walk: Hr. Day	Walk: Frequency
Drive: Hr. Day	Drive: Frequency

❏ **Group Exercise Instructor**

Position Title: Group Exercise Instructor

Position Description Summary:

The position of group exercise instructor is responsible for providing a safe and effective group exercise environment for club Members by providing instruction, coaching and supervision to the Members during scheduled group exercise activities.

Essential Accountabilities & Functions:

1. To provide group exercise instruction to Members that is safe and effective.

2. To provide a safe and motivating group exercise environment for the Members.

3. To connect Members to other Members through ongoing contact with the Members and promote other club activities.

Specific Job Accountabilities

1. To provide group exercise instruction for Members per the requirements and standards of the Club.

2. To insure that the group exercise studio is prepared to club standards for each class taught, including having the right equipment for the class, insuring that the classroom is properly cleaned, having the right music available and having the correct temperature.

3. To assist with any required job activity of the department, as may be needed, so as to insure Members are always served in accordance with the club's overall service philosophy.

4. To conduct oneself at all times in a manner of professionalism that aligns with the values, philosophies and standards of the club. This includes being in club-approved uniform and nametag and being on time for scheduled classes.

5. To attend all scheduled employee meetings.

Reporting Relationships:

Reports to: Fitness Director or Group Exercise Coordinator

Directly Supervises:

Indirectly Supervises:

Work Experience:
1. Minimum of one year's experience or 200 hours class instruction experience.

Education:
2. College Degree in health, fitness or recreation related field preferred, but not required.

Certification/License

1. Certification in CPR.
2. General group exercise certification from national organization such as AFAA or ACE.
3. For specialty classes such as Yoga, Pilate's, Group Cycling, Resist-a-Ball, etc., then certification from representative organization.

Working Conditions/Environment

(describe the club's specific facilities and general environment)

Specific Working Conditions

Squatting	Bending	Kneeling
Reaching	Twisting	Crawling
Ladder Climbing	Stair Climbing	Other Climbing
Walking on Rough Ground	Exposure to Temperature Change	Exposure to Dust, Fumes & Gas
Near Moving Machinery	Working from Heights	Cleaning/Scrubbing
Dialing	Collating	Filing
Opening/Closing	Sorting	Stamping
Stapling	Folding/Unfolding	Inserting/Removing

Max. Weight Lifted Occasional	State Weight Lifted if Above 100 lbs.
Max. Weight Lifted Frequently	State Weight Lifted if Above 100 lbs.
Max. Weight Carried Occasionally	State Weight Carried if Above 100 lbs.
Max. Weight Carried Frequently	State Weight Carried if Above 100 lbs.
Max. Weight Pushed Occasionally	State Weight Pushed if Above 100 lbs.
Max. Weight Pushed Frequently	State Weight Pushed if Above 100 lbs.
Max. Weight Pulled Occasionally	State Weight Pulled if Above 100 lbs.
Max Weight Pulled Frequently	State Weight Pulled if Above 100 lbs.
Sit: Hr. Day	Sit: Frequency
Stand: Hr. Day	Stand: Frequency
Walk: Hr. Day	Walk: Frequency
Drive: Hr. Day	Drive: Frequency

❏ **Massage Therapist**

Position Title: Massage/Spa Therapist

Position Description Summary:
The position of massage/spa therapist provides relaxing, soothing and effective bodywork treatments for Members and Guests that allows them to connect with themselves.

Essential Accountabilities & Functions:

1. To provide relaxing, soothing and beneficial bodywork treatments.

2. To provide warm greetings and an enriching environment within the context of the massage/spa work area.

3. To connect Members to other Members through ongoing contact with the Members and promotion of club activities.

Specific Job Accountabilities

1. To provide warm greetings and an enriching environment to all Members/Guests who you interact with.

2. To conduct relaxing, soothing, safe and beneficial bodywork treatments for Members and Guests in accordance with club standards.

3. To make sure that the massage/spa workspace is in compliance with standards and ready to be occupied by Member & guests. This includes having all equipment well maintained and cleaned, having the room cleaned and set-up, having all necessary information on the Member/guest that is needed, etc.

4. To assist with any required job activity of the department, as may be needed, so as to insure Members are always served in accordance with the club's overall service philosophy.

5. To conduct oneself at all times in a manner of professionalism that aligns with the values, philosophies and standards of the club. This includes being in club-approved uniform and nametag.

6. To attend all scheduled employee meetings.

Reporting Relationships:

     Reports to: Fitness Director and/or Spa Director
     Directly Supervises:
     Indirectly Supervises:

Work Experience:
Minimum of six month's experience providing massage/spa treatments.

Education:
1. Degree from accredited school of massage therapy if conducting bodywork treatments.
2. Degree from accredited cosmetology school if conducting services such as facials, manicures or pedicures.

Certification/License

1. State licensure in massage if conducting massage and bodywork treatments.
2. State licensure in cosmetology or similar if conducting manicures, pedicures and facials.
3. Certification in CPR.

Working Conditions/Environment

(describe the club's specific facilities and general environment)

Specific Working Conditions

Squatting	Bending	Kneeling
Reaching	Twisting	Crawling
Ladder Climbing	Stair Climbing	Other Climbing
Walking on Rough Ground	Exposure to Temperature Change	Exposure to Dust, Fumes & Gas
Near Moving Machinery	Working from Heights	Cleaning/Scrubbing
Dialing	Collating	Filing
Opening/Closing	Sorting	Stamping
Stapling	Folding/Unfolding	Inserting/Removing

Max. Weight Lifted Occasional	State Weight Lifted if Above 100 lbs.
Max. Weight Lifted Frequently	State Weight Lifted if Above 100 lbs.
Max. Weight Carried Occasionally	State Weight Carried if Above 100 lbs.
Max. Weight Carried Frequently	State Weight Carried if Above 100 lbs.
Max. Weight Pushed Occasionally	State Weight Pushed if Above 100 lbs.
Max. Weight Pushed Frequently	State Weight Pushed if Above 100 lbs.
Max. Weight Pulled Occasionally	State Weight Pulled if Above 100 lbs.
Max Weight Pulled Frequently	State Weight Pulled if Above 100 lbs.
Sit: Hr. Day	Sit: Frequency
Stand: Hr. Day	Stand: Frequency
Walk: Hr. Day	Walk: Frequency
Drive: Hr. Day	Drive: Frequency

❏ **Front Desk Attendant**

Position Title: Front Desk Attendant

Position Description Summary:
The position of front desk attendant is responsible for creating the first and last impressions of the club experience for Members by providing warm greetings and great service.

Essential Accountabilities & Functions:

1. To provide warm greetings and great service for members and guests..

2. To assist Members with the scheduling of appointments/reservations and the provision of information regarding club services and programs.

3. To connect Members to other Members through ongoing contact with the Members and promotion of club activities.

Specific Job Accountabilities

1. To provide warm greetings and great service to all Members/Guests who enter and leave the club.

2. To provide warm greetings and great service to all Members, guests and others over the telephone through compliance with the club'' phone etiquette standards.

3. To assist Members in scheduling appointments and reservations for club programs and services in accordance with club standards.

4. To assist in providing information to club Members about club facilities, programs and services.

5. To assist with any required job activity of the department, as may be needed, so as to insure Members are always served in accordance with the club's overall service philosophy.

6. To conduct oneself at all times in a manner of professionalism that aligns with the values, philosophies and standards of the club. This includes being in club-approved uniform and nametag.

7. To attend all scheduled employee meetings.

Reporting Relationships:

Reports to: Fitness Director/Front Desk Supervisor
Directly Supervises:
Indirectly Supervises:

Work Experience:
Minimum of six month's experience in the club or hospitality business in a similar capacity.

Education:
High School Diploma or Equivalent.

Certification/License

1. Certification in CPR.

Working Conditions/Environment

(describe the club's specific facilities and general environment)

Specific Working Conditions

Squatting	Bending	Kneeling
Reaching	Twisting	Crawling
Ladder Climbing	Stair Climbing	Other Climbing
Walking on Rough Ground	Exposure to Temperature Change	Exposure to Dust, Fumes & Gas
Near Moving Machinery	Working from Heights	Cleaning/Scrubbing
Dialing	Collating	Filing
Opening/Closing	Sorting	Stamping
Stapling	Folding/Unfolding	Inserting/Removing

Max. Weight Lifted Occasional	State Weight Lifted if Above 100 lbs.
Max. Weight Lifted Frequently	State Weight Lifted if Above 100 lbs.
Max. Weight Carried Occasionally	State Weight Carried if Above 100 lbs.
Max. Weight Carried Frequently	State Weight Carried if Above 100 lbs.
Max. Weight Pushed Occasionally	State Weight Pushed if Above 100 lbs.
Max. Weight Pushed Frequently	State Weight Pushed if Above 100 lbs.
Max. Weight Pulled Occasionally	State Weight Pulled if Above 100 lbs.
Max Weight Pulled Frequently	State Weight Pulled if Above 100 lbs.
Sit: Hr. Day	Sit: Frequency
Stand: Hr. Day	Stand: Frequency
Walk: Hr. Day	Walk: Frequency
Drive: Hr. Day	Drive: Frequency

G. Sample Compensation Agreements

<u>**COMPENSATION AGREEMENT**</u>
Fitness Director
(Employee)

The undersigned agrees to be employed in the position of Fitness Director ("Employee") of _____ ("Club"), effective _____, and shall continue for so long as Employee and Club both agree. This Compensation Agreement confirms our entire agreement concerning your employment compensation, which shall be based upon and subject to the following:

1. **Definitions**: The terms set forth shall have the following meanings:

   (a) "Fitness Department Net" shall mean the gross receipts from all fitness programs, services and retail merchandising minus any necessary expenses, including but not limited to all department expenses involved in the delivery of those programs, services and retail merchandise, but not limited to, promotional material, operational supplies, staff payroll and payroll costs, incentive items, etc.

   (b) "Membership Net" shall mean the amount of dues added, which is the additional dues from (i) new Members, and (ii) an increase in the amount of dues paid by Members, minus the dues lost from Members leaving the Club.

   (c) "Fitness Department Gross" shall mean the gross receipts from all fitness programs, services and retail merchandising, including but not limited to personal training, locker rental fees, massage, program fees, etc.

2. **Bi-Weekly Base Salary:** You will receive a bi-weekly salary of _____ to be paid out every two weeks in an amount equal to _____ (annualized amount equal to _____)

3. **Biweekly Performance Lesson Fee Rate**

   (a) Personal Training instruction taught by Employee shall earn a lesson fee rate equal to _____ _____ Dollars ($) for each lesson taught, up to a maximum of ten (10) lessons a week. The lesson rate earned will be the total compensation due Employee for each lesson.

   (b) Lesson fees shall be paid to you biweekly.

4. **Monthly Performance Bonus**:

   (a) A bonus of _____ Dollars ($) for meeting or beating budgeted Fitness Department Gross.

   (b) A bonus of _____ Dollars ($) for meeting or beating budgeted Fitness Department Net.

   (c) A bonus of _____ Dollars ($) for meeting or beating budgeted Membership Net.

   (d) Bonuses shall be calculated and paid to you within thirty (30) days following the end of each monthly accounting period.

   Employee must be employed on the last day of each monthly accounting period to receive the applicable period bonus.

Annual Performance Bonus

   (a) A bonus of _____ Dollars ($) for meeting or beating budgeted Fitness Department Net.

(b) Bonuses will be calculated and paid to you within thirty (30) days following the end of each calendar year.

5. **NO CONTRACT OF EMPLOYMENT: NEITHER THIS AGREEMENT NOR ANY OTHER COMMUNICATION SHALL BIND CLUB TO EMPLOY NOW OR HEREAFTER. THE EMPLOYMENT RELATIONSHIP BETWEEN YOU AND THE CLUB IS EMPLOYMENT AT WILL, AND THAT RELATIONSHIP MAY BE TERMINATED BY YOU OR BY CLUB FOR ANY REASON, AT ANY TIME, WITH OR WITHOUT NOTICE, AND WITH OR WITHOUT CAUSE. THE EMPLOYMENT AT WILL NATURE OF THIS RELATIONSHIP CANNOT BE ALTERED BY ANY STATEMENTS, ORAL OR WRITTEN, MADE BY ANYONE. IN THE EVENT OF TERMINATION, WEEKLY BASE SALARY AND COMMISSIONS/BONUSES SHALL BE PRORATED ON A DAILY BASIS TO THE DATE OF TERMINATION.**

6. Exempt Position: Your position as Fitness Director is an exempt position under the overtime provisions of the Fair Labor Standards Act and you are not entitled to overtime compensation. The compensation herein provided to you shall constitute full payment for the services rendered by you to Club.

7. Entire Agreement. This Agreement embodies the entire agreement and understanding of the parties relating to Employee's employment and supersedes all prior representations, agreements, and understandings..

If the foregoing accurately sets forth all of the terms of our agreement concerning your compensation, please indicate your acceptance by signing below.

EXECUTED this _____ day of _____, 20____.

Employee

Signature: _____

Print: _____

Club

Signature: _____

Title: _____

COMPENSATION AGREEMENT
(Personal Trainer/Fitness Instructor)

The undersigned agrees to be employed in the position of Personal Trainer ("Employee") by _____ ("Club"), effective _____,20____, and shall continue for so long as Employee and Club both agree. The purpose of this Agreement is to spell out the compensation for this position.

1. **Compensation**. The compensation paid to Employee will be comprised of the following:

   1.1 Employee shall earn a wage equal to _____ Dollars ($) for every member/guest paid one-hour personal training session that is conducted and appropriately recorded.

   1.2 Employee shall earn a wage equal to _____ Dollars ($) for every member/guest paid one-half hour personal training session that is conducted and appropriately recorded.

   1.3 Employee shall earn a wage equal to _____ Dollars ($) per hour for every fitness orientation, fitness test or other service that is provided by the Employee at the request of the Club.

   1.4 Time and one-half of Employee's Net Regular Rate will be paid to Employee for all hours worked over forty (40) in any one workweek.

2. **Duties**. Employee's duties shall include, but not be limited to, those described in Employee's job description.

3. **Full Compensation**. The compensation provided for Employee by this Agreement shall constitute full payment for the services rendered to Club. Employee shall not receive any additional compensation for any services performed unless such services and payment, prior to their rendition, are authorized in writing by the Club's General Manager. Employee expressly waives, discharges, and releases Club from any claims for such services performed unless authorized in writing in the manner provided above.

4. **THIS AGREEMENT IS NOT A CONTRACT FOR EMPLOYMENT FOR A FIXED TERM, INSTEAD, IT DESCRIBES THE TERMS UPON WHICH EMPLOYEE'S COMPENSATION IS TO BE BASED. EMPLOYEE UNDERSTANDS EITHER PARTY MAY TERMINATE THE EMPLOYMENT RELATIONSHIP AT ANY TIME, FOR ANY REASON, WITH OR WITHOUT CAUSE. THE EMPLOYMENT-AT-WILL NATURE OF THIS RELATIONSHIP CANNOT BE ALTERED BY ANY STATEMENTS, ORAL OR WRITTEN, MADE BY ANYONE. EMPLOYEE FURTHER UNDERSTANDS NO COMMISSIONS, BONUSES, OR OTHER FORM OF COMPENSATION ACCRUE AFTER EMPLOYMENT TERMINATES.**

5. **Entire Agreement**. This Agreement embodies the entire agreement and understanding of the parties relating to Employee's employment and supersedes all prior representations, agreements, and understandings, oral or written, relating to Employee's employment.

      EXECUTED this _____ day of _____,20____.

                                                  Employee:

      Signature: _____

      Printed Name: _____

                                                  Club:

      Signature: _____

      Title: _____

COMPENSATION AGREEMENT
SPA DIRECTOR
(Employee)

The undersigned agrees to be employed in the position of Spa Director ("Employee") by _____ ("Club"), effective _____, and shall continue for so long as Employee and Club both agree. This Compensation Agreement confirms our entire agreement concerning your employment compensation, which shall be based upon and subject to the following:

1. **Definitions**: The terms set forth shall have the following meanings:

    (a) "Spa Department Net" shall mean the gross receipts from all spa programs, services and retail merchandising minus any necessary expenses, including but not limited to all department expenses involved in the delivery of those programs, services and retail merchandise, but not limited to, promotional material, operational supplies, staff payroll and payroll costs, incentive items, etc.

    (b) "Spa Department Gross" shall mean the gross receipts from all spa programs, services and retail merchandising, including but not limited to hairstyling, massage, facials, pedicures, manicures, etc.

2. **Bi-Weekly Base Salary:** You will receive a biweekly salary of _____ to be paid out every two weeks in an amount equal to _____ (annualized amount equal to _____).

3. **Biweekly Performance Treatment Fee Rate**

    (a) Any spa service rendered by Employee shall earn a treatment fee rate equal to _____ Dollars ($) for each service rendered, up to a maximum of ten (10) treatments a week. The treatment fee rate earned will be the total compensation due Employee for each treatment performed.

    (b) Treatment Fee rate shall be paid to you biweekly.

4. **Monthly Performance Bonus**:

    (a) A bonus of _____ ($) for meeting or beating budgeted Spa Department Gross.

    (b) A bonus of _____ ($) for meeting or beating budgeted Spa Department Net.

    (c) Bonuses shall be calculated and paid to you within thirty (30) days following the end of each monthly accounting period.

    Employee must be employed on the last day of each monthly accounting period to receive the applicable period bonus.

5. **Annual Performance Bonus**

    (a) A bonus of _____ ($) for meeting or beating budgeted Spa Department Net.

    (b) Bonuses will be calculated and paid to you within thirty (30) days following the end of each calendar year.

6. **NO CONTRACT OF EMPLOYMENT: NEITHER THIS AGREEMENT NOR ANY OTHER COMMUNICATION SHALL BIND CLUB TO EMPLOY YOU NOW OR HEREAFTER. THE EMPLOYMENT RELATIONSHIP BETWEEN YOU AND THE CLUB IS EMPLOYMENT AT WILL, AND THAT RELATIONSHIP MAY BE TERMINATED BY YOU OR BY CLUB FOR ANY REASON, AT ANY TIME, WITH OR WITHOUT NOTICE, AND WITH OR WITHOUT CAUSE. THE EMPLOYMENT AT WILL NATURE OF THIS RELATIONSHIP CANNOT BE ALTERED BY ANY STATEMENTS, ORAL OR WRITTEN, MADE BY ANYONE. IN THE EVENT OF TERMINATION, WEEKLY BASE SALARY AND COMMISSIONS SHALL BE PRORATED ON A DAILY BASIS TO THE DATE OF TERMINATION.**

7. Exempt Position: Your position as Spa Director is an exempt position under the overtime provisions of the Fair Labor Standards Act and you are not entitled to overtime compensation. The compensation herein provided to you shall constitute full payment for the services rendered by you to Club. You shall not receive additional compensation for any services performed unless such services and payment therefor, prior to their rendition, are authorized in writing by, or on behalf of Club. Employee expressly waives, discharges and releases Club from any claims for such services performed unless the same are authorized in writing as provided above.

8. Entire Agreement. This Agreement embodies the entire agreement and understanding of the parties relating to Employee's employment and supersedes all prior representations, agreements, and understandings.

If the foregoing correctly sets forth all of the terms of our agreement concerning your compensation, please indicate your acceptance by signing below.

EXECUTED this _____ day of _____, 20____.

Employee

Signature: _____

Printed
Name:_____

Club:

Signature:_____

Title: _____

Printed
Name: _____

COMPENSATION AGREEMENT
(Group Exercise Instructor)

The undersigned agrees to be employed in the position of Group Exercise Instructor ("Employee") by _____ ("Club"), effective _____,20____, and shall continue for so long as Employee and Club both agree. The purpose of this Agreement is to spell out the compensation for this position.

1.　　**Compensation**. The compensation paid to Employee will be comprised of the following:

　　　1.1.　　Group Exercise Instruction by Employee to Members or Guests shall earn a class rate equal to_____ DOLLARS ($_____) for each class instructed that is forty-five minutes to one – hour in duration. The class rate earned will be the total compensation due Employee for the instruction;

　　　1.2　　Group Exercise Instruction by Employee to members or Guests shall earn a class rate equal to _____ DOLLARS ($_____) for each class instructed that is one – half hour to forty-four minutes in duration. The class rate earned will be the total compensation due Employee for the instruction.

　　　1.3　　A rate of _____ DOLLARS ($_____) per hour for all hours worked when not providing group exercise instruction (base pay). The stated hourly rate will be the total compensation due Employee for all hours worked when not providing group exercise instruction, including holiday, personal and vacation time;

　　　1.4.　　Time and one-half of Employee's Net Regular Rate will be paid to Employee for all hours worked over forty (40) in any one workweek.

　　　1.5　　Employee shall be paid every two weeks in an amount equal to what is earned based on 1.1, 1.2, 1.3 and 1.4 above.

2.　　**Duties**. Employee's duties shall include, but not be limited to, those described in Employee's job description.

3.　　**Full Compensation**. The compensation provided for Employee by this Agreement shall constitute full payment for the services rendered to Club. Employee shall not receive any additional compensation for any services performed unless such services and payment, prior to their rendition, are authorized in writing by the Club's General Manager. Employee expressly waives, discharges, and releases Club from any claims for such services performed unless authorized in writing in the manner provided above.

4　　**THIS AGREEMENT IS NOT A CONTRACT FOR EMPLOYMENT FOR A FIXED TERM, INSTEAD, IT DESCRIBES THE TERMS UPON WHICH EMPLOYEE'S COMPENSATION IS TO BE BASED. EMPLOYEE UNDERSTANDS EITHER PARTY MAY TERMINATE THE EMPLOYMENT RELATIONSHIP AT ANY TIME, FOR ANY REASON, WITH OR WITHOUT CAUSE. THE EMPLOYMENT-AT-WILL NATURE OF THIS RELATIONSHIP CANNOT BE ALTERED BY ANY STATEMENTS, ORAL OR WRITTEN, MADE BY ANYONE. EMPLOYEE FURTHER UNDERSTANDS NO COMMISSIONS, BONUSES, OR OTHER FORM OF COMPENSATION ACCRUE AFTER EMPLOYMENT TERMINATES.**

6.   **Entire Agreement**. This Agreement embodies the entire agreement and understanding of the parties relating to Employee's employment and supersedes all prior representations, agreements, and understandings, oral or written, relating to Employee's employment.

EXECUTED this _____ day of _____,20____ .

Employee:

Signature:_____

Printed Name: _____

Club:

Signature: _____

Printed Name: _____

Title: _____

COMPENSATION AGREEMENT
(Massage Therapist)

The undersigned agrees to be employed in the position of Massage Therapist ("Employee") by _____ ("Club"), effective _____,20____, and shall continue for so long as Employee and Club both agree. The purpose of this Agreement is to spell out the compensation for this position.

1.   **Compensation**. The compensation paid to Employee will be comprised of the following:

  1.1.   A rate of _____ DOLLARS ($_____) per forty-five minute to one-hour massage/body treatment that is delivered to a Member of Guest.

  1.2   A rate of _____ DOLLARS ($_____) per massage/body treatment of less than forty-five minutes duration.

  1.3   A rate of _____ DOLLARS ($_____) per hour for all hours worked when not providing massage/body treatments (base rate). The stated hourly rate will be the total compensation due Employee for all hours worked when not providing body massages. This base rate applies to all vacation, holiday and personal time;

  1.4   Time and one-half of Employee's Net Regular Rate will be paid to Employee for all hours worked over forty (40) in any one workweek.

  1.5   Employee shall be paid every two weeks in an amount equal to what is earned based on 1.1, 1.2, 1.3 and 1.4 above.

2. **Duties**. Employee's duties shall include, but not be limited to, those described in Employee's job description.

3   **Full Compensation**. The compensation provided for Employee by this Agreement shall constitute full payment for the services rendered to Club. Employee shall not receive any additional compensation for any services performed unless such services and payment, prior to their rendition, are authorized in writing by the Club's General Manager. Employee expressly waives, discharges, and releases Club from any claims for such services performed unless authorized in writing in the manner provided above.

4   **THIS AGREEMENT IS NOT A CONTRACT FOR EMPLOYMENT FOR A FIXED TERM, INSTEAD, IT DESCRIBES THE TERMS UPON WHICH EMPLOYEE'S COMPENSATION IS TO BE BASED. EMPLOYEE UNDERSTANDS EITHER PARTY MAY TERMINATE THE EMPLOYMENT RELATIONSHIP AT ANY TIME, FOR ANY REASON, WITH OR WITHOUT CAUSE. THE EMPLOYMENT-AT-WILL NATURE OF THIS RELATIONSHIP CANNOT BE ALTERED BY ANY STATEMENTS, ORAL OR WRITTEN, MADE BY ANYONE. EMPLOYEE FURTHER UNDERSTANDS NO COMMISSIONS, BONUSES, OR OTHER FORM OF COMPENSATION ACCRUE AFTER EMPLOYMENT TERMINATES.**

5. **Entire Agreement**. This Agreement embodies the entire agreement and understanding of the parties relating to Employee's employment and supersedes all prior representations, agreements, and understandings, oral or written, relating to Employee's employment.

EXECUTED this _____ day of _____,20____.

Employee:

Signature: _____

Printed Name: _____

Club:

Signature: _____

Title:_____

Printed Name: _____

Sample Job Offering Letter

CLUB LETTERHEAD

[Date]

[Name]
[Address]

Dear [Name]:

We are delighted to have you as the newest addition to our team. This letter outlines the terms of your agreement with [Entity] regarding your employment:

You will begin work at (Location) Club on [Date], as [Position] reporting directly to me. You will be paid at the biweekly Base rate of $[Rate] (annualized $[Base Amount]

You will also have the ability to earn income by giving lessons and/or providing training. The expectation is that those services will provide approximately $_____ in additional income which equates to approximately _____ hours per week/period. The Club and Employee agree that the number of lessons/sessions taught/given on an annual basis will not encumber the Employee's ability to manage all aspects of the golf/tennis/athletic operation, achieve his Performance Objectives and fulfill the requirements of his Job Description.

You will have an additional incentive potential of 30% of eligible base wages for the year _____ based upon the annual Club EBITDA Performance, the Department Financial Performance by period and your annual Individual Performance.

You will receive a Summary Plan Document that will provide detail regarding performance scales and earnings for the incentive potential component of your compensation.

You will be eligible to participate in the companies benefit plans upon completing six months of regular, full-time employment. Medical and dental coverage is also available for your dependents.

It is understood that you will move your personal belongings from
_____ to _____. Please submit receipts on your direct cost move, including travel expenses (gas, meals and lodging) to my office for approval prior to reimbursement by _____. (Include the relocation repayment agreement.)

Enclosed is a copy of the company handbook covering policies, procedures, and privileges with which you will want to become familiar. Be prepared to ask any questions you may have concerning the handbook during your orientation. You will need to bring it with you, as you will be asked to sign the receipt.

It is understood that nothing in this letter or in any previous or future communications is intended or should be construed to guarantee employment for any specified period of time. It is understood that either party, with or without cause may terminate this relationship at any time. It is likewise understood that the employment-at-will nature of this relationship cannot be altered by any statements, oral or written, made, or which may be made, contrary to the above.

If this is in agreement with discussions held, please sign and return one copy of this letter. Also, please complete the enclosed paperwork and be prepared to return it to the human resources department during your orientation at 9:00 am on your first day at work.

[Name], congratulations on your new responsibilities. We look forward to our mutual success.

If you have any questions or would like any assistance, please do not hesitate to call.

Sincerely,

[Name of Supervisor]
[Title]

Enclosures

Agreed to this_____day of _____, 2005

_____
(Name)

Appendix H: Sample Structured Interview Questioning Format for a Fitness Director Applicant

I. General Fitness

A. Please indicate what steps you normally take to insure that prospective exercisers receive a safe and effective exercise program when they first decide to begin exercising?

Key Elements of Response:

_____ Have individual complete a pre-activity screening such as health history, Par Q or similar.

_____ Have individual obtain medical clearance if high risk.

_____ Performa fitness test to obtain baseline information on physical abilities and fitness level.

_____ Complete an exercise prescription and then lead the individual through the actual prescription.

_____ Follow-up with the individual on a regular basis to insure that they are correctly following the program and to adjust if needed.

B. A significant portion of the exercising and non-exercising population at this club is over the age of fifty. What special precautions might you need to take when programming physical activity for a population of this age?

Key Elements of Response:

_____ Make sure that the individuals have received the appropriate screening, including medical clearance and screening when indicated.

_____ Make sure that the staff is familiar with the special physical requirements of this population and provide the necessary training if needed.

_____ Make sure that the activity programs are: lower impact, incorporate lower intensity activity, are monitored by qualified staff, include all components of the fitness spectrum (Flexibility, strength and cardiovascular) and are programmed at a time convenient for the individuals.

_____ Make allowances for more personal attention.

C. Please describe the critical elements involved in developing an exercise program for a forty five-year-old male who has been diagnosed as having type II diabetes. Assume that he has been cleared to exercise by his physician.

Key Elements of Response:

_____ Would make sure that he establishes a regular time to exercise each time he visits.

_____ Would make sure he exercises at lower intensity and for a longer duration versus high intensity and shorter duration.

_____ Would make sure that he consumes some carbohydrate before exercising (at least 60 minutes beforehand) and has some form of carbohydrate with him during the exercise.

_____ Would make sure to monitor performance and check for signs of fatigue, dizziness, etc.

D. According to the most recent literature, what are some key steps to assisting exercisers in maintaining their exercise program?

Key Elements of Response:

_____ Have the individual complete an interest questionnaire to obtain information about their goals, interests, support structure, etc.

_____ Establish realistic short term and long term goals (process and outcome) with the individual.

_____ Develop a behavioral contract that commits them and you to certain process goals and actions. Also establish a self-monitoring or tracking program.

_____ Make the exercise program progressive by starting out easy and gradually increasing.

_____ Establish a reward system to recognize achievement of process and reward goals.

E. What are the top four or five trends in the fitness/club industry today, including group exercise?

Key Elements of Response:

_____ Group Cycling

_____ Pilates

_____ Yoga and related

_____ Spa services such as massage and related

_____ Personal training

_____ Sports performance training

II. Employee Relations

A. You have just been hired as the fitness director, what steps would you take to insure that the employees under your responsibility are aware of your expectations and prepared to perform as a team?

Key Elements of Response:

_____ Would arrange to have a meeting with the entire group to provide an overview of expectations.

_____ Would meet one on one with each of the employees to get to know them and better understand their roles and needs.

_____ Would establish with the team some basic ground rules for performance.

_____ Would establish job descriptions and performance models for each employee.

_____ Would communicate with each on a regular basis through individual meetings, team meetings, etc.

B. You have an employee who is responsible for the group exercise program. Over the past month, you have noticed that the overall program is not being well received by the members. In addition, you have had complaints from members and employees about the quality of the program and their feeling that the individual in charge is not concerned about it. What steps would you take to address the perceived problem?

Key Elements of Response:

_____ Would meet with the employee to gather information from their perspective and share with them some of the concerns brought up by the members and fellow employees.

_____ Would set up an action plan for performance with some 30, 60 and 90-day goals. This plan would include expectations and actions to be taken for failure to meet expectations.

_____ Would provide additional coaching and training to address specific areas of need.

_____ Would meet with on a regular basis to review performance, counsel, redirect and hold accountable.

_____ Would inform others who expressed concern that things were being addressed and that you were dealing with the situation in a proactive manner.

III. Financial Management

A. Please describe the primary streams of revenue and the largest expense areas for a fitness department in a typical fitness and sports club?

Key Elements of Response:

_____ The primary sources of revenue would be personal training and program fees.

_____ The largest expenses would be payroll, commissions, program supplies, etc.

B. Please describe the primary steps you would take in preparing a budget for your department, including the difference between a zero-based budget and a trend line budget?

Key Elements of Response:

_____ Would gather information on existing financial performance and usage patterns.

_____ Would identify opportunities for revenue growth and expense control, including targets for specific revenue and expense areas.

_____ Would create a preliminary budget based on the historical information and projected targets.

_____ A zero based budget is when you start from scratch and build budget on projected targets and a trend line budget is when you project budget targets off of prior historical trends.

C. Your department net financial performance is 10% behind plan after the first six months of the year. Please describe briefly actions that you would take to get back on plan before the year was over.

Key Elements of Response:

_____ Would gather information on performance and identify specific strengths and weaknesses.

_____ Would identify revenue opportunities and set up action plans to achieve.

_____ Would identify expense control opportunities, particularly in payroll and then establish action plans for making the necessary changes.

_____ Would monitor each week and make necessary adjustments.

IV. Member Relations

A. Please describe from your perspective the key elements in creating great service and memorable experiences for members using the club?

Key Elements of Response:

_____ Make sure that all employees are trained in providing great service.

_____ Make sure members are greeted by name

_____ Make sure we provide programs and services that interest the members and fill their needs.

_____ Make sure that there is enough equipment and that it is in good working condition.

_____ Make sure that we monitor members programs and provide feedback.

_____ Listen to the members and try to meet or exceed their expressed expectations.

B. A member comes to you complaining that another member is making excessive use of the equipment and not allowing them to use the equipment when they are in the club. Furthermore, the member says the other member has been rude to them. The member says you should remove this other member. Please describe how you would address this member issue?

Key Elements of Response:

_____ Would listen to the members concerns and make note of them.

_____ Would let the member know that you would address the concern and get back with them.

_____ Would then meet with the other member and gather their perspective, without letting them know who had commented about them.

_____ Would determine the appropriate course of action, and then meet with the targeted member and let them know the action you feel needs to be taken.

_____ Would meet with the complaining member and let them know what action was taken.

V. **Marketing and Sales**

A. Please describe the strategies you would use to increase personal training participation and revenue?

Key Elements of Response:

_____ Would first gather information about current participation and why members either used or did not use personal training.

_____ Might use focus groups, survey or one on one discussion to gather information.

_____ Would establish targeted quotas for the department and each of the trainers. Would also monitor these targets on regular basis.

_____ Would package personal training to appeal to members, including having the right pricing.

_____ Would market using strategies such as pictures of the trainers with bios, a brochure on personal training, personal training bulletin board, etc.

_____ Would provide personal trainers with sales training.

B. What do you consider to be the most critical elements of promoting fitness programs to members so that participation levels are maximized?

Key Elements of Response:

_____ Making sure to communicate to members in advance the programs that are available (annual program calendar or monthly program calendar).

_____ Making sure that every employee is aware of the programs and talks it up with the members. Make each employee a sales person.

_____ Get members aligned with the programs and have them become spokespersons for the programs (committees, loyal members, etc.)

_____ Providing the right mix of promotional materials such as flyers, posters, statement stuffers, E-mail, etc.

Structured Interview Comparison & Ranking Form for Athletic Director

For each of the specified categories of structured interview questions, please indicate your rating for each category as follows:

1 = Response is unsatisfactory (candidate provides less than 50% of the expected key element responses)
2 = Response is satisfactory (candidate provides over 50% of the expected key element responses)
3 = Response is exceptional (candidate provides all of the expected key element responses)

Category						
I. General Fitness						
II. Employee Relations						
III. Financial Knowledge						
IV. Member Relations						
V. Sales & Marketing						
Total Score						

Additional comments:

_____
_____
_____
_____
_____
_____
_____
_____
_____
_____
_____
_____
_____
_____
_____
_____

Final Ranking: _____

Appendix I: Sample Strategic Planning Forms

Strategic Planning Worksheet

I. Mission (who do you serve, what is your product, how do you deliver it and its value)

```



```

II. Vision (what is it that your audience will see in 3 – 5 years)

```



```

III. Promise (what is it the member and/or employee will always experience)

```



```

IV. Core Values (the roots for every decision and action you take)

1	
2	
3	
4	
5	

V. Objectives & Goals (what is it you want to achieve and target)

Audience	Objectives	Target

VI. Strategies (the guidelines and general actions that will lead to achievement of the objectives)

Objective	Strategies

Strategic Plan
Action Worksheets

Objective:				
Target #:		Timeline:		
Strategy:				

#	Action Steps	Leader

Appendix J: Selected Front-of-the-House Operational Forms

OPENING REPORT

Name:_____   Date:_____

—   Turn on lights

—   Turn on radio; adjust volume. Set Television on desired channel.

—   Turn on computer in fitness testing room and front desk. Type in the club ID, date, and day of the week

—   Set up control desk:

- Pull out appointment book and turn to correct date
- Check on message from previous night
- Sharpen pencils if needed
- Rip day off of small calendar

—   Check out locker rooms and make sure they are clean, and supplies are replenished; roll out shower mats

—   Check out the fitness floor and make sure all equipment is turned on and ready to go (unplug cyclone charger)

—   Put away uniform bags

—   Fold towels

—   Put load in dryer

—   Read MOD log

—   Unlock fruit bar case

—   Check tires on Velodyne

—   Check all offices, aerobic room, and both locker rooms

—   Check free-weight area for footprints and note in MOD book

—   Call time before opening

—   Check all clocks before opening

—   Check temperature throughout club (thermostats on 68 degrees)

—   Make sure no light bulbs are burned out

—   Check ceiling tiles for leaks

—   Walk entire perimeter of the club

—   Check schedule and note activities, special events, and massage appointments

—   Turn on copier

—   Write cleaning inspection notes in log book

DEPARTMENTAL
CLOSING REPORT

Date:_____   Day:_____

Shift Supervisor:_____   Signature:_____

Control Desk

1. Report completed and attached   _____
2. All tickets completed/correct   _____   (control sheet attached)
3. Desk cleaned up   _____
4. TV and stereo off   _____
5. Lights out   _____

Fitness Floor

1. All weights, plates, etc., picked up   _____
2. Selectorized equipment set   _____
3. All electrical equipment off   _____
4. Exercise cards replaced/signed   _____
5. Floor cleaned   _____
6. Equipment cleaned   _____
7. Lights off   _____

Exercise Classroom

1. Attendance checked (#_____)   _____
2. Stereo off   _____
3. Equipment replaced   _____
4. Studio cleaned   _____
5. Lights off   _____

Locker Rooms and Laundry

1. All dirty towels/uniforms emptied   _____
2. Clean towels restocked   _____
3. All supplies restocked   _____
4. All cleaning completed   _____
5. Spa amenities checked   _____
   - Steam temperature   _____
   - Sauna temperature   _____
   - Whirlpool temperature   _____
   - Whirlpool pH   _____
   - Whirlpool chlorine   _____

6. Spa amenities turned off   _____
7. Massage linens emptied   _____
8. Massage room cleaned   _____
9. Laundry cleaned   _____
10. Dryers emptied   _____
11. Lights out   _____

Pool Area

1. Pool report completed and attached   _____
2. Equipment put away   _____
3. Pool area cleaned   _____
4. Pool temperature and chemistry okay   _____

Gym/Racquet Courts

1. Gym equipment away   _____
2. Gym cleaned   _____
3. Racquet courts cleaned   _____
4. Lights out in courts   _____
5. Lights out in gym   _____

Supervisor's Comments

_____

_____

_____

_____

_____

_____

_____

_____

_____

_____

Company Name and Address

Staff Name _____

Club Name _____

Department: _____

Purpose: _____

SS# or TAX ID # _____

DATE	AIR TRAVEL	AUTO EXPENSE		TAXI	LODGING	TRAVEL MEALS			TIPS	PARKING /TOLLS	TELEPH.	ENTRTNMNT (SCHLA)	Other Expenses		GRAND TOTAL
		MILES	RENTAL AMOUNT			BRKFST	LUNCH	DINNER					EXPLANATION	AMOUNT	
			$0.00												$0.00
			$0.00												$0.00
			$0.00												$0.00
			$0.00												$0.00
			$0.00												$0.00
			$0.00												$0.00
			$0.00												$0.00
			$0.00												$0.00
			$0.00												$0.00
			$0.00												$0.00
			$0.00												$0.00
			$0.00												$0.00
			$0.00												$0.00
			$0.00												$0.00
TOTAL	$0.00	0	$0.00	$0.00	$0.00	$0.00	$0.00	$0.00	$0.00	$0.00	$0.00	$0.00		$0.00	$0.00
															$0.00

TOTAL DUE EMPLOYEE

EXPLANATION OF ENTERTAINMENT EXPENSES

DATE	Supplier	BUSINESS PURPOSE	INDIVIDUALS ENTERTAINED	AMOUNT

EXPLANATION OF OTHER EXPENSES

DATE	TYPE OF EXPENSE	DESCRIPTION	AMOUNT

AUTHORIZATION

Supervisor Approval and Signature

I hereby indicate by my signature below that I have reviewed the expenses indicated in this report and hereby approve them as fully reimbursable.

Approved By _____ Date _____

Employee Signature

I hereby indicate by my signature below that the above listed expenses are legitimate expenses related to the performance of my job.

Employee Signature _____ Date _____

Chart of Account Numbers

	AMOUNT

Rev 5/1/98

Group Exercise
Class Attendance Sheet

Month: _____   Week: _____

Date/Day	Class Title	Time of Class	Instructor's Name	# of Participants in Class	Instructor Initials

LOST AND FOUND LOG SHEET

Item Found	Date	Day	Time	Staff Person	Member's Name if Known	Put in Closet

Share Your Experience
Member & Guest Comment Card

Date: _____   Time: _____

Experience you would like to share:

```
┌─────────────────────────────────────────────────┐
│                                                 │
│                                                 │
│                                                 │
│                                                 │
│                                                 │
└─────────────────────────────────────────────────┘
```

Overall how did you feel about your experience in the club today? Please indicate by checking of the appropriate response!

_____ Unsatisfactory (did not meet your expectations)

_____ Satisfactory (meet your expectations and needs)

_____ Delighted (exceeded your expectations, wow)

Would you like us to follow-up directly with you? _____ Yes _____ No
If yes, please provide us with your name and contact information.

Name (optional): _____

Contact phone #: _____   Contact email: _____

Thank you for sharing your feelings about your experience today.

ATHLETIC DEPARTMENT
TELEPHONE MESSAGE LOG

Period:_____
Week of:_____

Day/Date	Time	Who Called (Name) Who Called For (Name)	Message/Action	Staff Person's Initials

CLOSING REPORT

Name:_____   Date:_____

_____   Check laundry; make sure everything is on schedule

_____   Fill all supplies to the top of the label in both locker rooms and massage shower

(body wash, shampoo, conditioner, deodorant, hand soap, and lotion)

_____   Put away all uniforms

_____   Prop locker room doors open

_____   Restock towels, washcloths, paper towels, toilet paper, feminine napkins,

and hand soap

_____   Make sure boom box and lights are off in massage room

_____   Make sure all curling irons are off in the laudry room(s)

_____   Make sure fans throughout club are off

_____   Release Keiser air pressure

_____   Take half plates off all Cybex machines

_____   Readjust the volume in locker rooms and club

_____   Turn off lights, TV, VCR, DVD, CD and audio tape players

_____   Check stereo in aerobic room

_____   Check all thermostats in club to make sure temperature is correct (68 degrees);

aerobics studio (62 degrees)

_____   Put any problems or reminders for the next day in the MOD log

_____   Make sure exercise cards are signed and put away

_____   Lock fruit bar case

_____   Empty hampers in MLR and WL

_____   Turn computer off in F.Troom and front desk

_____   Complete recap sheet

_____   Lock up the club and recheck to make sure everything is finished

_____   Clean lint traps

_____   Turn off the copier

Day_____Date_____/_____/_____

Time					APPOINTMENTS			
6:00								
6:30								
7:00								
7:30								
8:00								
8:30								
9:00								
9:30								
10:00								
10:30								
11:00								
11:30								
NOON								
12:30								
1:00								
1:30								
2:00								
2:30								
3:00								
3:30								
4:00								
4:30								
5:00								
5:30								
6:00								
6:30								
7:00								
7:30								
8:00								
8:30								
9:00								
9:30								

Day_____Date_____/_____/_____

MEMBERSHIP ACTIVITY SHEET

Member Name	Member No.	Time	Pool	Classes	Weights	CV Equip.	RB/SQ	LRS	I-I's	Other

Appendix K: Selected Heart-of-the-House Operational Forms

Club Name

Check/Petty Cash Request Form

Staff person making request: _____

Position/title: _____

Signature: _____

Information Pertaining to Request

1. Requesting: _____ Check _____ Petty Cash

2. Amount being requested: _____

3. What are the funds being requested for (describe what the requested funds are for):

_____

_____

4. If a check is required, please provide the following information:

Check made out to: _____

Fed Tax ID or SS#: _____

Purchase order # (if applicable): _____

Day/date check needed: _____ Time needed: _____

5. If petty cash is being requested, the name of the staff person receiving the petty cash:

Name: _____ Position: _____

6. If petty cash requested, day/date and time needed: _____

Support information

Check Information

Check Number: _____ Amount of Check: _____

Date Check written: _____

Date Check cashed: _____

Receipt/invoice provided: _____ Yes _____ No

If yes, the invoice or receipt number was: _____

Product received: _____ Yes _____ No

Accounting signature: _____ Date: _____

Petty Cash Information

Amount of Petty Cash: _____

Date provided: _____

Receipt/invoice provided: _____ Yes _____ No

If yes, the invoice or receipt number was: _____

Amount of invoice/receipt: _____

Change returned: _____

Product received: _____ Yes _____ No

Staff person providing change and receipt: _____

Accounting signature: _____ Date: _____

Lost & Missing Item Report

Day and Date item reported: _____   Time: _____

I.   General Information on Person Reporting Lost/Missing Item

1. Person reporting lost/missing item (e.g. member, guest, employee, etc.)?	Name: Status: _____ member _____ guest _____ employee
2. Address of person reporting?	Street: _____ City/State/Zip: _____
3. Phone and email information on person reporting?	(H) _____ (B) _____ (C) _____ email: _____
4. If a member, provide their membership number:	

II.   Information on the Lost/Missing Item

1.   Description of lost/missing item:
2.   Location it was last seen:
3.   Time that it was last seen:

III.   Actions and Witness Information

Name: _____ Address: _____ _____ Phone: (B) _____ (H) _____ Email: _____	Name: _____ Address: _____ _____ Phone: (B) _____ (H) _____ Email: _____

IV.   **Club Action and Response**

Staff person responding: _____

Day/Date responding: _____ Time: _____

Action/response description: _____

_____

_____

Were the police contacted? _____ Yes _____ No

Did the police investigate? _____ Yes _____ No
If yes, please provide name, title and contact number for the officer.

Name: _____ Title: _____

Contact information: _____

Result of investigation? _____

_____

Did we follow-up with the person reporting the lost/missing item? _____ Yes _____ No

What was the nature of the club's follow-up? _____

_____

Staff person completing report: _____

Staff person signature: _____

Date completed: _____ Time completed: _____

Pool and Whirlpool
Weekly Report
Week of: _____

Date	Day	Time	Pool Chemistry	Whirlpool Chemistry
	Monday		pH level: Chlorine level: Alkalinity level: Temperature: Filter PSI:	pH level: Chlorine level: Alkalinity level: Temperature: Filter PSI:
	Tuesday		pH level: Chlorine level: Alkalinity level: Temperature: Filter PSI:	pH level: Chlorine level: Alkalinity level: Temperature: Filter PSI:
	Wednesday		pH level: Chlorine level: Alkalinity level: Temperature: Filter PSI:	pH level: Chlorine level: Alkalinity level: Temperature: Filter PSI:
	Thursday		pH level: Chlorine level: Alkalinity level: Temperature: Filter PSI:	pH level: Chlorine level: Alkalinity level: Temperature: Filter PSI:
	Friday		pH level: Chlorine level: Alkalinity level: Temperature: Filter PSI:	pH level: Chlorine level: Alkalinity level: Temperature: Filter PSI:

Date	Day	Time	Pool Chemistry	Pool Chemistry
	Saturday		pH level: Chlorine level: Alkalinity level: Temperature: Filter PSI:	pH level: Chlorine level: Alkalinity level: Temperature: Filter PSI:
	Sunday		pH level: Chlorine level: Alkalinity level: Temperature: Filter PSI:	pH level: Chlorine level: Alkalinity level: Temperature: Filter PSI:

Purchase Order Request

Staff completing purchase order request: _____

Day and Date of Request: _____   Time of Request: _____

Signature of staff person making request: _____

Supplier/Vendor Information

Name: _____

Address: _____

_____

Contact person: _____

Phone number: _____   Email: _____

Federal Tax ID #: _____

Have we purchased from this supplier in the past?   _____ Yes   _____ No

Payment terms: _____

Purchase Order Request Detail (attach any applicable forms from supplier)

Item Being Requested	Amount of Item
1.	
2.	
3.	
4.	
5.	
Sub- total	
Freight	
Taxes	
Total Amount of Purchase Order	

Purchase Order Approval Information

Person approving the purchase order: _____

Signature of person approving: _____

Date of approval: _____Purchase Order # Assigned: _____

Date Purchase order placed: _____

Purchase Order and Invoice Verification

Purchase order #: _____ Purchase order amount: _____

Invoice #: _____ Invoice order amount: _____

Variance between purchase order and invoice: _____

Explanation of variance: _____

_____

Person verifying purchase order to invoice: _____

Signature: _____ Date: _____

Maintenance and Repair Service Request Form

Service Order Request Number: _____ Date of Request: _____

Staff Person Requesting Service: _____ Position/title: _____

Signature of staff person requesting service: _____

I.   Description of Service being Requested (completed by person requesting service):

1. Area of the facility:	
2. Piece of equipment (if applicable):	
3. Description of repair/service/work needed:	
4. When repair/service/work needs to be completed:	Day: _____ Date: _____ Time: _____

Please submit this form to the staff person in charge of facilities and equipment and keep a record for the files.

II.   Results of Request (completed by staff person completing the repair/service/work):

1. Name of staff person completing work:	
2. Day, date and time work completed:	
3. Signature of staff person completing work:	

After work is completed, place form in the appropriate file and return copy to the staff person who originally requested the work.

Appendix L: Sample Design and Construction Checklist

I.   FACILITY DESIGN

_____ Select an architect

_____ Complete Agreement with Architect (AIA document B 141 Standard Form of Agreement between Owner and Architect).

_____ Have initial meeting with architect and share strategic conversation and marketing information. Complete architect program questionnaire.

_____ Architect will do Three phases of planning, schematic design, design development and construction documents.

_____ Team should meet with architect once during each of the phases. All plans should be reviewed and signed off on before the next phase begins. Last sign-off is at 90% construction documents.

_____ Identify with architect the need for additional specialists such as landscape architect, civil engineer, acoustical engineer, etc. (Architect provides mechanical, electrical, plumbing, and structural engineers).

_____ Any changes in architect services are to be handled through AIA ASP Form signed by architect and owner.

_____ Architect will work with owner to identify contractors for bidding documents. Bidding should take about three weeks.

_____ Architect and owner should interview each contractor before selecting the final contractor.

_____ Contractor will be selected by owner and architect.

II.   CONSTRUCTION

_____ Once the contractor is selected, a pre-construction meeting is held to review and clarify plans, clarify contract terms and responsibilities, establish timelines, etc.

_____ Sign legal agreement with contractor (AIA Document A101 Standard Form of Agreement between Owner and Contractor for where the Basis of Payment is a Stipulated Sum).

_____ Owner and architect should meet with contractor at least once a month. If club/owner has a construction manager, then the construction manager should meet with the contractor weekly. Meetings should focus on work progress, schedules, delays, inspections, change orders, etc.

_____ Contractor will meet with subs on a weekly basis. Owner should get relevant notes and pictures from meetings.

_____ All clarifications on construction documents are done between architect's construction administrator and contractor's construction manager. Often, contractor will issue a request for Information (RFI) as part of the process.

_____ Any changes to project scope, whether a credit or cost is handled through change orders. Only the architect requests a change order after talking with the owner and contractor. A change order, to be completed, must be approved by both architect and owner. Recommend keeping a change order log.

_____ Contractor will submit monthly pay applications (in triplicate) using standard AIA form. To be paid, the pay application must be notarized, signed by contractor and approved by architect.

_____ Contractor will submit partial lien waivers starting with the second pay application. The liens must match up with previous pay application before current pay application is processed.

_____ Each pay application will have retainage taken out, usually equal to 10% until 50% of the project is completed, after which retainage is reduced to 5%.

_____ Final pay application will be for retainage and must be accompanied by final lien waivers.

_____ Contractor must submit letter of substantial completion when to work at 95% to 98% completed and prior to punch list. All warranties are effective this date.

_____ At completion of construction a punch list is done with architect, owner and contractor. The punch list should be done off the approved construction documents.

_____ Contractor, as part of closing project must conduct an HVAC balance report.

_____ Prior to final contract payment, contractor must provide three sets of closing documents. These contain:

- ❑ As-built construction drawings.
- ❑ All subcontractor warranties on work.
- ❑ All equipment manuals.
- ❑ All permits and certificates.
- ❑ All final lien waivers.
- ❑ Signed punch list and balance report.

Appendix M: Sample Construction Project Budget

Project Phase		Budget		%		Actual
General Construction		**$1,632,292**		**69.9%**		**1,645,400.00**
Construction		$1,522,229				1,522,229.00
Landscape Allowance		$54,825				77,946.00
Contingency/CO's		$55,238				45,225.00
Price per square foot		**$131**				
Fees & Consultants		**$246,048**		**10.5%**		**223,771.00**
Architect and Engineers		$220,000				177,569.00
Permits & Related		$0				12,919.00
CCF&G Fees		$0				0.00
Consultants		$12,000				20,235.00
Landscape architects		$13,048				13,048.00
Marketing & Membership		$0				0.00
Models and Boards		$1,000				
Soft Costs		**$50,088**		**2.1%**		**49,821.00**
Reimbursables		$50,088				49,821.00
FF&E		**$373,118**		**16.0%**		**349,277.00**
Cardiovascular		$69,656				74,780.00
Resistance Circuit		$24,008				24,008.00
Ground Zero		$10,485				10,485.00
Freeweights		$25,240				10,334.00
Spa Equipment		$7,099				16,308.00
Child Care Areas		$6,706				6,847.00
Group Exercise Equipment		$9,647				13,469.00
Office/Business		$5,336				5,026.00
Café & Kitchen		$26,584				29,118.00
Audiovisual Equipment		$30,800				30,724.00
Spa Lounge/Relax		$0				497.00
Lobby furniture		$1,876				2,130.14
Control Desk		$532				512.00
Teen Center		$750				750.00
Women's Locker Room		$0				478.00
General Fitness		$14,185				32,407.00
Computers/phones		$46,394				49,932.00
Freight		$44,595				30,744.00
Tax		$20,810				14,347.00
Laundry		$18,000				18,000.00
Contingency		$10,415				-21,619.14
Miscellaneous Fees		**$32,091**		**1.4%**		**26,586.00**
Start-up Supplies		$32,091				26,586.00
Pre-Opening		$0				0.00
Miscellaneous		$0				0.00
Total Phase One Budget		***$2,333,637***				***2,294,855.00***
Balance Remaining						**$38,782**

Appendix N: Sample Member Satisfaction Survey

2005 Member Satisfaction Survey

DECATHLON CLUB

Please tell us how the following areas of the club are meeting your needs and expectations.
Please rate only those areas that you have experienced personally, otherwise check the "no experience" box.

	Strongly Disagree	Disagree	Neutral	Agree	Strongly Agree	No Experience
Sports Desk						
Greeting is friendly, warm and sincere	1	2	3	4	5	○
Staff is well-trained	1	2	3	4	5	○
Information is readily available	1	2	3	4	5	○
Staff is able to problem solve effectively	1	2	3	4	5	○
Staff is service-oriented	1	2	3	4	5	○
Locker Rooms						
Locker room is kept clean, well-stocked and maintained	1	2	3	4	5	○
Steam room and sauna are kept clean and in working order	1	2	3	4	5	○
Spa is clean and well maintained	1	2	3	4	5	○
Showers are clean and well maintained	1	2	3	4	5	○
Staff is service-oriented	1	2	3	4	5	○
Café						
Quality of food meets expectations	1	2	3	4	5	○
Variety of food meets expectations	1	2	3	4	5	○
Café is kept clean and well maintained	1	2	3	4	5	○
Speed of service meets expectations	1	2	3	4	5	○
Value for your money meets expectations	1	2	3	4	5	○
Staff is service-oriented	1	2	3	4	5	○
Dining Room for Lunch						
Quality of food meets expectations	1	2	3	4	5	○
Variety of food meets expectations	1	2	3	4	5	○
Dining room is kept clean and well maintained	1	2	3	4	5	○
Speed of service meets expectations	1	2	3	4	5	○
Value for your money meets expectations	1	2	3	4	5	○
Staff is service-oriented	1	2	3	4	5	○
Club Activities and Programs						
Club sponsored events are valuable to me	1	2	3	4	5	○
I am satisfied with the parties offered	1	2	3	4	5	○
I am satisfied with the social/athletic outings offered	1	2	3	4	5	○
Programs are effectively promoted	1	2	3	4	5	○
I would like the club to offer more social events	1	2	3	4	5	○

	Strongly Disagree	Disagree	Neutral	Agree	Strongly Agree	No Experience
Business Office						
Staff is professional, knowledgeable and helpful	1	2	3	4	5	○
Staff is able to problem solve effectively	1	2	3	4	5	○
Staff is service-oriented	1	2	3	4	5	○
Tennis						
Tennis courts and surrounding areas are kept clean and well maintained	1	2	3	4	5	○
Pro staff is knowledgeable, enthusiastic and available	1	2	3	4	5	○
I would like the department to offer more social events	1	2	3	4	5	○
The department effectively promotes its programs	1	2	3	4	5	○
I am satisfied with the USTA league structure	1	2	3	4	5	○
I recommend the department to others	1	2	3	4	5	○
Aquatics						
Pool deck and surrounding area are kept clean and well maintained	1	2	3	4	5	○
Water quality in pool and spa meets expectations	1	2	3	4	5	○
I am satisfied with the adult aqua classes	1	2	3	4	5	○
I would like the department to offer more classes, clinics, programs	1	2	3	4	5	○
Staff is service-oriented	1	2	3	4	5	○
Spa						
Massage staff are professional, knowledgeable and helpful	1	2	3	4	5	○
Skin care staff are professional, knowledgeable and helpful	1	2	3	4	5	○
Value for your money meets expectations	1	2	3	4	5	○
Group Exercise Program						
Studios and equipment are kept clean and well maintained	1	2	3	4	5	○
I am satisfied with the variety of classes and programs offered	1	2	3	4	5	○
Staff is knowledgeable, enthusiastic and friendly	1	2	3	4	5	○
The department effectively promotes programs and communicates class changes	1	2	3	4	5	○
Fitness						
The fitness center and equipment are kept clean and well maintained	1	2	3	4	5	○
I am satisfied with the variety of equipment offered	1	2	3	4	5	○
Availability of fitness equipment meets expectations	1	2	3	4	5	○
Staff is knowledgeable, enthusiastic and friendly	1	2	3	4	5	○
Staff is service-oriented	1	2	3	4	5	○
Children's Center						
The center and equipment are kept clean and well maintained	1	2	3	4	5	○
Staff is knowledgeable, enthusiastic and friendly	1	2	3	4	5	○
The security/safety of the center meets expectations	1	2	3	4	5	○
I would like the department to offer more programs	1	2	3	4	5	○

	Strongly Disagree	Disagree	Neutral	Agree	Strongly Agree	No Experience
Squash						
The squash courts and surrounding area are kept clean and well maintained	1	2	3	4	5	○
Pro staff is knowledgeable, enthusiastic and available	1	2	3	4	5	○
I am satisfied with the variety of programs offered	1	2	3	4	5	○
The department effectively promotes its programs	1	2	3	4	5	○
I recommend the department to others	1	2	3	4	5	○
Pro Shop						
Staff is friendly, knowledgeable and enthusiastic	1	2	3	4	5	○
The Pro Shop carries merchandise that meets my needs	1	2	3	4	5	○
Staff is service-oriented	1	2	3	4	5	○
Gymnasium						
The gymnasium is kept clean and well maintained	1	2	3	4	5	○
I am satisfied with the variety of programs offered	1	2	3	4	5	○
Decathlon Club Overall						
I am satisfied with the overall club appearance	1	2	3	4	5	○
The club is kept clean and well maintained	1	2	3	4	5	○
Repairs and maintenance are completed quickly and efficiently	1	2	3	4	5	○
Staff is knowledgeable, friendly and enthusiastic	1	2	3	4	5	○
Value for your money meets expectations	1	2	3	4	5	○
The club meets my needs and expectations	1	2	3	4	5	○
Staff is service-oriented	1	2	3	4	5	○

Please share with us your experience with other Decathlon Club programs and services.

	Aware of		Have Tried		Will Try		Not Interested	
	Yes	No	Yes	No	Yes	No	Yes	No
Pilates								
Individual	○	○	○	○	○	○	○	○
Group Allegro	○	○	○	○	○	○	○	○
Group Mat	○	○	○	○	○	○	○	○
Personal Fitness Training								
Individual	○	○	○	○	○	○	○	○
Group	○	○	○	○	○	○	○	○
Bay Sport								
Physical Therapy	○	○	○	○	○	○	○	○
Executive Physical Exam	○	○	○	○	○	○	○	○
Cholesterol Screening	○	○	○	○	○	○	○	○
Complimentary Injury Check	○	○	○	○	○	○	○	○

	Aware of		Have Tried		Will Try		Not Interested	
	Yes	No	Yes	No	Yes	No	Yes	No
Adult Swim Classes								
Individual	○	○	○	○	○	○	○	○
Group	○	○	○	○	○	○	○	○
Nutrition Consultation w/Dietician	○	○	○	○	○	○	○	○
Yoga Classes	○	○	○	○	○	○	○	○
Gymnasium								
Basketball Leagues	○	○	○	○	○	○	○	○
Badminton Individual Lessons	○	○	○	○	○	○	○	○
Badminton Group Lessons	○	○	○	○	○	○	○	○
Social/Athletic								
Golf outings	○	○	○	○	○	○	○	○
Club seminars	○	○	○	○	○	○	○	○
Club parties	○	○	○	○	○	○	○	○
Electronic Funds Transfer	○	○	○	○	○	○	○	○

(Automatic payment from your checking account)

The following questions are for classification purposes only:

Gender: _____Male _____Female   Age: _____   Please indicate the year you joined DC: _____

How many visits to the Club do you make during a typical week? _____

What time of day do you most frequently utilize the Club? _____before 9:00am _____9–12:00pm _____12:00–4:00pm _____4:00–8:00pm _____8:00pm–close

What type of membership do you have? _____Individual _____Family _____Racquet _____Fitness

Please circle your two most preferred methods for the Club to communicate with you about programs and events.

Special Mailing	Statement Insert	Email	Sports Desk Bulletin
Club Bulletin Boards/Posters	Newsletter	DC Website	Activity Information Center

What one improvement would make visiting the Club a significantly better experience for you?

_____

_____

Please share any additional comments you may have.

_____

_____

Optional: We may wish to contact you about a comment or suggestion that you've made.

Name: _____   Member number: _____

Email address: _____

Thank you for your comments! Please return completed survey by December 31, 2005.

Appendix O: Sample Corporate Sales Checklist

Step 1   Decide What It Is You Are Going To Sell

        _____ Memberships
        _____ Brown bags
        _____ Seminars
        _____ HRAs
        _____ Testing

Step 2   Develop A Presentation Package That Can Be Used During Any Initial Contacts

        _____ Industry data on savings achieved
        _____ Pamphlet and/or sheet on services
        _____ Club brochure
        _____ Business cards
        _____ Generic Sales Presentation

Step 3   Target Your Companies

        _____ Companies already using Club or with Member in the Club
        _____ Local Chamber business listing
        _____ Utilize specific criteria outlined in handbook and prioritize!

Step 4   Learn All You Can About The Companies

        _____ Interviews with Members
        _____ Check with PR departments
        _____ Library
        _____ Chamber information

Step 5   Decide What It Is You Want To Accomplish With Your First Contact

        _____ Make a sale
        _____ Get an appointment to introduce your services
        _____ Get them to visit the club

Step 6   Getting the First Appointment

        _____ Get current Member to arrange Appointment
        _____ Write a short letter as outlined
        _____ Include with you letter a nice reminder item (book, etc.)
        _____ Make sure you will follow-up with a call; give day and
                  time period (Tuesday through Thursday)
        _____ Make the follow-up phone call.
        _____ Send a thank you after scheduling appointment
        _____ Follow-up regularly and include small gift

Step 7   The First Appointment: Make It Work For You

        _____ Get them to the Club if you can
        _____ Bring a generic presentation package
        _____ Make sure you bring your homework on the company
        _____ Arrive early

_____ Bring a partner
_____ Keep presentation short and to the point
_____ Get a commitment for a next step
_____ Listen for needs

Step 8 <u>Immediate Appreciation Is A Hallmark Of Any Appointment</u>

_____ Send a brief handwritten thank you upon returning to the Club
_____ Express appreciation for their time and let them know when your proposal will arrive

Step 9 <u>Get Your Proposal In The Person's Hands</u>

_____ Customize your proposal and include

• Executive Summary
• Services/products you will provide
• Delivery system for services
• Timetable
• Benefits
• List of clients
• List of Members who work for that company
• Fees and schedules

_____ Deliver your proposal in person. Try to hand it to the person who makes the decision.
_____ Send proposal only if delivering in person is impossible. Your proposal must be accompanied by a cover that outlines your next step, including date(s) of follow-up.

Step 10 <u>Follow-Up Your Proposal With A Call</u>

_____ Allow two or three weeks before you call
_____ Find out their feelings toward the proposal
_____ Answer any questions
_____ Try to schedule an appointment
_____ Continue to follow-up

Step 11 <u>Taking Your Proposal To An Agreement</u>

_____ Make your next appointment effective by being prepared for further questions
_____ Realize that you may have to make additional presentations before signing
_____ Have an agreement prepared ahead of time in the event you have a chance to sign
_____ Realize it might take six to twelve months to finalize

Step 12 <u>Service the Sale</u>

_____ Deliver what you promise
_____ Provide regular feedback to the company
_____ Maintain contact with company representatives
_____ Perform evaluation of their services

Appendix P: Selected Health/Fitness Industry Programming Practices

The programs featured in this appendix are examples of programming that has been conducted successfully in various clubs in the health/fitness industry.

❑ **4th of July Member Classic**

I. Program Overview
- 5K & 1 mile races through community

II. Program Specifics

A. Program Goals:
- Gain exposure for the club in the community; the local paper includes articles on it which can lead to new members and revenue leads
- Promote wellness in the club; help increase retention

B. Equipment/Facility Needs:
- 5K & 1 mile courses, timing system, pace vehicle

C. Number of Members/Guests Participating:
- 140—50% of which were members

D. Marketing/Promotion Actions:
- Running magazines
- Newsletter/e-mail blasts
- Past-participants
- Banners & fliers throughout the community and club
- Registration at www.active.com

E. Fee Charged:
- $18/$16/$13 (per member)
- $18/$16/$13 (per guest)

F. Number of Staff Involved:
- 7-10 staff involved

III. Revenue & Expense = Profitability

A. Program Revenues:
- # of participants: 140
- Revenue per participant (fee): Approximately $15 per person
- Sponsorship: Donated food items and $1000
- Total revenues: $3,410

B. Program Expenses:
- Marketing promotions: $100
- Supplies: $50
- Awards: Trophies for the overall winner and for each age division; T-shirts, food, and drinks after the race for participants—$900 total
- Payroll (average time & average payroll dollars): $200
- Total expenses: $1,250

C. Program Net: $1,850

IV. The Keys That MADE IT WORK
- Good advertising using websites and running magazines

- Flexible staff—staff takes pride in gaining exposure for the club
- Good location for course—private gated community
- Active community—relatively young community with health conscience people
- Past successes—runners enjoy the race and return each year

❑ 5k Club

I. Program Overview

This club was designed to take the hassle out of running in 5K races. We pick certain 5K races to run every month and advertise the 5K throughout the club. Members are able to register for the race here at the club and can charge the registration fee to their membership account. We pick up the race packets for them and make them available at the pro shop five days before the race. After each race on Saturday mornings, members that participated come back to the club for breakfast. This program gets great reception because it's easy for members to participate in the races and it gives them a chance to meet other members interested in running.

II. Program Specifics

A. Program Goals:
- Achieve member-to-member connections through 5K race and breakfast participation
- Make it convenient for the members to participate in 5K races that support community events and charities

B. Equipment/Facility Needs:
- Club dining facility

C. Number of Members/Guests Participating:
- 15-20 people per race

D. Marketing/Promotion Actions:
- Each 5K that we participate in is posted in the club newsletter
- Different 5K club fliers for each race are posted throughout the club
- Message on hold phone system advertising the 5K club

E. Fee Charged:
- Members are charged $5 above the cost of the race registration. This club does not generate a lot of revenue, but it is a great retention tool.

F. Number of Staff Involved: 2

III. Revenue & Expense = Profitability

A. Program Revenues:
- # of Participants: About 15-20 members
- Revenue per Participant (fee): $5
- Sponsor dollars (if any): $0
- Total revenues: $5 per person

B. Program Expenses:
- Marketing promotions: We print fliers in-house and post throughout the club. We also put information in the newsletter and on the message on hold system
- Supplies: $5 per person covers the food cost for the breakfast that we serve after each race
- Total expenses: $5 per person

C. Program Net:
- Program does not generate any revenue but rather serves as a member retention tool

❏ After-School Activity Camp

I. Program Overview
- A fun-filled day of outdoor activities, arts, crafts, and lunch for the kids.

II. Program Specifics

A. Program Goals:
- Gain recognition in community
- Grow membership
- Generate revenue – generated $85,000 in first year

B. Equipment/Facility Needs:
- Areas for activities: Open field, swimming pool, basketball court, etc.

C. Number of Members/Guests Participating:
- About 150 different children participate in some degree; 80% are children of members

D. Marketing/Promotion Actions:
- Local neighborhood paper
- Folders at the local elementary school
- Fliers/e-mail blasts
- Personal phone calls
- Newsletter

E. Fee Charged:
- $115/$145 (per member)
- $145/$195 (per guest)

F. Number of Staff Involved: 2-8 people involved

III. Revenue & Expense = Profitability

A. Program Revenues:
- # of participants: 150
- Revenue per participant (fee): $115-$195
- Sponsor dollars (if any): Food items are donated
- Total revenues: $85,000

B. Program Expenses:
- Marketing Promotions: $200 for local paper
- Supplies: Food/art supplies = $1,000/yr
- Payroll * (average time & average payroll dollars): $42,000/yr.
- Total Expenses: $43,000/yr.

C. Program Net: $42,000

IV. The Keys That MADE IT WORK
- The hard work of our youth program coordinator who takes pride in his work
- Flexible, consistent staff
- Great promotions—mail database has helped a great deal
- Active community—a young working community with lots of young kids
- Location—elementary school target market is nearby

❏ **Anniversary Gala**

I. Program Overview

In November 2001, the Club hosted a gala in celebration of the 20th anniversary of the club. For the occasion, we had eight sports celebrities serve on an honorary committee as well as the Stanley and the Grey Cup on hand. The club invited approximately 4,000 people (including current & past members and the business community at large). Over 1,900 invitees attended the event that was featured live on KRDS (TV) with a lot of publicity provided via the press for days both before and after the event.

II. Program Specifics

A. Program Goals:
- Generate membership leads through exposure to the club
- Generated press for the club

B. Equipment/Facility Needs:
- A stage, sound system, giant screens, bars, DJ, coat check/racks, decoration, red carpet, outside light system, limo, etc.

C. Number of Members/Guests Participating: 1,900

D. Marketing/Promotion Actions:
- Traditional invitations, e-mail invitations and a media kit were produced and sent delivered. Posters, banners were prominent throughout the club
- Follow-up phone calls to all guests, members, and media
- Sponsored gift to everyone (sponsored by Roots). Business cards were collected for door prizes (and for follow-up of course).
- Along with their gift they received a guest pass, and an invitation to "Save $150.00 on Initiation Fees!"
- Link to a referral program in December, January, and February

E. Fee Charged: $0

F. Number of Personnel Involved: Approximately 50 people (staff and volunteers)

III. Revenue & Expense = Profitability

A. Program Revenues:
- # of participants: 1,900
- Revenue per participant (fee): $0—but we had at least 85 tours linked to the event, and approximately 50 new members signed-up in the following months ($50,000).
- Sponsor dollars (if any): Over $30,000 in money and supplies, and another $100,000 in free media publicity
- Total revenues: $50,000 to date

B. Program Expenses:
- Marketing promotions: $5,000
- Supplies: $15,000
- Awards: 0
- Payroll (average time & average payroll dollars): $2,000 (with over 40 volunteers)
- Total Expenses: $20,000

C. Program Net: $30,000 to date

IV. The Keys That MADE IT WORK

- The unique positioning of the club in this market place
- The strong names on the honorary committee
- Our contact list of sponsors and suppliers and VIP's
- Very strong, creative visuals
- Staff working on making it happen

❑ Birthday Parties & Sleepovers

I. Program Overview

Birthday parties and sleepovers at the club are a huge success due to the careful planning and an enthusiastic team to execute the parties. We cater to every party need and provide a high-energy party that all will remember. We are as flexible as the member needs us to be and always set out to offer the best Member service possible.

II. Program Specifics

A. Program Goals:
- To offer a party that both the parents and kids will remember forever. To cater to all member needs and be as flexible as possible, without losing the profit margin
- To constantly reevaluate the party structure and consistently offer the best parties possible

B. Equipment/Facility Needs:
- Party room with decorations—gift table, food table, soft seating area for parents
- A cozy and high-energy party atmosphere

C. Number of Members/Guests Participating:
- 15 - 20 children; 2 - 6 adults - birthday parties
- 20 -120 children; 25 adults – sleepovers

D. Marketing/Promotion Actions:
- Fliers around the club. Information in the newsletter
- Targeted Girl Scouts—promoted through direct contact with troop leaders
- Word of mouth
- Parties in a visible location for self-promotion
- Discounts in newsletter for parties

E. Fee Charged:
- $20 to $35 per person, depending on the type of party (A $300 facility fee is assessed for sleepovers)

F. Number of Staff Involved:
- 1 – 5 depending on the size of the party and the number of participants

III. Revenue & Expense = Profitability

A. Program Revenues:
- # of participants - Birthday party (minimum of 10 participants), sleepovers (minimum of 15 participants), adults (1-25 participants)
- Revenue per participant (fee): $20-$35/ per person
- Total revenues: Varies, based on the size of the party

B. Program Expenses:
- Marketing promotions: Paper cost
- Supplies equipment costs: all products for party—paper products, décor, food

- Awards: $0
- Payroll: Average $7 per hour, per extra person—3-4 hours for birthday parties; 13 hours for sleepovers
- Total expenses: Between $50 and $100 per birthday party and from $600 - $800 for sleepovers

C. Program Net:
- Varies; usually about a 50-60% profit for both types of programs. Most of the sleepover revenue is generated during hours we are usually closed.

IV. The Keys That MADE IT WORK

- PROMOTION
- Enthusiastic extra personnel to work every party
- Planner with the resources to handle all party needs
- Planning and preparation
- Flexibility

❑ Boxing Night

I. Program Overview: Amateur boxing night; 10 bouts – 3 minutes each; roast beef dinner; awards

II. Program Specifics

A. Program Goals:
- Sell out the event
- Ensure that participants get their money's worth

B. Equipment/Facility Needs:
- Boxing ring
- Awards and trophies
- Referees
- Physician on standby

C. Number of Members/Guests Participating:
- 200 participants total (including guests)

D. Marketing/Promotion Actions:
- Found a sponsor (La Queue de Cheval)
- Posters
- Billing statement stuffer
- Word of mouth advertising
- Staff promotion

E. Fee Charged:
- $50 per member or $60 per table
- 8 people per table; 20 tables

F. Staff Involved:
- F&B staff, logistics staff, maintenance.

III. Revenue & Expense = Profitability

A. Program Revenues:
- # of participants - 160

- Revenue from Fees: $12,000
- Sponsor dollars (if any): $1,000
- Total revenues: $13,000

B. Program Expenses:
- Supplies: $3,500
- Awards: $500
- Payroll: $720
- Total expenses: $4,720

C. Program net: $8,280

IV. The Keys That MADE IT WORK
- Good concept
- Strong marketing and visuals
- Fits within the club's environment
- Teamwork
- Flawless execution

❏ Cross-Training Challenge

I. Program Overview
To offer a fun, current, and educational approach to group exercise.

II. Program Specifics

A. Program Goals:
- To encourage members to cross-train throughout the club
- Increase group-exercise participation

B. Equipment/Facility Needs:
- Dumbbells, bands, tubing, steps, spin bikes, mats, jump ropes, medicine balls

C. Number of Members/Guests Participating:
- 120 sign-ups; 86 participants

D. Marketing/Promotion Actions:
- Prizes
- Posters
- Word of mouth
- Professionalism
- Fliers

E. Fee Charged: None

F. Staff Involved: All group-exercise staff (approximately 25)

III. Revenue & Expense = Profitability

A. Program Revenues:
- Sponsor dollars: $500 for prizes

B. Program Expenses:
- Awards (t-shirts) $500
- Total expenses $500

C. Program Net: $0

IV. The Keys That MADE IT WORK
- Staff & participant enthusiasm
- Following current trends
- Education of staff
- Teamwork
- Prizes

❑ Fibromyalgia Seminar

I. Program Overview
We teamed up with our physical therapy staff to produce a seminar on fibromylagia. The staff brought in a physician to speak on the subject and the club supplied wellness professionals from different areas, including massage, personal training, yoga, and aquatics.

II. Program Specifics
A. Program Goals:
- Educate members and guests concerning fibromyalgia
- Provide an opportunity to give relief to those afflicted by symptoms of this syndrome
- Generate revenue (future and immediate) for the club in potential Membership growth and through non-member class enrollment

B. Equipment/Facility Needs:
- Large group-exercise room and seven tables, 35-40 chairs

C. Number of Members/Guests Participating:
- Approximately 20 members/20 guests came to the seminar. Three people signed up for the water therapy class (12 sessions for $40.00). Ten people requested to be contacted about membership.

D. Marketing/Promotion Actions:
- Sign on the marquee
- Pass out interest sheets (e.g., who would be interested in...)
- Fliers mailed to everybody who replied to interest sheets
- Club newsletter article
- Promotional pamphlets placed in strategic locations throughout the club, at public places, and other affiliated health offices

E. Fee Charged: $0

F. Number of Staff Involved:
- One personal trainer, one massage therapist/yoga instructor, four physical therapists

III. Revenue & Expense = Profitability

A. Program Revenues:
- # of participants: 35
- Revenue per participant (fee): $0
- Sponsor dollars (if any): $0
- Total revenues: Three people signed-up for the class we offered in conjunction with the seminar (water therapy Class) $120.00 + 10 leads for membership.

B. Program Expenses:
- Marketing Promotions: One ream of paper for fliers
- Supplies $0
- Awards: $0
- Payroll: 1-hour meetings at lunch and outside lunch prep time, 20 hrs. @ avg. of 10.00 per hour
- Total expenses: $206

IV. The Keys That MADE IT WORK

- Dedicated health and wellness professionals with a genuine concern for the
- participants
- Ability of fitness staff to work with physical therapy staff to reach target market
- Being aware of the membership growth opportunity provided through marketing this type of seminar to non-members. If and when they join, these new members are then already aware of some of the services we offer that can help them as an individual.
- Recording/polling interests of the participants at the seminar allows us to find out if they want the club to contact them with further information about membership.
- Partnering local healthcare professionals with personal trainers, massage therapists, etc. Many people are asked by their physicians/physical therapists to maintain lifestyle changes but are left on their own to find a medium to accomplish this. By bringing this seminar to our club, we market ourselves attractively as a place where these people can help facilitate a change in their lives and have a positive experience in an inviting environment.

❏ Fitness Holiday

I. Program Overview
A holiday-style program emphasizing healthy living. Included are many activities (indoor and outdoor) that exercise and educate the client. In addition, there is also a daily cooking course complete with a chef where clients learn how to prepare healthy, delicious meals.

II. Program Specifics
A. Program Goals:
- Provide clients with a healthy week of exercise and diet
- Educate clients on healthy living
- Everything should be fun and social

B. Equipment/Facility Needs:
- A chalet rental in Whistler, Canada. All exercise equipment such as bikes, skis, extra would be rented.

C. Number of Members/Guests Participating: 12 clients

D. Marketing/Promotion Actions:
- Signage throughout the club
- Articles and advertisement in newsletter
- Informational seminars
- Encouragement from personal trainers

E. Fee Charged: $4,500 per week

F. Staff Involved: Two fitness staff and chef

III. Revenue & Expense = Profitability

A. Program Revenues
- # of Participants: 12
- Revenue per participant (fee): $4,500
- Total revenues: $54,000

B. Program Expenses
- Marketing promotions: $1,000
- Supplies; accommodations and rentals: $15,000
- Flights: $9,000
- Payroll (average time & average payroll $): $5,000
- Total Expenses: $30,000

C. Program Net: $24,000

IV. The Keys That MADE IT WORK
- Great idea
- Organization
- Quality staff
- Great location

❏ Hell Week is Back Again

I. Program Overview

A program not for the weak of mind or body—Hell Week is Back Again! This military boot camp-style class, lead by our top instructor, challenges anyone who dares to take it. Each participant is take to their limit and loves it. The week is made up of five mornings each with 1-hour workout sessions. Workouts are group-oriented and physically challenging. Each workout begins with a 2-3 mile jog, followed by a total-body workout. The end of "Hell Week" ends with 15-20 minutes of games and other team activities. All participants receive a "Hell Week" T-shirt. There is a $40 charge for this "Mission Impossible!" Proceeds benefit St. Jude's Children's Hospital.

II. Program Specifics

A. Marketing/Promotion Actions:
- Fliers entitled, "Hell Week is Back Again!" were made and placed strategically throughout the fitness center.
- A large poster was made featuring a picture of the instructor in full military fatigues and face paint with the slogan;—"We Want You!"—placed in the reception area.
- All fitness specialists were asked to suggest this class to their clients.
- Featured in our monthly newsletter

B. Fee Charged: $40 per member

III. Revenue & Expense = Profitability

A. Program Revenues: Total revenues $600

B. Program Expenses: Total expenses $410

C. Program Net: $190

☐ Introduction to Hot Stone Therapy

I. Program Overview

Hot stone therapy has become extremely popular in the spa/massage marketplace. The use of heated basalt lava stones allows for a therapeutic, yet profoundly relaxing massage. The introduction of this service to members has expanded the club's scope of massage services it provides. Where members may have gone elsewhere to receive this service previously, they now are now able to enjoy (and pay for access to) Hot Stone Therapy at SMC.

II. Program Specifics

A. Program Goals:
- Expand clubs massage services, appeal to a wider scope of members
- Create a volume and rate variance above and beyond past budgets

B. Equipment/Facility Needs:
- Existing rooms are used. Additions include roasters, stones, and cleaning supplies.

C. Number of Members/Guests Participating:
- Out of the total number of massages over the last month, hot stone therapy has been utilized by 3% of members taking advantage of massage program.

D. Marketing/Promotion Actions
- Signage and fliers
- Mini - demonstrations with hot stones to membership and staff
- Front-desk staff prompting members when they call for an appointment

E. Fee Charged: $ 85 (member), $ 95 (guest)

F. Number of Staff Involved:
- Initially one therapist; subsequently, four therapists will be able to provide service.

III. Revenue & Expense = Profitability

A. Program Revenues:
- Total revenues: $850

B. Program Expenses:
- Total expenses: $414

C. Program Net:
- After payroll, the club has broken even after just 10 sessions.

IV. The Keys That MADE IT WORK
- Increased availability by therapists
- Education and exposure to new service
- Quality, consistent service

PROGRAM BEST PRACTICES
BENCHMARK FORM

Club Name:_____   Contact Name:_____

Telephone:_____   Fax:_____

Email:_____

I.   Program Title:

II.   Program Overview (limit one paragraph):

III.   Program Specifics

      A.   Program Goals:

      B.   Equipment/Facility Needs:

      C.   Number of Members/Guests Participating (if personal training list # sessions weekly and % of total membership)

D. Marketing/Promotion Actions (list specific actions you took to market the program and sign-up of participants

1.	
2.	
3.	
4.	
5.	

E. Number of Staff Involved

IV. Revenue & Expense = Profitability

Revenues		Expenses & Net	
# Participants		Payroll	
Fee Charged		Commissions	
Revenue from Fees		Other Expenses	
Other Revenue (sponsor)		Total Expenses	
Total Revenue		Program Net	

V. The Five Keys That MADE IT WORK

1.	
2.	
3.	
4.	
5.	

Please attach any marketing materials or related materials used in delivering and marketing your program.

Appendix Q: Selected Risk Management Forms*

Club Name
Authorization for Release of Protected Health information

I, _____, hereby authorize _____
to release the following health information:

[ ]

and forward it to the following person/facility:

Name or person or facility: _____

Address (street, city, state and zip code): _____

[ ]

Phone #: _____ Email: _____

This information is for the purpose of:

[ ]

This authorization is in effect until _____, when it expires.

I understand that by signing this authorization:

- o I authorize the use or disclosure of my individually identifiable health information as described above for the purpose listed. I understand that authorization is voluntary.
- o I understand the notice of Privacy Practices provides instructions should I choose to revoke my authorization.
- o I understand that if the organization I have authorized to receive the information is not a health plan or health care provider, the released information may no longer be protected by federal privacy regulations.
- o I understand that I have the right to receive a copy of this authorization.
- o I understand that I am signing this authorization voluntarily and that treatment, payment, or eligibility for my benefits will not be affected if I do not sign this authorization.

I DECLARE UNDER PENALTY OF PERJURY THAT THE INFORMATION ON THIS FORM IS TRUE AND CORRECT.

SIGNATURE: _____ **DATE:** _____

*Because the selected risk management forms in this appendix can represent a form of legal document, before using, them legal counsel should reivew them concerning their application to state and local laws, which can vary from location to location.

ACTIVITY RELEASE AND INDEMNITY AGREEMENT - ADULT

THIS RELEASE AND INDEMNITY AGREEMENT ("Release") is made by the undersigned adult (the "Participant"), to release and indemnify _____, a _____ corporation, its parent company, affiliated or subsidiary companies, and all their respective officers, directors, agents, contractors, employees, heirs, successors, and assigns (collectively, the "Club"), as set forth below.

1. **Activity**. Participant, on Participant's own behalf and on behalf of the other members of Participant's family, including Participant's spouse, parents, children, heirs, and assigns, (singularly and collectively referred to as "Participant") hereby grants to the Club this full release and indemnification as consideration in exchange for permitting Participant to participate in the following athletic or physical activity which may utilize Club premises and/or equipment (the "Activity"): _____.

Participant is entering into this Release after (i) having viewed or having had the opportunity to view Club premises and/or equipment; (ii) if there is an instructor, having reviewed or having had the opportunity to review the instructor's qualifications; (iii) having had the scope of the services and/or the associated risks explained to Participant; and/or (iv) having had an opportunity to ask questions regarding the services and/or the risks associated with the Activity.

2. **Release and Indemnity**.

- PARTICIPANT IS VOLUNTARILY PARTICIPATING IN THE ACTIVITY WITH FULL KNOWLEDGE, UNDERSTANDING AND APPRECIATION OF THE RISKS OF INJURY INHERENT IN ANY PHYSICAL EXERCISE, MASSAGE OR THERAPY PROGRAM, PHYSICAL ACTIVITY OR ATHLETIC ACTIVITY AND EXPRESSLY ASSUMES ALL RISKS OF INJURY AND EVEN DEATH WHICH COULD OCCUR BY REASON OF PARTICIPANT'S PARTICIPATION.

- PARTICIPANT RELEASES CLUB FROM ANY LIABILITY AND AGREES NOT TO SUE CLUB WITH RESPECT TO ANY CAUSE OF ACTION FOR BODILY INJURY, PROPERTY DAMAGE, OR DEATH OCCURRING TO PARTICIPANT AS A RESULT OF PARTICIPATING IN THE ACTIVITY.

- PARTICIPANT HEREBY ASSUMES FULL RESPONSIBILITY FOR RISKS OF BODILY INJURY, PROPERTY DAMAGE OR DEATH TO PARTICIPANT DUE TO THE ORDINARY NEGLIGENCE OR GROSS NEGLIGENCE OF THE CLUB AND THE ORDINARY NEGLIGENCE, GROSS NEGLIGENCE, OR WILLFUL MISCONDUCT OF ANY THIRD PARTY INCLUDING OTHERS PARTICIPATING IN THE ACTIVITY.

- PARTICIPANT AGREES TO INDEMNIFY, DEFEND, AND HOLD HARMLESS, AT PARTICIPANT'S SOLE COST, THE CLUB FROM ANY AND ALL CLAIMS ARISING OUT OF PARTICIPANT'S PARTICIPATION IN THE ACTIVITY.

- ALL PERSONAL PROPERTY BROUGHT TO THE ACTIVITY, IS BROUGHT AT THE SOLE RISK OF PARTICIPANT AS TO ITS THEFT, DAMAGE, OR LOSS.

3. **Medical**. Participant consents to emergency medical care and transportation in order to obtain treatment in the event of injury to Participant as the Club may deem appropriate. This Release extends to any liability arising out of or in any way connected with the medical treatment and transportation provided in the event of an emergency.

4. **Severability**. Participant expressly agrees that the terms of release and indemnity contained herein are intended to be as broad and inclusive as is permitted by the laws of the state in which Club operates its business. Any provision or portion of this Release found to be invalid by the courts having jurisdiction shall be invalid only with respect to such provision or portion. The offending provision or portion shall be construed to the maximum extent possible to confer upon the parties the benefits intended thereby. Said provision or portion, as well as the remaining provisions or portion hereof, shall be construed and enforced to the same effect as if such offending provision or portion thereof had not been contained herein.

PARTICIPANT HAS READ AND VOLUNTARILY SIGNS THIS RELEASE AND INDEMNITY AGREEMENT.

PARTICIPANT:

_____
Signature

_____
Printed Name

_____
Date

ACTIVITY RELEASE AND INDEMNITY AGREEMENT - MINOR

THIS RELEASE AND INDEMNITY AGREEMENT ("Release") is made by the undersigned adult, as parent or legal guardian (the "Representative") of the below listed minor(s) (the "Participant"), to release and indemnify _____, a _____ corporation, its parent company, affiliated or subsidiary companies , and all their respective officers, directors, agents, contractors, employees, heirs, successors, and assigns (collectively, the "Club"), as set forth below.

1. **Activity**. Representative, on Participant's behalf and on behalf of the other members of Representative's family, including Representative's spouse, parents, children, heirs, and assigns, (singularly and collectively referred to as "Representative") hereby grants to the Club this full release and indemnification as consideration in exchange for permitting Participant to participate in the following athletic or physical activity which may utilize Club premises and/or equipment (the "Activity"): _____.

Representative, on Participant's behalf, is entering into this Release after (i) having viewed or having had the opportunity to view Club premises and/or equipment; (ii) if there is an instructor, having reviewed or having had the opportunity to review the instructor's qualifications; (iii) having had the scope of the services and/or the associated risks explained to Participant; and/or (iv) having had an opportunity to ask questions regarding the services and/or risks associated with the Activity.

2. **Release and Indemnity**.

   • **REPRESENTATIVE PERMITS PARTICIPANT TO PARTICIPATE IN THE ACTIVITY WITH FULL KNOWLEDGE, UNDERSTANDING AND APPRECIATION OF THE RISKS OF INJURY INHERENT IN ANY PHYSICAL EXERCISE PROGRAM, MASSAGE OR THERAPY PROGRAM, PHYSICAL ACTIVITY OR ATHLETIC ACTIVITY AND EXPRESSLY ASSUMES ALL RISKS OF INJURY AND EVEN DEATH WHICH COULD OCCUR BY REASON OF PARTICIPANT'S PARTICIPATION.**

   • **REPRESENTATIVE RELEASES CLUB FROM ANY LIABILITY AND AGREES NOT TO SUE CLUB WITH RESPECT TO ANY CAUSE OF ACTION FOR BODILY INJURY, PROPERTY DAMAGE, OR DEATH OCCURRING TO PARTICIPANT AS A RESULT OF PARTICIPATING IN THE ACTIVITY.**

   • **REPRESENTATIVE HEREBY ASSUMES FULL RESPONSIBILITY FOR RISKS OF BODILY INJURY, PROPERTY DAMAGE OR DEATH TO PARTICIPANT DUE TO THE ORDINARY NEGLIGENCE OR GROSS NEGLIGENCE OF THE CLUB AND THE ORDINARY NEGLIGENCE, GROSS NEGLIGENCE, OR WILLFUL MISCONDUCT OF ANY THIRD PARTY INCLUDING OTHERS PARTICIPATING IN THE ACTIVITY.**

   • **REPRESENTATIVE AGREES TO INDEMNIFY, DEFEND, AND HOLD HARMLESS, AT REPRESENTATIVE'S SOLE COST, THE CLUB FROM ANY AND ALL CLAIMS ARISING OUT OF PARTICIPANT'S PARTICIPATION IN THE ACTIVITY.**

   • **ALL PERSONAL PROPERTY BROUGHT TO THE ACTIVITY, IS BROUGHT AT THE SOLE RISK OF PARTICIPANT AS TO ITS THEFT, DAMAGE, OR LOSS.**

3. **Medical**. Representative on Participant's behalf, consents to emergency medical care and transportation in order to obtain treatment in the event of injury to Participant as the Club may deem appropriate. This Release extends to any liability arising out of or in any way connected with the medical treatment and transportation provided in the event of an emergency.

4. **Severability**. Representative expressly agrees that the terms of release and indemnity contained herein are intended to be as broad and inclusive as is permitted by the laws of the state in which Club operates its business. Any provision or portion of this Release found to be invalid by the courts having jurisdiction shall be invalid only with respect to such provision or portion. The offending provision or portion shall be construed to the maximum extent possible to confer upon the parties the benefits intended thereby. Said provision or portion, as well as the remaining provisions or portion hereof shall be construed and enforced to the same effect as if such offending provision or portion thereof had not been contained herein.

REPRESENTATIVE HAS READ AND VOLUNTARILY SIGNS THIS RELEASE AND INDEMNITY AGREEMENT.

PARTICIPANT(S):   **REPRESENTATIVE**:

_____   _____
Printed Name   Signature

_____   _____
Printed Name   Printed Name

_____   _____
Printed Name   Date

IDENTIFYING INFORMATION

_____ Copy of identification attached.

Type of identification: _____
(e.g. driver's license, birth certificate, passport, federal ID card, managed care card, etc.)

Number on identification: _____

IF NO IDENTIFICATION IS ATTACHED, YOUR SIGNATURE MUST BE NOTARIZED.

Notarized by: _____

On: _____

Notary Public Number: _____

NOTARY MUST STAMP IN THE SPACE PROVIDED

Cardiovascular Health Pre-Activity Screening

For each of the following questions, please place a check by each item that has direct application to you..

_____   Age: Men>45   Women>55

_____   Family History: MI or sudden death before 55 years of age for father or other first degree male
                   Relative or 65 years of age for mother or female first degree relative.

_____   Cigarette Smoker: (Current or have quit in the previous 6 – months)

_____   Dyslipidemia: Blood cholesterol>200 mg/dl
                (one or more of the   LDL cholesterol>130 mg/dl
                Following)   HDL<40 mg/dl
                                        LDL/HDL ratio>3 to 1
                                        Triglycerides>150

_____   Hypertension: Blood Pressure – systolic $\geq$ 140 or diastolic $\geq$90
                                           on blood pressure medication.

_____   Impaired Fasting Glucose: Fasting glucose $\geq$ or presence of diabetes

_____   Sedentary lifestyle: Do not participate in at least 30 minutes of moderate physical
                                         activity at least 3x a week.

_____   Obesity: BMI > 30,
                                      Waist circumference > 102 cm for men and > 88 cm for women

---

Place a check the appropriate category that applies to this indivudal.

_____   **Low Risk:**   Men < 45 years of age and women < 55 years of age who are asymptomatic and have no more
                                than one risk factor as indicated above..

_____   **Moderate Risk:**   Men > 45 years of age and women > 55 years of age or those who have two or more
                                risk factors as indicated above.

_____   **High Risk:**   Individuals with one or more symptoms of cardiovascular disease or known cardiovascular,
                                metabolic or pulmonary disease.

Any individual classified as either moderate risk or high risk needs to receive a physician's clearance prior to participating in a program of structured physical activity.

** Physician's Note Required**   Date Contacted: _____

Emergency Medical Authorization
Adult

I hereby give consent, in the event I am incapacitated and unable to provide such consent and approval for a situation requiring medical attention and action for the administration of any treatment or care deemed necessary, and my designated representative, _____ can not be reached in a reasonable period of time to extend such consent and approval on my behalf for attention and action for the administration of any treatment and/or care deemed necessary for the listed above by Dr. _____, or any of his/her associates, the preferred physician, or Dr. _____, or any of his/her associates, the preferred dentist, or in the event the appropriate preferred physician, dentist or other identified healthcare professional is not available, by another qualified physician, dentist or healthcare professional; and the transfer of myself to _____ hospital, the preferred hospital, or any hospital reasonably accessible.

This authorization does not cover non-emergency medical situations or non-emergency major surgery unless the opinions of at least two other licensed physicians, dentists or healthcare professionals concurring in the necessity of such emergency medical action are obtained prior to the performance of such emergency medical action/surgery and unless all reasonable attempts to obtain my approval and in the event I am incapable of providing such approval then efforts to contact my designated representative have been exhausted, defining such period for non-emergency medical action/surgery as 24 hours.

The following information is being released by me in the event that the physician, dentist, healthcare professional or hospital is unable to access my medical history;

Allergies:

Medications:

Physical limitations/restrictions:

Other critical information (e.g. blood type, health conditions, etc.):

Insurance coverage:

Insurance provider		Policy number	

I the undersigned, hereby agree appoint and constitute the club, and its duly authorized representative(s), namely _____, for the period of _____, 20____, through and including _____, 20____, and do hereby authorize them to obtain any x-ray examination, anesthesia, medical or surgical diagnosis or treatment, and hospital care to be provided for me in the event I am unable to provide approval and my designated representative can not be reached for approval in a reasonable period of time, under the general and special supervision, and on the advice of a licensed physician, dentist, or other qualified health care professional acting under their supervision.

Signature: _____

Name (print): _____

Club representative (witness) signature: _____

Club representative name (print): _____

Date: _____   State of _____

Country of _____

Club Name
Incident Report Form

I. General Incident Information

Month Day Year Time of Incident	Club Member	Club Name:
A.M. P.M.	_____ Yes _____ No	Club Location:

	First M.I. Last	Hospital/EMS or Physician Notified? _____ Yes _____ No
Name of Injured Person:		
Street Address:		Name of Caller: _____
		Time of Initial Call: _____
		Time of any Follow-Up Calls: 1. _____
State/City/Zip:		2. _____ 3. _____
		Time of EMS arrival: _____
Phone #'s:		Time of EMD departure: _____
		Hospital taken to: _____
Email address:		Name of EMS contact: _____

II. General Description of the Incident

Description of Incident:

_____

_____

_____

_____

Bleeding related injury?   _____ Yes _____ No

Visible injury?   _____ Yes _____ No

Not outwardly noticeable injury, but person expressed pain?   _____ Yes _____ No

If an eye injury, was eye wear/protection being worn?   _____ Yes _____ No

III. Incident Details, including Club Response to the Incident

Description of the injury/injuries:	Description of club response/first aid:

IV. Responder, Supervisor and Witness Information

First Responder (name):

Responders position/title;

CPR certified? _____ Yes _____ No   AED certified? _____ Yes _____ No

First Aid certified? _____ Yes _____ No

Signature:

Manager on Duty (name):

Manager on Duty position/title:

CPR certified? _____ Yes _____ No   AED certified? _____ Yes _____ No

First Aid certified? _____ Yes _____ No

Signature:

Witness (name):

Witness address: _____

Witness phone: (B) _____   (H) _____   (C) _____

Witness email: _____   Signature: _____

Witness (name):

Witness address: _____

Witness phone: (B) _____   (H) _____   (C) _____

Witness email: _____   Signature: _____

V. Details on Location of Incident

1. Specific location: _____ fitness center   _____ studio   _____ gymnasium

   _____ pool   _____ tennis court   _____ locker rooms

   _____ spa   _____ lobby/circulation area

   _____ children's area   _____ steam/sauna/whirlpool (circle)

   _____ outside

2. Please describe the conditions of the environment during the time of the incident (e.g. was it a wet surface, was it extremely hot, etc.)

3. Other comments

VI. Miscellaneous

1. Did the police investigate? _____ Yes _____ No   If yes, please give name, rank and contact information on the lines below.

Name: _____   Rank: _____

Contact phone number: _____

2. Did another agency investigate (fire department, etc.) _____ Yes _____ No
If yes, please give name, rank and contact information on the lines below.

Name: _____   Rank: _____

Contact phone number: _____

Report submitted by: _____   Signature: _____

Date and time submitted: _____

Please make multiple copies, including one for the person's file, the club's incident files, the insurer and the individual involved in the incident.

Appendix R: Suggested References

- *2002 Profiles of Success; Industry Data Survey.* Compiled by the International Health, Racquet and Sportclub Association and Industry Insights, Inc. Boston, MA. 2002.

- *2003 Profiles of Success; Industry Data Survey.* Compiled by the International Health, Racquet and Sportclub Association and Industry Insights, Inc. Boston, MA. 2003

- *2004 Profiles of Success; Industry Data Survey.* Compiled by the International Health, Racquet and Sportclub Association and Industry Insights, Inc. Boston, MA. 2004

- *2004 ISPA Consumer Trends Report.* Complied and prepared by the International Spa Association and the Hartman Group, Inc. Lexington, KY. 2004.

- *22 Immutable Laws of Branding: How to Build a Product or Service into a World Class Brand.* Al Reis and Laura Reis. Harper Collins. New York. 1998.

- *A Study of Consumer Attitudes Toward Physical Fitness and Health Clubs.* American Sports Data, Inc. Hartsdale, NY. 2002.

- *A Study of Former Health Club Members.* Conducted for IHRSA by American Sports Data, Inc. Hartsdale, NY. 1998.

- *ACSM's Health/Fitness Facility Standards and Guidelines.* 3rd Edition. Steve Tharrett, Kyle McInnis, and James A. Peterson. Human Kinetics. Champaign, IL. 2006.

- *AED Position Paper.* ClubCorp Internal Document. Dallas, TX. 2002.

- "Best of HBR on Leadership; It is Hard Being Soft." *Harvard Business Review.* Boston, MA. 2001.

- *Best Programming Best Practices.* ClubCorp Internal Document. Dallas, TX. 2003.

- *Beyond the Universe.* Bill Pearl. Bill Pearl Enterprises, Inc. Agni Press. New York. 2003.

- *Building Membership Best Practices.* IHRSA Publication. Boston, MA. 2000.

- *ClubCorp Athletic Operations Manual.* ClubCorp Internal Document. Dallas, TX. 1998.

- *ClubCorp Standards of Operation for Athletics and Tennis.* ClubCorp Internal Document. Dallas, TX. 2003.

- *Discovering the Soul of Service.* Leonard Berry. The Free Press. New York. 1999.

- *Employee Compensation and Benefits Survey Results for the Commercial Health and Fitness Industry.* IHRSA and Industry Insights. Boston, MA. 2002 and 2003.

- *The Experience Economy.* Joseph Pine, II, and James Gilmore. Harvard Business School Press. Boston, MA. 1999.

- *Fitness American Style: a Look at How and Why Americans Exercise.* Prepared for IHRSA by Roper Starch Worldwide. Boston, MA. 2001.

- *Guidelines 2000 for Cardiopulmonary Resuscitation and Emergency Cardiovascular Care.* International Consensus on Science Part III: Adult Basic Life Support. Circulation 2000. American Heart Association in collaboration with International Laison Committee on Resuscitation. Dallas, TX. 2000.

- *Health and Fitness Club Review.* Granville Baird Ltd. London, England. 2000.

- *Health/Fitness Management.* Grantham, Patton, York and Winnick. Human Kinetics. Champaign, IL. 1998.

- *IHRSA/ASD Health Club Trend Report (1987 – 2003).* American Sports Data, Inc. Hartsdale, NY. 2004.

- *IHRSA European Market Report: The Size and Scope of the Health Club Industry.* Compiled by the International Health, Racquet and Sportclub Association. Boston, MA. 2005.

- *IHRSA's Guide to Lenders and Investors.* 2nd edition. IHRSA. Boston, MA. 2004.

- *King of Clubs. Grow Rich in More than Money.* Robert Dedman with Debbie Deloach. Taylor Publishing. Dallas, TX. 1999.

- *Leadership and the One-Minute Manager.* Ken Blanchard, Patricia Zigarmi and Drea Zigarmi. William Morrow and Company, Inc. New York. 1985.

- *Legal Aspects of Preventative and Rehabilitative Exercise Programs.* 2nd Edition. Herbert and Herbert. Professional Reports Corporation. Canton, OH. 1989.

- *Marketing Health and Fitness Services.* Richard Gerson. Human Kinetics. Champaign, IL. 1989.

- *Marketing for Results. A Common Sense Approach for Health Clubs.* Brenda Abdilla. CBM Books. Fort Washington, PA. 1996.

- *Marketing Outreach Techniques for Clubs.* Management Vision, Inc. Internal Document. New York. 2002.

- *Muscletown USA.* John Fair. Pennsylvania State University Press. University Park, PA. 1999.

- *Raving Fans.* Ken Blanchard and Sheldon Bowles. William Morrow and Company, Inc. New York. 1993.

- *Spa Industry Survey.* Conducted and prepared by Price Waterhouse Coopers for the International Spa Association. Lexington, KY. 2002.

- *Sports Club Bell Notes.* ClubCorp Internal Document. Dallas, TX. 2003.

- *Sports and Fitness Programming Manual.* ClubCorp Internal Document. Dallas, TX. 1999.

- *State of the Health Club Industry: Global Report.* Compiled by the International Health, Racquet and Sportclub Association. Boston, MA. 2003.

- *State of the Health Club Industry: Global Report.* Compiled by the International Health, Racquet and Sportclub Association. Boston, MA. 2004.

- *State of the Health Club Industry: Global Report.* Compiled by the International Health, Racquet and Sportclub Association. Boston, MA. 2005.

- *The One Minute Manager Builds High Performing Teams.* Ken Blanchard, Don Carew and Ernie Parisi-Carew. William Morrow and Company. New York. 1990.

- *The Seven Habits of Highly Effective People.* Stephen Covey. Fireside Publishing. New York. 1989.

- *Trends in Physical Fitness Behavior (1987 – 2002).* American Sports Data, Inc. Hartsdale, NY. 2003.

- *Uniform System of Accounts for the Health, Racquet and Sportclub Industry.* Copyrighted by the Educational Institute of the American Hotel and Motel Association. Lansing, MI. 1998.

- *Winning the Retention Battle: Parts One through Four.* Conducted by the Fitness Industry Association and Leisure Industry Week with assistance from Gladstone MRM. London, England. 2001.

- *Why and Where People Exercise.* An IHRSA study conducted by American Sports Data, Inc. Hartsdale, NY. 1995.

- *Why People Quit.* An IHRSA Study conducted by American Sports Data, Inc. Hartsdale, NY. 1998.

- *Why People Stay: Health Club Member Retention Research and Best Practices.* IHRSA Publication. Boston, MA. 2000.

Stephen Tharrett, M.S., is currently a management consultant and public speaker in the health/fitness club industry, providing club owners with an extensive array of services that include strategic planning, business planning, employee development programs, marketing and facility design and development. Prior to entering the consulting field in late 2004, Stephen spent just over 20 years working with ClubCorp, a billion-dollar Dallas, Texas-based company that owned and operated private clubs, including business clubs, country clubs, resorts and sports clubs. From 2002 to 2004, he was a senior vice president of athletics, golf and tennis, with responsibility for the educational systems, operating systems and revenue programs for the athletic, golf and tennis lines of business (over $250 million in annual revenues). From 1994 to 2002, he was the vice president of athletics and tennis and from 1987 to 1994 as the director of athletics. During his tenure with ClubCorp, Stephen's responsibilities ranged from the development and management of over $30 million in construction projects, opening clubs in both the U.S. and overseas, developing company-wide operating systems, chairing the athletic, golf and tennis committees, and serving on the company's leadership cabinet and business-planning committee.

Stephen has been involved in the fitness and sport industry for over 26 years. He has served on the Board of the International Health, Racquet and Sportclub Association (IHRSA) from 1994 to 1997 and as IHRSA president from 1996 to 1997. Stephen has also been a member of IHRSA's membership committee. He has served as a contributing editor for the *American College of Sports Medicine's (ACSM) Health/Fitness Facility Standards and Guidelines, 1st edition* and as the co-editor for *ACSM's Health/Fitness Facility Standards and Guidelines 2nd edition* released in 1997 and the 3rd edition of the same publication which is being released in 2006. Stephen has also served the American College of Sports Medicine in several capacities, including chairing the committee on Health & Fitness Facilities, chair of the marketing sub-committee for the education and certification committees and on the Association's certification committee. Stephen has been a member of the advisory boards for Star Trac and StairMaster. He has also served as a member of the editorial advisory board for *ACSM's Health and Fitness Journal*. He has been a keynote speaker and feature speaker at numerous national and international conferences. Finally, he has served an adjunct professor at the University of Texas at Arlington and a lecturer at the IHRSA Institute of Professional Management.

On the personal side, Stephen and his wife of 29 years, Denise, have two children, Alyssa, an architect with Ohlson Lavoie Collaborative in Denver, CO, and Travis, a lead computer animator and artist with Terminal Reality, a Dallas, Texas-based video game company. Stephen's interests include golf, martial arts (in which he holds two black belts), and bonsai.

James A. Peterson, Ph.D., FACSM, is a sports medicine consultant who resides in Monterey, California. A fellow of the American College of Sports Medicine, he was a faculty member at the United States Military Academy at West Point from 1971-1990. From 1990 to 1995, he served as the director of sports medicine for StairMaster Sports/Medical Products, Inc. He has written or co-authored over 80 books and 200 articles on a variety of sports, health, and wellness topics. He holds two FDA-approved patents on back pain management measures. Since 1997, he has been a contributing editor to *ACSM's Health & Fitness Journal* ("Take 10" column). He served as the co-editor of both the second and the third editions of *ACSM's Health/Fitness Facility Standards and Guidelines*. He has appeared on several national television shows, including ABC's Good Morning America, the CBS Evening News, and ABC's Nightline. Since 1992, he has served as a fundraiser for the Make-A-Wish Foundation®. Jim and his wife, Susan, have been married for 38 years.